PREVENTION AND CURE

THE LONDON SCHOOL OF HYGIENE & TROPICAL MEDICINE

Here is a history of the London School of Hygiene and Tropical Medicine - from its beginnings as "Manson's Tropical School" in the late 1890s through its development in the 1920s into an international school of public health and its present position as a centre of education and research in the biomedical sciences in the context of world health. Within the tropical disciplines, many of the early pioneers, who spent long periods in the tropics before the introduction of vaccines and other effective control measures, have survived well into their eighties and nineties and have generously supplied personal reminisces and unique information concerning past events.

Lady Lise Wilkinson, educated at the University of Copenhagen and at the University of California, Berkeley, has previously published works in the field of medical history with a focus on the history of virology and aspects of comparative medicine and pathology. She is Senior Research Fellow at the Wellcome Institute, London.

Anne Hardy lives at Oxford.

keganpaul.com

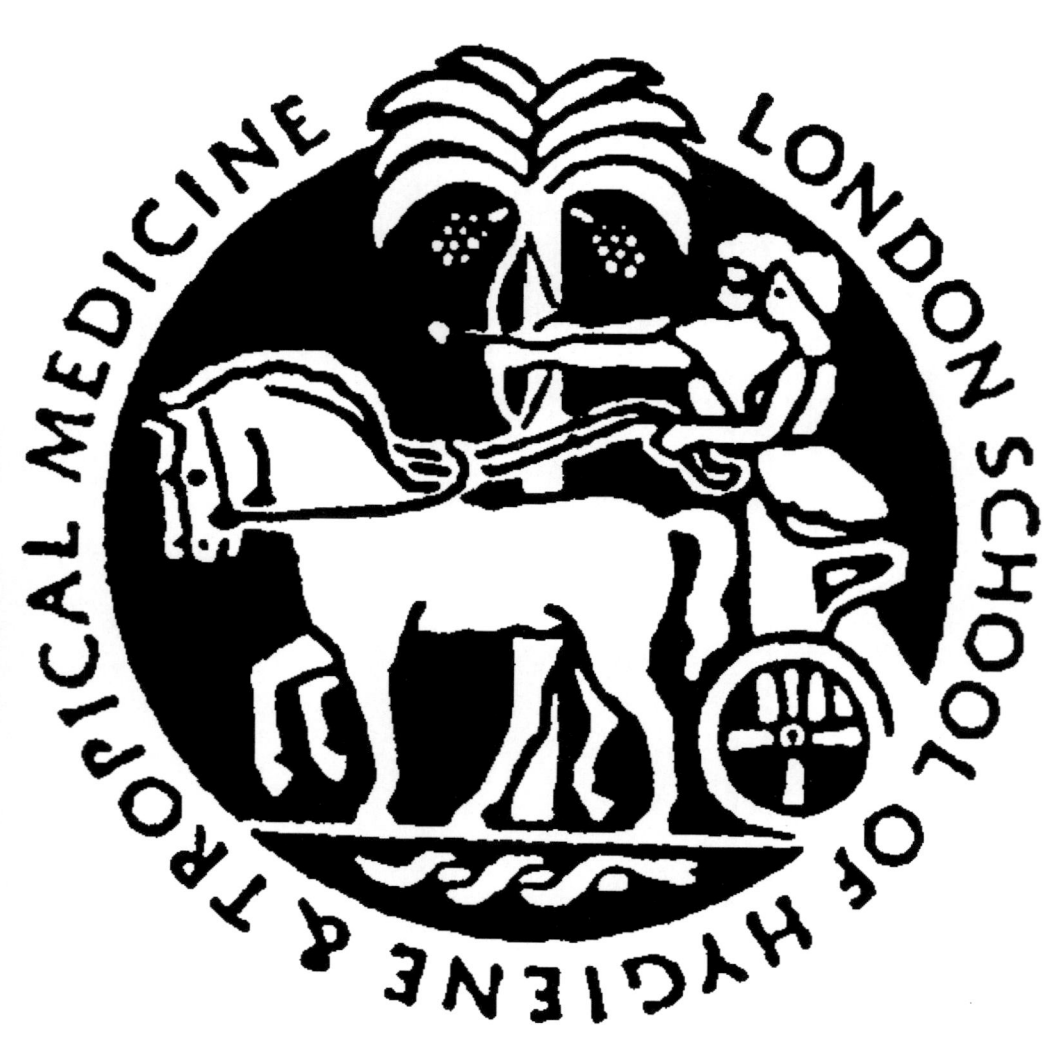

PREVENTION AND CURE

THE LONDON SCHOOL OF HYGIENE & TROPICAL MEDICINE

A 20TH CENTURY QUEST FOR GLOBAL PUBLIC HEALTH

Lise Wilkinson and Anne Hardy

KEGAN PAUL
London • New York • Bahrain

First published in 2001 by
Kegan Paul Limited
UK: P.O. Box 256, London WC1B 3SW, England
Tel: 020 7580 5511   Fax: 020 7436 0899
E-Mail: books@keganpaul.com
Internet: http://www.keganpaul.com
USA: 61 West 62nd Street, New York, NY 10023
Tel: (212) 459 0600   Fax: (212) 459 36780
Internet: http://www.columbia.edu/cu/cup
BAHRAIN: bahrain@keganpaul.com

Distributed by:
Turpin Distribution
Blackhorse Road
Letchworth, Herts. SG6 1HN
England
Tel: (01462) 672555 Fax: (01462) 480947
Email: books@turpinltd.com

Columbia University Press
61 West 62nd Street, New York, NY 10023
Tel: (212) 459 0600   Fax: (212) 459 36780
Internet: http://www.columbia.edu/cu/cup

© Lise Wilkinson and Anne Hardy, 2001

Printed in Great Britain, IBT Global London

All Rights reserved. No part of this book may be reprinted or reproduced or utilised in any form or by any electric, mechanical or other means, now known or hereafter invented, including photocopying or recording, or in any information storage or retrieval system, without permission in writing from the publishers.

ISBN: 0-7103-0624-5

British Library Cataloguing in Publication Data
A catalogue record for this book is available from the British Library.
Library of Congress Cataloging-in-Publication Data
Applied for.

ACKNOWLEDGEMENTS

The idea of a history of the School and the development of its diverse disciplines over the years until its centenary in 1999 was first put by the late C.E.Gordon Smith in the year of his retirement in 1989, after nearly twenty years as its Dean. It was realised with the help of Professor W.F.Bynum of the Wellcome Institute for the History of Medicine and University College, and in part supported by a grant from the Wellcome Trust. Bill Bynum has also heroically read through and commented on the MS.

We are also indebted to Gordon Smith's successors as Deans, in the last decade, R.G.A.Feachem and Harrison Spencer; and especially to B.S.Drasar, acting Dean 1995, and D.J.Bradley, Director of the Ross Institute for almost 20 years and Professor of Tropical Hygiene, both of whom take a lively interest in the history of the School and of their respective subjects. Their unflagging interest and encouragement have been invaluable throughout the years of writing.

Very many current and former members of staff of the School have generously given of their time to answer questions, volunteer information, and comment on parts of the MS. Their numbers make it impossible to list all the names here, but their contributions appear in the text and their names in the references. We are grateful to them all.

The scarcity of surviving archive material at the School has been mitigated by much helpful advice from the Librarian Brian Furner and the Bibliographer Mary Gibson and all the library staff. Additional material has been found in the Contemporary Medical Archives Centre (CMAC) collections, with the help of archivists Julia Sheppard and Lesley Hall, and at the Public Record Office at Kew. A number of illustrations are also from the Wellcome collections.

Paula Stanley has patiently and efficiently typed and word-processed the MS and inevitable changes over the years; we have also enjoyed the support of Phoebe Roome and Joanne Bent in the Dean's Office. Our thanks to all who helped.

Lise Wilkinson and Anne Hardy   July 1998.

CONTENTS

Acknowledgements

1. The London School of Tropical Medicine 1899–20: Background and Beginnings
2. Protagonists of a medical specialty: Parasites, Vectors, and Exotic Life-cycles
3. Transition 1919–29: from Tropical Medicine to Global Public Health
4. Epidemiology and Medical Statistics
5. Bacteriology and Immunology, and the Public Health Laboratory Service
6. Public Health and its coming of age: from MOH and DPH to 'Social Medicine' and 'Community Medicine'
7. The wider spectrum of Public Health: basic research in developing biochemistry; and applied science and statistics in Occupational Health
8. Feeding the hungry, balancing the diet: Nutrition and Public Health
9. Winches Farm: from agricultural comparative parasitology to LSHTM field station
10. A many-faceted subject: tropical medicine in a changing world 1919–89
11. Malaria: a century of advances and reversals in the fight against an intractable threat
12. Towards the Millennium: Back to the Future

Biographical Appendix A
Biographical Appendix B
Chronological Table LSHTM

1

THE LONDON SCHOOL OF TROPICAL MEDICINE:
1899–1920:
BACKGROUND AND BEGINNINGS

In 1999, on the eve of the twenty-first century, the London School of Hygiene and Tropical Medicine (LSH&TM) will celebrate its centenary. In historical perspective, the date of 1899, when it opened as the London School of Tropical Medicine (LSTM), is crucial to the decisive role it has played in the development of preventive medicine in the twentieth century. Its long and complex history falls into two distinct parts: for an initial quarter of a century the Schools' teaching and research facilities were devoted exclusively to tropical medicine; from the early 1920s it began a period of development into an institution concerned with research and teaching of public health in general, of preventive medicine and hygiene on a global scale and including all latitudes and climates, tropical and temperate alike. In this form, as a national and international school of public health, it has become the European counterpart to the Johns Hopkins School of Hygiene and Public Health in Baltimore, founded during World War I in an effort to co-ordinate and professionalise training in public health in the United States.[1] On the face of it, the forces that shaped the original London School of Tropical Medicine and the Johns Hopkins School were very different; only gradually did the similarities emerge and comparison become justified.

It is a truism that public health movements in the past have had their origin in the need to preserve and conserve manpower for manual labour: in times of peace for working the land, and later for industrial tasks, in times of war for the armed forces. Orchestrated concern with public health and preventive medicine in general terms has relatively recent origins. Apart from early crisis measures developed in response to the great epidemics of smallpox and of bubonic plague – quarantine regulations and isolation hospitals, often water-borne or situated on the edge of rivers[2] – serious attempts to introduce formal means of, and policies for, preserving and improving the health of entire populations, belong to the nineteenth century and the aftermath of the cholera years.[3]

Whereas early actions taken against plague and pestilence reflected enforced concern with public disease rather than public health, serious consideration of the impact of disease on society and of the means which might be made available to combat it and even prevent it, began with the era of exploration and colonisation by European powers. It was the adverse effects on European travellers, and later on troops and civil servants abroad, of long sea voyages and of exotic climates and diseases once distant goals were reached, which inspired the medical profession, and political and economic authorities, to recognise the importance of preventive as much as of curative measures. Bodies of men, in the armed services and on board ship for long voyages, constituted ready-made groups for early, empirical, forerunners of 'controlled trials'. Knowledge of scurvy in particular benefited from such fortuitous isolation of groups of men on board ship, and off ships in extreme circumstances, although in this case claims and counter-claims continued to obscure results for a very long time.[4]

Throughout the eighteenth century, concern had been growing for the health of seamen and military personnel serving in increasingly far-flung possessions acquired by a number of European powers. 'Fevers', still inadequately characterised, brought death and disabilities to many, and financial losses to their employers.[5] Britain and France in particular reflect in their medical literature in the later eighteenth century the concerns forcefully imposed by the head-on collision of expanding empires and their employees with hitherto unknown diseases prevailing in tropical and subtropical climates. In their attempts to come to terms with problems abroad, the authorities were to some extent and unknowingly laying the foundations for much later health policies at home.

When William Hillary sailed for Barbados in the West Indies in 1747,[6] 'tropical diseases' was a term not yet in general use. In his *Observations*, published in London in 1759, he referred to 'Diseases... indigenous or endemial, in the West India Islands or in the Torrid Zones.'[7] Bynum has emphasised the impact of geographical expansion on the growing volume of literature on fevers, and on the consequent heightened public consciousness of the inherent dangers of life in hot climates abroad.[8] When John Hunter, MD, and J.F.Lafosse[9] in the last decades of the eighteenth century recommended moving troops and officials away from the fever-ridden lowlands of West Indian islands to camps at higher altitudes, they were striking a blow for measures later to become part and parcel of preventive medicine in the tropics; but the diseases they described were referred to as diseases 'of the army' or of 'the inhabitants of the colonies'. Even if not in general use, the term 'tropical diseases' was occasionally used in the eighteenth century, earlier than the date given by the *Oxford English Dictionary:* Benjamin Moseley published *A treatise on tropical diseases* in the late 1780s.[10]

The first journal to use the term 'tropical medicine' in its title was short-lived. It belonged to what Chernin has called the 'prehistory of the journals of tropical medicine', and was appropriately enough devoted to 'the experience of the Medical Officers of her Majestys' armies and fleets in all parts of the world'. Published in London in 1863, its editor was anonymous and it did not survive beyond its first volume.[11]

If terms such as 'tropical diseases' and 'tropical medicine' were not in general use until later in the nineteenth century, the concept of exotic diseases prevailing in hot climates was of increasing concern to those responsible for the health and welfare of the growing proportion of European populations living and working abroad in tropical and subtropical areas from the mid-eighteenth century onwards. They included soldiers, sailors, officials of companies trading in Africa, India and the Far East; and later growing numbers of officials and administrators employed in the colonial services.

Determined attempts to formulate public health policies began in Britain only in the nineteenth century in the wake of epidemics, especially of cholera, with appointments of the first Medical Officers of Health, William Henry Duncan (1805–63) in Liverpool in January, 1847 (following the Liverpool Sanitary Act of 1846), and of John Simon (1816–1904) in London in October, 1848. Medical Officers attached to colonial outposts, to the East India Company, and to the armed services, had by then also provided an empirical basis for the study of spread of infections at home and in other climates abroad.[12]

At the end of the eighteenth century, the Napoleonic Wars erupted into an atmosphere of quiet progress in knowledge of the nature and geography of diseases prevailing in other climates, and on board ships bound for such climates. Inevitably, the wars interrupted progress; concern with the health of fighting men in Europe became paramount. Early in the wars, less than six months after Nelson had defeated the French in the Battle of the Nile, a surgeon who had served on two East Indiamen had written to the Directors of the East India Company, drawing their attention to the need for 'Rules and regulations for the more effectual preservation of health' in the Company's ships.[13] Problems on board ships directly involved in the European conflict doubtless included a higher proportion of gunshot wounds and other injuries in addition to more everyday questions of cleanliness and diet.

At the end of the wars, after the final fall of Napoleon, sailors returning home, often after years at sea, had more acute problems: problems of their very survival. In many cases they had lost touch with their families; employment was difficult to find, and even if found, pay was less generous than in war-time. Some were ill, most were rootless, and many were roaming the streets of unfamiliar London with nowhere to go, ill equipped to cope with life on *terra firma*. Their precarious existence in the capital was a hazard to themselves, and to their more established fellow citizens. It was an obvious case for early nineteenth century charity; and William Wilberforce (1759–1833), no stranger to philanthropy, and his brother-in-arms against slavery, Zachary Macauly (1768–1838), decided to take action in 1816.[14] An appeal for subscriptions for 'the relief of distressed seamen' was launched at a meeting at the City of London Tavern on January 5th, 1818.[15] Response was immediate. Major financial contributions came from Trinity House and the East India Company; the Marine Society offered to clothe one hundred destitute seamen. By January 8th, two hundred 'distressed seamen' had already been supplied with food and temporary lodgings.

After three years of work on an *ad hoc* basis, Wilberforce's Committee for the Relief of Distressed Seamen realised the need for a more permanent organisation. This was to include a 'floating hospital' which could offer assistance to sick, and otherwise helpless, seamen, to treat their illnesses and to help them to re-establish themselves after their discharge from the hospital.[16]

Under Royal Patronage, the Committee became the Seamen's Hospital Society, supported by voluntary subscriptions, on March 8th, 1821. Two weeks later, the Admiralty had agreed the loan of the 48 - gun ship *Grampus* as the Society's hospital ship. Ten years later the *Grampus* was replaced by the larger *Dreadnought*,[17] a name adopted for subsequent ships and, eventually, for the hospital buildings at Greenwich to which patients were moved in 1870, when on-shore facilities were at last deemed preferable to moorings on the increasingly crowded river. It was here, and in the Society's Branch Hospital at the Albert Dock across the Thames, opened in 1890, that teaching and research in tropical medicine began in London in the 1890s. And it was on the premises of the Albert Dock Branch Hospital that the London School of Tropical Medicine was founded at the end of the century.

The seeds had been sown when in May, 1892, Patrick Manson (1844–1922) was appointed physician to the Branch Hospital.[18] He was 47 years old; three years earlier he had returned to his native Scotland after more than twenty years in the Far East, first at Amoy (now Hsiamen) on the Chinese mainland, and later at Hong Kong. With James Cantlie (1851–1926, Sir James from 1918), who was subsequently to join him at the Albert Dock, he had founded a medical college there, and achieved a considerable reputation for his discoveries, above all his identification of the microfilariae of elephantiasis and the demonstration of their transmission by mosquitoes.[19] Having also along the way accumulated reasonable private means, he came home with the intention of retiring to gentlemanly pursuits in Aberdeenshire. It proved to be the wrong moment. The Chinese dollar was depreciating; what had seemed a comfortable fortune was no longer so. Manson was forced back to work, and chose to practise in London. His reputation secured him a continuing supply of blood specimens to sustain his scientific observations on exotic parasites and their life-cycles. In 1892 his appointment to the Seamen's Hospital Society's Branch Hospital at Albert Dock was unanimous in spite of the equally 'high qualifications and recommendations' of his fellow applicants for the post.[20]

As mentioned above, Manson had in the 1880s played a major role in establishing a medical school in Hong Kong. He had seen the need there for local educational facilities for native doctors. Ten years later, back in London, he recognised the need there for centralised instruction in tropical medicine for British Medical Officers sent to serve abroad in outposts of the Empire. Manson's biographer has called his work room ('the muck room') at the top of his house in Cavendish Square the 'nucleus of the future London School of Tropical Medicine'.[21] But Manson would have got nowhere without the support of the other driving forces behind the project: the Seamen's Hospital Society, and the British Colonial Office under Joseph Chamberlain (1836–1914) and his able Private Secretary, Herbert Read (1863–1949).

Chamberlain had chosen the office of Colonial Secretary when in 1895 he had joined Lord Salisbury's government. His belief in trade with the Crown Colonies as an essential factor in economic development both at home and abroad had intensified over the years. Now consideration of the potential of Egypt and the African possessions, and of the West Indies, if sympathetic government help were forthcoming, led to a re-thinking of the responsibilities of the Colonial Office. Already research projects at Kew were aimed at improvements in West Indian agriculture; such policies could now be extended to serve the rest of the Empire, in the hope that it would ultimately become self-sufficient. Nor was this Chamberlain's first brush with medical and biological sciences. In 1886, when President of the Local Government Board, he had agreed to Sir Henry Roscoe's suggestion that a commission be formed to investigate the merits of Pasteur's anti-rabies treatment. The commission's favourable verdict fifteen months later led to calls for a medical research institute in London and eventually resulted in the establishment of the British Institute of Preventive Medicine, amalgamated with the College of State Medicine in December, 1893, and later known as the Lister Institute.[22] In his analysis of the East Coast fever controversy of 1902–4, Paul Cranefield examined the development of Chamberlain's motives and political attitudes before and during his time at the Colonial Office (1895–1903). It was a period which covered that controversy as well as the Boer War and the creation of the London and Liverpool schools of tropical medicine.

It is also a period which, in the second half of the twentieth century, has been included in a growing volume of examination of socio-economic and political aspects of health policies pursued by Britain and other colonial powers in the nineteenth and early twentieth century. Cranefield discussed the way in which Chamberlain's belief in a powerful empire supported by the discoveries of new agricultural and medical research reached its climax during these years. He also pointed out the subsequent gradual overshadowing of these early ideals of radical reform by Chamberlain's alarmed realisation of the potential threat to the Empire represented by the growing naval and industrial powers of Germany and of the United States.[23]

Certainly until the end of the century Chamberlain's reforming spirit and genuine concern for the health problems throughout the Empire remained undiminished. He was also influenced by awareness that a major natural enemy to the creation of a strong economy was an ever present threat to the health of native workers and to officials sent to serve abroad: a high risk of contracting tropical diseases. Malaria, yellow fever, and sleeping sickness, were only the most prominent among a host of other debilitating diseases taking a higher toll in hot climates, even those not unknown elsewhere. When Manson became medical adviser to the Colonial Office in July, 1897, Chamberlain was more than ready to accept lobbying for education and research to combat tropical diseases.

Manson had declared an interest in the inclusion of the subject of tropical diseases in the curriculum of English medical schools as early as 1894. The then Dean of St.George's Hospital, Sir Isambard Owen, was receptive to Manson's ideas, and arranged for him to give an annual course of lectures to students there.[24] In the same year Sir William MacKinnon (1830–97), head of the Army Medical Department, had pointed to the need for special training for future colonial Medical Officers of Health. MacKinnon proposed to institute a three months' course at the Army Medical School at Netley, already attended by officers of the Indian Medical Service.[25] It was an idea which was to cause controversy in the following years, until the new London School of Tropical Medicine could finally open its doors on the site of the Albert Dock Branch Hospital of the Seamen's Hospital Society in October, 1899.

On October 1st, 1897, Manson began his annual course for students at St.George's with a lecture 'On the necessity for special education in tropical medicine'.[26] Less than three months earlier he had, almost by chance, succeeded Sir Charles Gage Brown (1826–1908) as medical adviser to the Colonial Office. The Seamen's Hospital Society noted the appointment of their visiting physician to the post with approval;[27] in their turn, the Colonial Office lost no time in reacting to Manson's seminal lecture. On December 2nd, 1897, H.J.Read, as Chamberlain's mouthpiece, issued a memorandum on the need for special education in tropical medicine, along the lines of Manson's proposals.[28] It proved to be a policy-making document of considerable impact, and not only in London.

Manson's predecessor, Gage Brown, had endorsed his proposals immediately, setting out various options for training. They included attendance at Manson's lectures at St.George's, instruction at Netley, and as a third possibility, instruction at the local Head Quarter's hospital of individual colonies. Read added that 'at least two other medical schools have arranged lectures on tropical diseases' (in Edinburgh, Andrew Davidson had lectured on tropical diseases; and John Anderson (1840–1910) lectured at St.Mary's, see G.C.Cook note 36). Thus the scene was set for the bureaucratic arguments which, together with financial problems, were to delay the realisation of plans for a specialise London School of Tropical Medicine for long enough to enable a rival school, privately funded at Liverpool, to open six months before its London counterpart.[29]

The Liverpool School of Tropical Medicine owed its existence to the initiative of Rubert Boyce (1863–1911), and very much to the private funds of Alfred Jones (1845–1909), one of many successful merchants contributing to the healthy economy of that city in the late nineteenth century. Importing nuts and bananas from West Africa and the Canary Islands, Jones had a vested interest in the promotion of knowledge and control of tropical diseases, which frequently threatened the health of his employees abroad, and the crews serving his shipping line. Although the ideas put forward in Liverpool were conceived later than those for a London School – were in fact the result of Chamberlain's circular to Colonial Governors in May, 1898 – Jones's business acumen and his private means, together with the tireless organisational talents and fund-raising activities of Boyce, Professor of Pathology at Liverpool's University College, smoothed the path to completion in Liverpool.[30]

In contrast, the planning and eventual completion of the London School were subject to all the obstacles and delays which the bureaucracy of officialdom, and the tedium of endless committee work, could throw in its way. For the creation of the London School of Tropical Medicine was one of a handful of examples, at the turn of the century, of slowly progressing, but ultimately successful, negotiations resulting from a growing understanding and collaboration between enlightened politicians and an emerging breed of medically oriented scientists.[31]

Manson's lecture at St.George's on education in tropical medicine in 1897 is sometimes seen as the formal introduction of the concept into the consciousness of those who were to take the subject into the realm of academic medicine in the following years. Rather it was, like Jenner's paper on cowpox vaccination a hundred years before, a definitive formulation of tentative ideas and policies which had been abroad for some time. Manson himself had helped to establish a medical school in Hong Kong; Andrew Davidson (1836-1918) had written on diseases in Madagascar and, back in Edinburgh, had lectured on tropical diseases and written two standard works, *Geographical Pathology* and *Hygiene and Diseases of Warm Climates*. The latter was a forerunner of Manson's enduring *Manual of Tropical Diseases,* and of Leonard Rogers' *Fevers in the Tropics,* and of the later *Tropical Medicine* by Rogers (1868-1962) and J.W.D.Megaw (1874-1958).[32] In his original preface to *Tropical Diseases* Manson included Davidson, and also Laveran, among the 'systematic writers' in the field, whose treatises were more complete and elaborate, but of a less 'handy size... for exigencies of travel and tropical life...' than his own manual. The confidence Manson displayed in his firm call for new policies for education in tropical medicine in 1897 owed more than a little to the positive support already extended to his plans by P.J.Michelli (1853-1935), Secretary of the Seamen's Hospital Society, and its able chairman, Sir Perceval Nairne (1841-1921), and of course by Joseph Chamberlain himself.

A particular concern of the Colonial Office, reflected in Read's memorandum of December, 1897, was the exceptionally high mortality rate in the West African dependencies on the Gold Coast. He wrote:

> ... there seems to be little doubt that the *East African* Protectorates are, on the whole, healthier than our possessions in West Africa.
> ... One advantage of the proposed arrangement will be that officers who are *unable to stand the West Coast* any longer will have a chance to transfer to the East Coast, & vice versa, officers who have been to the East Coast will have been acclimatised and probably better able to stand the West than a man sent direct from this country, as at present. I believe that Dr.Manson concurs in this view. [authors' italics]

The vision conjured up of the overwhelming unhealthiness of the Gold Coast compared to other areas in Africa is underlined by the list of salaries offered to medical personnel: salaries in West Africa exceeded those in the East African protectorate by twenty to one hundred per cent.[33] Read also adopted Manson's suggestion of the introduction of health sheets to facilitate the keeping of continuous records of the health of all officers; other ranks were not mentioned.

Manson's lecture and Read's memorandum had immediate results. Read had noted Manson's preference for the Seamen's Hospital at Greenwich as a more suitable place than Netley for the teaching of specialised courses in tropical medicine. At Netley, so Manson claimed, 'our officials' would 'not see a sufficient variety of tropical diseases, particularly of the diseases of the natives'. Moreover, they would be 'lost in the crowd of other students and feel themselves aliens and interlopers'. Although Netley had the immediate advantage of accommodation for large numbers of students, the Albert Dock Branch of the Seamen's Hospital was to be enlarged, and also had room for a new building.

Two months later, the Colonial Office wrote to the Seamen's Hospital Society to enquire about the possibility of their participation in such a scheme. The response, signed by Michelli, was favourable, and included an estimate of expenses:

Cost of the New Wing to the Albert Dock Hospital
and School Buildings £13,000
Current expenditure £ 3,047

A sum equivalent to interest at 3 per cent per annum on a
capital sum not exceeding £100,000

Maintenance of 6 students for 10 months of the year at
4 guineas per week equalled approximately £1,000 per annum

The proposed fees for a course of not less than four weeks:

Residents per week £ 4.4.0
Non resident students £2.12.6

Michelli's letter[34] reached the Colonial Office in April; a month earlier, Chamberlain had addressed the General Medical Council on the desirability of extending the teaching of tropical medicine in a memorandum circulated to all medical teaching institutions. He followed this up at the end of May with the circular to Colonial Governors, stressing the importance of research into the causes of malaria, and the need for a school to provide specialised training for medical officers bound for the colonies. The document also emphasised the necessity to offer regular supplementary up-to-date information to physicians already in service overseas during their homes leaves.[35]

The joint initiative of Manson and Chamberlain led directly to the creation of the London School of Tropical Medicine; but not before a number of difficulties had been overcome. Senior physicians at the main Seamen's Hospital at Greenwich complained that they had not been adequately consulted; some of London's larger teaching hospitals feared a possible loss of clinical cases and teaching to a specialised school; the spectre of Netley also remained a threat to Manson's plans; finally, some of his opponents even stooped to personal attacks.[36] In the end, the arguments and the committee work, largely undertaken by the Management Committee of the Seamen's Hospital Society, assisted by a special Advisory Committee under the auspices of the Colonial Office, dragged on for nearly two years. Not until October, 1899, could the London School of Tropical Medicine open its doors in a new building at Albert Dock.

The eleven students registered as the first intake by the Seamen's Hospital Society and the School were all male and English or Scottish, with the exception of one German, employed by the Rhenish Missionary Society. Most were bound for West Africa, one for the West Indies, and two for India. One Staff Surgeon R.N., P.W.Bassett-Smith (1861–1927), then in his late thirties, attended the course in the interests of his teaching responsibilities as lecturer on tropical medicine and bacteriology (1900–12) at Haslar. A founder member of the Society of Tropical Medicine and Hygiene in 1907, he was later knighted and became Consultant in tropical diseases, based in Harley Street. The second class, which began in January, 1900, included three young women in their twenties, going to work as medical missionaries in India and China. They were preceded in the School Register by 27-year-old George Carmichael Low (1872–1952), later Superintendent at the School and Director of the Clinical Division at the Hospital for Tropical Diseases. In the Register his destination was described as 'The Campagna Rome Malaria Expedition'. Three years later, in January, 1903, the new intake of students included one 'A.L.Barton, age 30'. Alberto Barton was the son of British immigrants to Peru; after supplementing his training with a course at Manson's School, he was later to give his name to *Bartonella bacilliformis*, the causative agent of Carrión's disease.[37]

By comparison with London, events leading to the opening of the

Liverpool School had followed an easier course. Chamberlain's circulars to the General Medical Council and the Colonial Governors had not gone unnoticed in the rest of the country. In Liverpool, the combined talents of Rubert Boyce and Alfred Jones, referred to above, helped by the city's economic climate at the end of the century, put plans for education in tropical medicine into practice with much less delay than was experienced in London. Liverpool at the end of the nineteenth century possessed a flourishing business community, much of its trade based on its busy port. Jones was an exponent of the healthy enterprise of this community. He had risen from modest beginnings to take control, in his early thirties, of Messrs Elder, Dempster, one of the most important of the city's shipping lines. Nor did his ambition stop there; he had wider aims, and was soon to take over competing lines, British and foreign, with a view to establishing a monopoly of West African ports.

In the 1880s, his attention had been drawn to the Canary Islands, then on the verge of bankruptcy. Establishing a coaling station at Las Palmas (he owned mines in South Wales producing steam coal), he encouraged commercial growing of bananas, which he brought to Britain in his ships under carefully controlled conditions. He even began a tourist trade with the islands, and established sanatoria there for officers invalided from the West African colonies. Later he was to develop trade with the British West Indies; a branch of his firm, which promoted Jamaican bananas in England, incorporated the name Fyffes.[38]

With an eye to commercial success, and also genuinely concerned for the health of his employees and his ships' crews, British or African, Jones, already prompted by Rubert Boyce, reacted in November, 1898, to Chamberlain's appeals with an offer to Liverpool's Royal Southern Hospital of an annual contribution of £350 for three years, 'for the study of tropical diseases'. Accepting the offer, the President of the hospital, William Adamson wrote:

> ... The laboratory part of the work would be well handled at the University College, but the proximity of the Southern Hospital to the Docks, especially your steamers, points to this Institution as being the one where the clinical part must be done if the safety of the patients is to be considered.[39]

The latter argument echoed those used on behalf of the Albert Dock as the ideal position for a London School. In London, many patients coming through the Albert Dock came off ships engaged in trade with China, India, and the far East; in Liverpool, most incoming steamers and their crews, ill or well, came from Africa and the West Indies.

With commendable speed a committee, headed by Alfred Jones, was formed little more than a week after acceptance of his offer. Its most influential member was Rubert Boyce, then already active in University College politics, and in the movement to transform the College into the University of Liverpool, a goal reached when the University Charter was granted on July 15th, 1902. The movement had had its origins in another famous Liverpool partnership: in 1891 Richard Caton (1842–1926), pioneer electrophysiologist, physician at Liverpool's Royal Infirmary, and first holder of its part-time Chair of Physiology, had persuaded George Holt, a member of another family of Liverpool shipowners, to endow a full-time Chair of Physiology at University College.[40] In the manner of Manson and Chamberlain in London, Boyce and Jones were the driving forces behind the creation of the Liverpool School. With the generous funding of Jones, and with Boyce's boundless energy and expert handling of administration and further fund-raising, the Liverpool School was officially opened in April 1899, well in advance of the London School's opening in October of the same year.[41] Alfred Jones's first offer of financial help had been received on November 12th, 1898; the three-way negotiations between Patrick Manson, the Colonial Office, and the Seamen's Hospital Society, formal and informal, had then been under way for more than a year.[42]

The reliance on substantial private support from interested individuals at Liverpool, especially from representatives of the Ship Owner's Association and of the Chamber of Commerce, some of whom served on the Managing Committee of the new school, remained essential for the work of the school over the years. Boyce was an inspired fund-raiser; one obituary stated that his 'success as a beggar was marvellous', resulting in a wide-ranging and steadily growing list of subscribers. When Boyce died in 1911, the Liverpool School had an annual income of £8,000, in addition to its fully endowed Chair of Tropical Medicine. The latter was funded by Alfred Jones and held by Ronald Ross (1857–1932) from 1902 until, a Nobel Prize and a knighthood in turn, he left for London and his tireless, but vain and increasingly paranoid, search for what he regarded as his due financial reward, in 1912. He lectured on tropical sanitation at Liverpool for another five years; aspects of his career associated with the London School will be discussed in later chapters.[43]

Local philanthropy also defrayed much of the cost of the numerous expeditions organised by the Liverpool school: between July, 1899, when Ronald Ross sailed for West Africa in search of 'malaria mosquitoes', accompanied by representatives of the School, the British Museum, and the Belgian Government, soon to establish a tropical medicine institute of its own,[44] and August, 1905, no less than sixteen expeditions left Liverpool for various parts of the globe. Two months after the outbreak of war in 1914, the School's 32nd expedition left for Sierra Leone to study sleeping sickness; it was also to report on possible sites for a permanent laboratory on the west Coast of Africa, to be established with a sum specified in the will of Alfred Jones. A suitable site was found on a hill overlooking Freetown. The plans for the laboratory, on the site leased from the War Office, were finally approved in 1920.[45]

During the same period, the travels undertaken by staff members from the London School were fewer in number and, with the exception of named travelling scholarships such as were endowed by Sir Henry Burdett and by J.G.Craggs, and a bequest from the estate of Lord Wandsworth, they were supported by outside, official bodies. These included the Royal Society's Commission on Sleeping Sickness (1902), the Colonial Office which sent W.J.R.Simpson to West Africa in 1908, and which also lent its support to the School's crucial malaria experiment in the Roman Campagna in 1900; and the War Office which sent R.T.Leiper and associates to the Far East to investigate schistosomiasis in December, 1914.[46] Collaboration between the two schools was rare. The Malaria Commission, jointly sponsored by the Royal Society and the Colonial Office, was appointed in 1898, before opening of the schools. J.W.W.Stephens (1865–1946) and S.R.Christophers (1873–1978) represented the Royal Society, and C.W.Daniels (1862–1927) the Colonial Office. Only afterwards did Stephens become associated with the Liverpool School, and Daniels with the London School.[47]

Compared to the funds raised by the Liverpool School, the financial position of the London School remained precarious throughout its early years. The Seamen's Hospital Society had made a generous initial contribution, and continued to be responsible for maintenance of the buildings. Government grants accounted for £3,550 in the first twelve years of the School's existence; smaller contributions were sought from individual colonies by Chamberlain's successor, Alfred Lyttelton (1857–1913). Private benefactors made donations towards scholarships, prizes, and specific research projects. Finally, the banquets which had been arranged by Joseph Chamberlain at the Hotel Cecil in 1899 and in 1905 added another £23,000 to the always hard-pressed finances.[48]

When at last the buildings and arrangements at the Albert Dock Hospital were ready for the first students in the autumn of 1899, problems still remained for the official opening of the School. It had been planned initially as a major occasion, with an inaugural address by a doyen of the profession. One after another, Alphonse Laveran (1845–1922), William Osler (1849–1919), and Guido Baccelli (1832–1916), declined the invitation.[49] Having finally decided in favour of a less formal opening, Manson himself was indisposed on the day, and his welcoming address to the students was read by James Cantlie (1851–1926), his friend and associate from the China years, who played an influential role in the School and the Hospital, and in the Society of Tropical Medicine and Hygiene. Cantlie had also founded, and funded, the *Journal of Tropical Medicine* in 1898. The address reiterated the need, so forcefully put by Manson at St.George's two years earlier, for special training in tropical medicine, and defended the choice of the Albert Dock Hospital for this purpose. Manson also underlined the distinction between the 'cosmopolitan' bacterial diseases, 'acquired anywhere and everywhere', and the entozoal, parasitic diseases with a 'limited geographical range'. This distinction, and its corollary, was to be reflected in both teaching and research at the London School in its early years and throughout the troubled period of World War I. Manson put it bluntly in October, 1899:

> The discovery of the bacterial cause of many diseases concentrated too exclusively for a time the medical mind on that particular class of germ. To-day the protozoon and the helminth, at all events as regards tropical pathology, are in the ascendant. In this school, although the bacterium will not be neglected, necessarily a large share of your time will be occupied with animal parasites...[50]

It did not mean that bacteriology was neglected at Manson's School before 1914; rather that it assumed a low profile in comparison with the enthusiasm surrounding the subjects of helminthology and parasitology in general, with their emphasis on the varying and complex life-cycles unravelled by research teams at home and abroad. It is possible that the position of bacteriology in the eyes of the students was not helped by the teaching offered in this discipline. Lecturer in bacteriology at the School from its inauguration, Richard Tanner Hewlett (1865–1940) also held a Chair at King's College, London, from 1901. He had no tropical experience, and it was said that he lectured competently if somewhat colourlessly, on bacteria of tropical importance throughout his thirty years at the School. Only with the transformation of the School in the 1920s, and the arrival of W.W.C.Topley (1886–1944) and of Graham Wilson (1895–1987), did bacteriology assume its rightful importance there.[51]

Manson was nevertheless prepared to spread the honours evenly between bacteria and the larger parasites when it came to his 'sanitary creed' for himself, for his School, and for the students about to enter it. He chose diseases from different classes to make his point about the importance of prevention rather than belated attempts at cure. He wrote graphically:

> For the prevention of *cholera* the facts indicate the policy of a *pure water supply*; for the prevention of *malaria* the policy of drainage, cultivation and other methods of *mosquito extermination;* for the prevention of *plague* the policy of the *rat-catcher*... But ... these measures must be employed in anticipation. When our springs are polluted with cholera vibrios, when the house is full of malaria-charged mosquitos, when the rats are tumbling about the floors drunk with plague, it is *too late for general prophylaxis*. Then we must fall back on ... personal prophylaxis; for cholera the *teakettle;* for malaria the *mosquito net* and *quinine bottle*; for plague, *Haffkine's injections*.[52] [authors' italics]

From the very first, emphasis at the School was indeed on policies of prevention. For twenty-five years, that theme was to provide an ideal background, first to cooperation with the Rockefeller initiative and the Johns Hopkins School in the hookworm campaign;[53] and from the early 1920s onwards for the extension of work, in teaching and research, for the School's new existence as a national and international school of public health. Its concerns from then on was to be with all aspects of public health, at home as well as abroad, in tropical and temperate climes.

From its very beginnings, the life of Manson's School, its struggles and its successes, were reflected in not just the carefully compiled Minute Books of the Seamen's Hospital Society, but also in reports issued by the School Committee. Until graduates became too numerous for inclusion they were listed, by name, qualifications, and eventual destination, in these reports, as well as in the handwritten registers.[54] The distribution between various services of Medical Officers trained at the School in its first two years, was listed as follows:

	1st year	2nd year
Colonial Service	42	57
Foreign Service	4	8
Navy	2	2
Army (RAMC & IMS)	5	6
Missionary	16	21

Foreign Governments, Railways, Trading Corporations, Private	27	50
Total	96	144

Eleven of the first year's total were described as 'Lady Graduates'; of these, four had obtained their medical qualifications in Ireland, two in Edinburgh, one in Melbourne to which she returned, two in London, and two in Brussels.[55] Their destinations place them in the 'Missionary' category. By January, 1903, the total number of students who had attended the School's courses had more than doubled. Among them were several who would later leave their mark on academic tropical medicine. They included Aldo Castellani (1877-1971), whose controversial role in the investigations of sleeping sickness in the first decade of the twentieth century did not prevent his long association with British tropical medicine, nor his eventual position as Director of Mycology at the Ross Institute upon its amalgamation with the LSH&TM in 1934.[56] Also prominent among the early graduates was Andrew Balfour (1873-1931), who became Director of the Wellcome Research Laboratories at Khartoum the following year. On the eve of World War I he transferred to London as Director-in-Chief of the Wellcome Bureau of Scientific Research.[57] There he stayed for nearly ten years until the autumn of 1923, when he was appointed Director of the newly established London School of Hygiene and Tropical Medicine, then under construction, with support from the Rockefeller Foundation, in Keppel Street.

    In London (as in Liverpool), appointment of teachers in the School had been under way well before the official opening date. In July, 1899, the organising committee had approved the appointments of Louis Westenra Sambon (1865-1931) and of W.J.Ritchie (later Sir William) Simpson (1855-1931). At the same meeting, it was decided to advertise the School, at weekly intervals, in *The Times, Nature, The Lancet,* the *British Medical Journal,* the *Indian Medical Gazette,* the *Journal of Tropical Medicine,* and a 'Missionary Paper'. Not long afterwards the Seamen's Hospital Society *Minutes* mention 'certain documents' from the London University Commission recognising the School as part of the newly reconstituted University of London.[58] The University also recognised James Cantlie, Andrew Duncan (1850-1912), Tanner Hewlett, Patrick Manson, and Ritchie Simpson, as teachers. With the exception of Simpson, they were all on the staff of the Albert Dock Hospital, and all were described as 'lecturers' at the School. Only Simpson carried the title of 'professor', dating from his appointment to the Chair of Hygiene at

King's College, London, in 1898. R.T.Leiper (1881-1969), a younger fellow Scot appointed by Manson as the first specialist helminthologist at the School in 1905, later became London's first University Professor of Helminthology in 1919.[59]

Initially, teaching at the School took the form of three annual sessions of three months each. The courses combined clinical teaching in the hospital with lectures and laboratory studies in the adjacent new School building.[60] The proximity of School to Hospital, and the doubling of clinical staff as School lecturers, promoted an easy and fruitful relationship between clinical medicine and laboratory analyses and studies which was at that time by no means to be taken for granted elsewhere. This special relationship at the School and Hospital was to some extent also a corollary of Manson's early and continuing enthusiasms and working methods: the larger parasites were so much easier to identify under the microscope (sometimes even with the naked eye) than bacteria, let alone viruses, and hence could more easily and definitively be linked to specific clinical diseases. Now, as the School nears it centenary, its courses have in a sense come full circle: what is now a full-time one year M.Sc. course is offered by the Department of Medical Parasitology jointly with the Department of Clinical Sciences; and a popular 'Short Course' is taught in 'Advanced Laboratory Diagnosis of Parasitic Diseases'. A growing demand for student places testified to the success of the new school and its policies in the early years of the century; it also introduced a need for periodic expansion of teaching facilities, and of student accommodation in this relatively remote corner of London. Leiper's appointment in 1905 signalled more teaching emphasis on specialist subjects, and more involvement of School staff in research expeditions abroad. From quite an early date the School had had a reciprocal arrangement with the Royal Veterinary College which allowed veterinary graduates to follow its courses, while medical graduates in turn had access to the College's courses. It was an arrangement which acknowledged the close connection between animal and human parasitology; and also the need for flexibility in the further education of Veterinary and Medical Officers 'likely to be stationed abroad' where they might be required to stand in for each other in remote areas.[61]

The initial teaching staff was recruited from the Hospital's physicians and surgeons. All had the title of 'Lecturer'; even Manson himself never assumed any more imposing title. Until 1912 he lectured twice a week for the first five weeks of every twelve weeks' course. From then on, in semi-retirement, he continued to deliver a few lectures 'by arrangement'.[62]

Short reports were published at the end of each of the School's first three years. They contained only scant details of the teaching, described as receiving 'chief attention'. There was no printed syllabus or timetable for lectures until 1907. Responsible for the curriculum and the syllabus in 1899 was David C.Rees (1868–1917), first Superintendent and Medical Tutor, who left after only one year to join the South African plague service.[63] The syllabus initially made no attempt to define specialised courses, and according to Manson-Bahr (1881–1966), who attended the three-month course in the summer of 1909, 'the lectures included ... protozoological and helminthological aspects of tropical diseases in so far as these were known at that time. Entomology hardly existed as a separate science; ...'.[64]

A more structured approach began with the arrival of Leiper as helminthologist and Charles Morley Wenyon (1878–1948) as protozoologist, in 1905. It was a year of change in the structure and direction of the School, and in its relations with the University of London, which was to influence developments in the future. In January, the University approved and granted an application from the London School of Tropical Medicine to be included as a branch of its MD examination in addition to the existing five of medicine, pathology, mental diseases, midwifery and diseases of women, and state medicine. Not surprisingly, this was shortly followed by a similar application from the Liverpool School, granted in October of the same year.[65]

Also in 1905, Manson's School was admitted a School of the University in the Faculty of Medicine, with the stipulation that this be in *tropical medicine* only, and that the School must improve and extend its laboratory accommodation. Less than four months later the Lister Institute was likewise admitted into the University's Medical Faculty, 'for the purpose of *research, hygiene and pathology*'.[66] When E.A.Minchin (1866–1915) was appointed University Professor of Protozoology the following March, the two newly recognised schools competed for the privilege of housing the Chair. It was established specifically as a research chair, with no teaching commitment, and not formally 'assigned to any particular School'. Minchin chose to be based at the better equipped Lister Institute;[67] a fact which may to some extent explain why, in 1909, the Council of the University declined to support applications for formal recognition of Leiper as teacher of helminthology and Wenyon as teacher of protozoology in the School, although Fleming Mant Sandwith (1852–1918) had been recognised as teacher of tropical medicine two years earlier at the same time as A.W.Alcock was similarly approved as teacher of medical zoology.[68] Judging by examples of the School's printed syllabus and prospectus, missing University approval did not interfere with the teaching activities of Leiper and of Wenyon; but only after Minchin's early death, and the end of World War I, was Leiper finally appointed the School's first University Professor, in helminthology, in 1919.[69]

With the appointments of Leiper, Wenyon, and Alcock at the School, with Minchin as University Professor, and with G.H.F.Nuttall (1862–1937) at Cambridge, specialisation was taking another turn. 'Tropical medicine' was acquiring sub-divisions; and influenced by Nuttall and Manson, the University of Cambridge established in 1904 the first Diploma in Tropical Medicine and Hygiene.[70] In London, staff at the Hospital for Tropical Diseases continued to lecture on a variety of diseases, supported by clinical demonstrations of cases in the wards of the hospital. In the laboratories of the adjoining school, the focus was on the parasites, the vectors, and the life-cycles, studied in new courses in helminthology, protozoology, and emerging medical entomology.

At the same time, extension and diversification spawned a need for greater coherence, and in 1907 this need found practical expression in the formation of the Society for Tropical Medicine and Hygiene. The founder members were a representative cross-section of those involved in building up the subject of tropical medicine in London, Liverpool, and Cambridge.[71] Among its most enthusiastic supporters were Cantlie and Simpson, who had edited the *Journal of Tropical Medicine,* the first issue of which had been published in August, 1898, with financial support from Cantlie himself. The *Transactions* of the new society began appearing shortly after its ordinary meeting in June, 1907. Less successful was a journal of the London School, established in 1911 as a forum for work by the School's staff and students, past, present, and future. It proved to be a needless addition to the existing journals, and ceased publication at the conclusion of its second volume in 1913.[72]

From 1909 onwards, the School's prospectus included detailed diaries specifying each lecturer's weekly teaching commitment. Only Manson lectured twice a week; the nine other regular lecturers gave a maximum of one lecture per week.[73] First available in 1907, the printed prospectus contained a 10-page syllabus of all the lectures offered in each course by ten respective lecturers. Following this, the practical laboratory course was described in detail in 8 pages; it was supervised by C.W.Daniels. The somewhat casual, *ad hoc* arrangements in the early years of the School are well illustrated by the frequent changes in position of Daniels, who had briefly succeeded David Rees as Superintendent, and then after only three years at the Straits Settlement's research laboratory at Kuala Lumpur had returned to the Albert Dock Hospital and teaching. He also resumed the post of Superintendent in a series of exchanges with G.C.Low. In 1909 Daniel's title was changed to 'Director', before he resigned the following year to concentrate on teaching and clinical work in the hospital. Frequent exchanges of staff between the London School and research laboratories abroad was a favourite policy ideal of Manson's which never quite came to fruition. The decision to abolish the post of 'Superintendent' was perhaps not unrelated to the fact that the School's first Dean had been appointed in 1903. Sir Francis Lovell (1844–1916) had retired from the Colonial Service in 1901, and then took an interest in the fledgling School, expressed in successful fund raising in the Far East, including in Hong Kong and in Japan, and also across the Atlantic in Canada. In addition, he succeeded in initiating a collaborative arrangement with the Institute of Medical Research in Kuala Lumpur (although this did not ultimately survive). When he was appointed Dean in 1903, his firm and considerate working relationship with students and staff stood the School in good stead until his death in 1916. His successor, Sir (Richard Henry) Havelock Charles (1858–1934), lacked Lovell's easy-going personality, bearing all the hallmarks of his former career in the IMS. Bemedalled and aloof, he was in his element running committees and receiving VIPs, but remained uneasy in daily life inside the School. Replaced by Andrew Balfour when the School was restructured in 1924, he then 'vanished to a great extent' in the words of Sir Philip Manson-Bahr.[74]

In 1907, W.J.Simpson's lectures on 'Hygiene of the Tropics' were described in little more than two pages of the prospectus. Over the next few years, Simpson succeeded in proving the importance of his subject. By 1914, although those original lectures were retained as part of the basic course, a new specialised course had been added to the curriculum, with wider terms of reference, and involving eight other lecturers in addition to Simpson himself.[75] At the same time, advanced courses were introduced in protozoology, helminthology, and entomology. Protozoology under Wenyon and helminthology under Leiper (in that first year, the prospectus flatly stated that 'No advanced classes will be held in this subject until the Helminthologist returns from Foreign Service early in 1915') were designed as practical courses. The entomology course consisted of lectures, based on demonstrations, given by Alfred William Alcock (1859–1933).

Alcock had joined the School at Manson's instigation in 1907, as part of the new policy of specialisation begun with Leiper and Wenyon. He was then a marine zoologist, with no experience of entomology. Over a period of twenty-five years, Alcock built up the discipline of medical entomology in the School, organising the teaching programme and writing the influential textbook *Entomology for Medical Officers*. In March, 1920, he was appointed the University of London's first Professor of Medical Zoology.[76]

It was specialists such as Leiper, Wenyon, and Alcock, and their students and associates, who were to consolidate the tropical school's position, and to continue and extend Manson's legacy of excellence and achievement in the study of medically important exotic parasites and their life-cycles. From a strong position as an internationally recognised authority on helminthology, Leiper also played a crucial role in the development of relations with the Rockefeller Foundation and its hookworm campaign.[77] For it was the central position of the humble hookworm, and the disease it causes, in that campaign which led, directly and indirectly, to the re-emergence in the 1920s of Manson's School as the London School of Hygiene and Tropical Medicine.

Abbreviations in Notes

CO – Colonial Office papers, Public Record Office (Kew)

MH – Ministry of Health papers, Public Record Office (Kew)

SHSMB – Seamen's Hospital Society Minute Books

ULSM – University of London Senate Minutes

LSHTM – London School of Hygiene and Tropical Medicine, Reports and manuscript papers.

NOTES

[1] Elizabeth Fee, *Disease and Discovery A history of the Johns Hopkins School of Hygiene and Public Health* 1916-39, Baltimore & London, The Johns Hopkins University Press, 1987.
[2] C.-E.A.Winslow, *The conquest of epidemic diseases,* Madison WI, University of Wisconsin Press, 1980, esp. pp.115-16.
[3] Anne Hardy, *The Epidemic Streets,* Oxford University Press, 1993.
[4] Kenneth Carpenter, *The history of scurvy and vitamin C,* Cambridge University Press, 1986.
[5] W.F.Bynum and V.Nutton, eds, *Theories of fever from antiquity to the Enlightenment, Medical History*, Supplement No.1, London Wellcome Institute for the History of Medicine, 1981.
[6] Christopher C.Booth, *Doctors in Science and Society*, Cambridge University Press for the *British Medical Journal*, 1987, chapter 3, or *Medical History* 1963, 7:297-316.
[7] William Hillary, *Observations on the Changes of the Air and the Concomitant Epidemical Diseases in the Island of Barbados;...* London, C.Hitch and L.Hawes, 1759.
[8] W.F.Bynum, 'Cullen and the study of fevers in Britain 1760-20', in: *Theories of fever...,* op.cit. note 4, pp.135-47.
[9] J.Hunter, *Observations on the diseases of the army in Jamaica,* London, J.Johnson, 1788. On Hunter see L.Wilkinson, ' "The other" John Hunter, MD, FRS (1754-09)'..., *Notes and Records R.Soc.Lond.* 1982, 36:227-41;
J.F.Lafosse, *Avis aux habitants des colonies, particulièrement a ceux de l'isle S.Domingue,* Paris, Royez, 1787.
Much of the early literature is mentioned by Michael Worboys in 'Science and British Colonial Imperialism', Ph.D. thesis, Sussex University, 1979, chapter on 'Tropical medicine and colonial imperialism 1895-1914', pp.83-142.
[10] Benjamin Moseley, *A treatise on tropical diseases, and on the climate of the West Indies,* London, T.Cadell, 1787.
[11] Anon.ed., *Annals of military and naval surgery and tropical medicine and hygiene*, London, John Churchill & Sons, 1864 (for the year 1863), vol.1;
Eli Chernin, 'The early British and American journals of tropical medicine and hygiene: an informal survey', *Medical History* 1992, 36:70-83.
[12] W.M.Frazer, *Duncan of Liverpool,* London, Hamilton Medical, 1947; Royston Lambert, *Sir John Simon 1816-1904 and English Social Administration,* London, MacGibbon & Kee, 1963.

John Hunter, MD (note 9 above) for example was Superintendent of military hospitals 1881–3, and the East India Company employed their own surgeons.

[13] *Gentleman's Magazine,* 1799, *69*(i):53.

[14] A.G.McBride, *The history of the Dreadnought Seamen's Hospital at Greenwich,* Greenwich, Seamen's Hospital Management Committee, 1970, pp.7–8;
A short 'illustrated history' has recently appeared:
Jane Matthews, *Wellcome aboard: the story of the Seamen's Hospital Society and the Dreadnought,* Buckingham, Baron, 1992. A comprehensive recent study of the institution which became the Hospital for Tropical Diseases is: G.C.Cook, *From the Greenwich Hulks to Old St.Pancras,* London, Athlone Press, 1992.

[15] *Gentleman's Magazine.* 1818, *88*(i):79.

[16] SHSMB *1*, entry 8 March 1821 ('Founder's Day').

[17] *ibid.*, 20 March 1821; also McBride, and G.C.Cook, n.14 above.

[18] *ibid.*, 12, pp.136–9, May 1892.

[19] P.Manson, 'Report on haematozoa', and 'Further observations on *Filaria sanguinis hominis* in the mosquito', China Customs Medical Reports, September 1877; also *Proc.Linn.Soc.* March 1878;
idem, 'The metamorphosis of *Filaria sanguinis hominis* in the mosquito', *Trans.Linn.Soc.* 1884, 2:367–88;
Ian A.McGregor, 'Patrick Manson 1844–1922: the birth of the science of tropical medicine', *Trans.Roy.Soc.Trop.Med.Hyg.,* 1995, *89*:1–8;
Anon., 'Sir James Cantlie', *Lancet,* 1926, *i*:1121–2;
J.C.Stewart, *The quality of mercy: the lives of Sir James and Lady Cantlie,* London, Allen and Unwin, 1983 (cf.note 72).

[20] SHSMB *12*, p.136, May 1892.

[21] Sir Philip Manson-Bahr, *History of the School of Tropical Medicine in London (1899–1949),* LSHTM Memoir No.11, London, H.K.Lewis & Co.Ltd., 1956, pp.3–14. This 'History' is largely anecdotal and suffers from lack of notes, references, and index, but benefits from a number of period photographs;
P.H.Manson-Bahr and A.Alcock, *The life and work of Sir Patrick Manson,* London, Cassell & Co.Ltd., [1927], pp.84–103.

[22] H.Chick, M.Hume and M.Macfarlane, *War on Disease: a history of the Lister Institute,* London, Andre Deutsch, 1971, p.23.

[23] Paul Cranefield, *Science and Empire,* Cambridge University Press, 1991, pp.135–6; examples of recent multi-author volumes are: Roy MacLeod and Milton Lewis (eds), *Disease, Medicine and Empire,* London and New York, Routledge, 1988; and David Arnold (ed), *Imperial*

medicine and indigenous societies: disease, medicine and empire in the nineteenth and twentieth centuries, Manchester and New York, Manchester University Press, 1988.
24 Manson-Bahr, op.cit. note 22, p.28.
25 *Memorandum* by Read, 2 December 1897, CO 885/7/119, No.1, p.2.
26 Patrick Manson, 'On the necessity for special education in tropical medicine', *Lancet* 1897, *ii*:842–5; also quoted by Manson-Bahr (note 22) pp.31 and 41–2, and referred to in Read's *Memorandum;* CO 323/425/22442 pp.392–5.
27 SHSMB *13*, p.1, 13 August 1897.
28 H.J.Read, *Memorandum*, op.cit. note 25;
Eli Chernin, 'Sir Patrick Manson: physician to the Colonial Office, 1897–1912', *Medical History* 1992, 36:320–30.
29 [J.J.Stephens, W.Yorke, B.Blacklock], *Liverpool School of Tropical Medicine. Historical Record 1898–1920,* Liverpool University Press, 1920;
Helen J.Power, *Tropical Medicine in the Twentieth Century: a history of the Liverpool School of Tropical Medicine 1898–1990,* London and New York, Kegan Paul International, 1998.
30 *ibid.*;
C.S.S. [Sherrington], 'Sir Rubert Boyce (1863–1911), *Proc.Roy.Soc.B* 1911, *84*:iii–x; Anon., 'Sir Rubert William Boyce', *Lancet* 1911, *ii:*59–60;
Obituaries of Sir Alfred Jones, *Lancet* 1909, *ii:*1838; *Br.med.J.* 1909, *ii:*1770;
DNB, Supplement 1901–11;
also biographies cited in note 38.
31 Another example was the eradication of rabies in Britain by 1902, following the successful, but heavily contested and protracted, campaign by Victor Horsley and Walter Long.
32 Andrew Balfour, 'Some British and American pioneers in tropical medicine and hygiene', *Trans.Roy.Soc.Trop.Med.Hyg.* 1925–6, *19*:189–231;
P.Manson, *A manual of tropical diseases*, London etc., Cassell and Co.Ltd., 1898 (many later editions; 19th ed., P.E.C.Manson-Bahr and D.R.Bell eds, Bailliere, Tindall Ltd, 1987);
Leonard Rogers, *Fevers in the tropics: their clinical and microscopical differentiation,* Oxford Med.Publ., 1907 (2nd ed. 1910).
Leonard Rogers and J.W.D.Megaw, *Tropical Medicine*, London, J.and A.Churchill, 1930 (6th ed. 1952).
33 Read, note 25 above, pp.2 and 3. A footnote flatly states that 'there are

a few other medical appointments filled by natives, and not so well paid'.
[34] SHSMB *13*, pp.56–7, draft letter to Under Secretary of State, April 1898. Details of teaching and student life at Netley in the 1890s, when Leonard Rogers attended, may be found in a biographical chapter on Rogers in: Helen Power, A study of Sir Leonard Rogers, FRCP, FRS (1868–1962) Ph.D.thesis, London University, 1993.
[35] *Liverpool School of Tropical Medicine,* note 29 above, p.4; and CO 885/7/119, Nos. 12–25.
[36] Manson–Bahr, op.cit. note 22, p.39;
G.C.Cook, 'Doctor Patrick Manson's leading opposition in the establishment of the London School of Tropical Medicine: Curnow, Anderson and Turner', *J.Med.Biogr.,* 1995, *3:*170–7.
[37] LSTM School Register, book 1;
SHSMB *13*, p.207, 13 October 1899;
T.B.Shaw, 'Sir Percy Bassett–Smith', *Trans.Roy.Soc.Trop.Med.Hyg.,* 1927–8, *21:*435–8;
N.H.F., 'George Carmichael Low', *ibid.,* 1952, *46:*571–3;
Louis Sambon and George C.Low, 'Report on two experiments on the mosquito–malaria theory instituted by the Colonial Office and the London School of Tropical Medicine', *Med.Chir.trans.,* 1901, *84:*497–536. The work in the Roman Campagna is described in detail in Manson-Bahr, op.cit. note 22, pp.98–103; and also in *Br.med.J.,* 1900, *ii:*847–8;
Myron G.Schultz, 'A history of bartonellosis (Carrión's disease), *Am.J.trop.Med.hyg.,* 1968, *17:*503–15;
Marcos Cueto, 'Tropical medicine and bacteriology in Boston and Peru: studies of Carrion's disease in the early twentieth century', *Med.Hist.,* 1996, *40:*344–64.
[38] Obituaries and *DNB,* Supplement 1901–11, op.cit. note 30;
P.N.Davies, *Sir Alfred Jones,* London, Europa Publications, 1978, cited by Worboys in *Disease, Medicine and Empire,* op.cit. note 23, p.35;
Peter N.Davies, *Fyffes and the Banana: Musa Sapientium. A centenary history 1888–1988,* London and Atlantic Highlands, NJ, 1990.
[39] *Liverpool School of Tropical Medicine*, op.cit. note 29, p.5.
[40] *ibid.,* p.28;
Boyce obituaries, op.cit. note 30;
Anon., 'Richard Caton', *Lancet,* 1926, *i:*102;
Lord Cohen, 'Richard Caton (1842–1926) pioneer electrophysiologist', *Proc.Roy.Soc.Med. (Section Hist.Med.),* 1959, *52:*645–51;
June Jones, 'Science, utility and the 'second city of the empire': the sciences and especially the medical sciences at Liverpool University 1881–1925', Ph.D. thesis, University of Manchester, 1989.

[41] As note 39, see footnotes pp.4 and 5.
[42] SHSMB *13,*p.35-7, Colonial Office to SHS, dated 2 February, 1898; reply, SHS to Col.Off., 16 April, 1898, CO 885/7/119, no.17.
[43] G.H.F.N.[Nuttall], 'Sir Ronald Ross 1857-1932', *Obit.Not.Fell. Roy.Soc.* 1932-5, *1:*108-14;
C.M.Wenyon, 'Colonel Sir Ronald Ross', *Trans.Roy.Soc.Trop.Med.Hyg.* 1932-3, *26*:473-8.
[44] Following the creation of the London and Liverpool schools, Hamburg acquired its *Institut für Schiffs-und Tropenkrankheiten* in 1900; in 1906, the Congo State Government established an institute offering instruction for Belgian colonial medical officers; France, already well provided with Pasteur Institutes abroad, added an institute for 'colonial medicine' in Paris, and Holland followed suit in 1910: The Calcutta School of Tropical Medicine, crowning achievement of Leonard Rogers in India, opened in 1920.
F.M.Sandwith, 'A visit to the tropical school at Hamburg', *J.Trop.Med.Hyg.* 1907, *10*:397-9.
A.de Mets, 'L'Institut de Médecine Tropicale Prince Léopold', Anvers, Éditions St.-Jacques, [1934];
N.H.Swellengrebel. 'De afdeeling voor tropische hygiene van het Kolonial Institut te Amsterdam', Amsterdam, J.H.de Bussy, 1916;
J.W.D.Megaw, *A short account of the Calcutta School of Tropical Medicine, I.M.S., 1921;*
R.Knowles, *The Calcutta School of Tropical Medicine 1920-33,* Alipore, Bengal Government Press, 1934; also Helen Power thesis, note 34 above.
[45] *Liverpool School of Tropical Medicine* op.cit. note 29, pp.55-6.
[46] Manson-Bahr, op.cit. note 22, on Roman Campagna experiment pp.98-103; on expeditions until the outbreak of war in 1914, pp.267-78; also early School Reports.
[47] Details of expeditions in obituaries:
S.R.Christophers, 'John William Watson Stephens 1865-1946',
Obit.Not.Fell.Roy.Soc. 1945-8, 5:525-40;
H.E.Shortt and P.C.C.Garnham, 'Samuel Rickard Christophers 27 November 1873-19 February 1978', *Biogr.Mem.Fell.Roy.Soc.* 1979, 25:179-207;
A.Alcock, 'In memoriam Charles Wilberforce Daniels 1862-1927', *Trans.Roy.Soc.Trop.Med.Hyg.* 1927-8, *21:*249-55.
[48] Manson-Bahr, op.cit. note 22, 'Diary of the School', pp.267-72. Between 1902 and 1913, the School received regular contributions from a number of overseas dependencies, including Hong Kong, the Federated Malay States, the Bahamas, Jamaica, Brit.Guiana, Brit.Honduras, etc.,

LSHTM MSS FA: D3 (12); only the Falklands, admittedly non-tropical, refused to contribute, see Governor to Colonial Office, CO 885/9/170, No.54.

[49] SHSMB: *13*, p.181, Laveran, 16 June 1899; p.191, Osler, 14 July 1899; p.197, Baccelli, 11 August 1899; p.206.

[50] P.Manson, 'The need for special training in tropical diseases', *Br.med.J.* 1899, *ii*: 922–6, p.925.

[51] Manson-Bahr, op.cit. note 22, p.138;
M.Greenwood, 'William Whiteman Carlton Topley 1886–1944', *Obit.Not.Fell.Roy.Soc.* 1944, *4*:699–712;
E.S.Anderson and Sir Robert Williams, 'Graham Selby Wilson 10 September 1895–5 April 1987', *Biogr.Mem.Fell.Roy.Soc. 1988, 34*:887–919.

[52] Manson, op.cit. note 50, p.925, (authors' italics).

[53] For details of the American hookworm campaign from the Sanitary Commission to the Rockefeller Foundation see John Ettling, *The germ of laziness,* Cambridge, Mass., Harvard University Press, 1981, pp.189–90; Ettling mentions contacts with the Colonial Office in London in 1913, and between Wickliffe Rose and Sandwith, but does not refer to Leiper (cf.following chapters).

[54] Seamen's Hospital Society, *The London School of Tropical Medicine.* Report for the year 1899–1900, pp.15–16; *ibid.,* 2nd year 1900–1, pp.18–20; *ibid., January* 1903, pp.19–23; LSTM School Register, cf.pp.14–15 above and note 37.

[55] *ibid.*

[56] Anon., 'Sir Aldo Castellani', *J.Trop.Med.Hyg.*, 1971, *74*:233–7; P.C.C.Garnham, 'Aldo Castellani 1877–1971', Pontifica Academia Scientiarum, *Commentarii*, vol.ii.no.45:1–36, Vatican City, 1972; Sir John Boyd, 'Sleeping sickness. The Castellani-Bruce controversy', *Notes and Records Roy.Soc.* 1973, *28*:93–110;
A.J.Duggan, 'Bruce and the African trypanosomes', *Am.J.Trop.Med.Hyg.,* 1977, *26*:1080–3;
cf. also chapter 8 on the Ross Institute below.

[57] Anon., 'Sir Andrew Balfour', *J.Trop.Med.Hyg.*, 1931, *34*:63–4; also cf. chapter 3.

[58] SHSMB *13*, p.191, and 243–4, 14 July 1899.

[59] ULSM ST 2/2/35, No.3517, 23 July 1919;
a recent study of Simpson's contributions to tropical hygiene is:
Mary Preston Sutphen, 'Imperial hygiene in Calcutta, Cape Town and Hong Kong: the early career of Sir William John Ritchie Simpson (1855–1931)', Yale University Ph.D. thesis, 1995.

[60] School Reports 1899–1900 and 1900–1; also Manson-Bahr op.cit. note 22, p.45. Photographs in Manson-Bahr and in LSHTM *Prospectus,* from 1907 onwards.
[61] Manson-Bahr, op.cit. note 22, 'Diary of the School', pp.272–8; LSTM *Report*, 1904, p.6.
[62] 'Diary of Lectures in the School', LSTM *Prospectus*, 1909 and 1914.
[63] 'David Charles Rees', obituaries in *Lancet*, 1917, *ii:*549 and *Br.med.J.*, 1917, *ii:*469–70.
[64] Manson-Bahr, op.cit. note 22, p.267.
[65] ULSM ST 2/2/21, Nos.757–9, 25 January 1905; *ibid.,* ST 2/2/22, No.155, 25 October 1905.
[66] ULSM ST 2/2/21, Nos.1065–6, 22 February 1905; *ibid.,* No.1917, 7 June 1905.
[67] ULSM ST 2/2/21, No.1441, 28 March 1906; *ibid.,* Nos. 1849–52.
[68] ULSM ST 2/2/25, Nos.3242, 3268, 3269, 21 July 1909; *ibid.,* ST 2/2/23 No.2529, 24 July 1907.
[69] ULSM ST 2/2/35, No.3517, 23 July 1919.
[70] G.S.Graham-Smith, 'George Henry Falkiner Nuttall', *J.Hyg.*, 1938, *38*:129–40.
[71] G.Carmichael Low, 'The history of the foundation of the Society of Tropical Medicine and Hygiene', *Trans.Roy.Soc.Trop.Med.Hyg.*, 1928, *22:*197–202.
[72] J.C.Stewart, *The quality of mercy: the lives of Sir James and Lady Cantlie*, London, Allen and Unwin, 1983, chapter 11; *Journal of the London School of Tropical Medicine,* 1911–13, 1–2.
[73] 'Diary of Lectures in the School', LSTM *Prospectus,* 1909–24.
[74] Manson-Bahr op.cit. note 22, pp.162–5 and 174–6; Alcock's obituary of Daniels, op.cit. note 47.
[75] LSTM *Prospectus*, 1907, pp.14–16; 1914, pp.27–33. On advanced courses, pp. 34–7.
[76] Manson-Bahr op.cit. note 22, pp.234–7; W.T.C. and S.W.K., 'Alfred William Alcock 1859–1933', *Obit.Not.Fell.Roy.Soc.,* 1932–5, *i:*119–24; Alcock biographical papers, LSHTM MSS FA:D1 (14).
[77] Donald Fisher, 'Rockefeller philanthropy and the British Empire: the creation of the London School of Hygiene and Tropical Medicine', *Hist.Educ.,* 1978, *7:*129–43, p.132. This connection will be further explored in subsequent chapters.

2

PROTAGONISTS OF A MEDICAL SPECIALTY: PARASITES, VECTORS, AND EXOTIC LIFE-CYCLES

As briefly mentioned above, much attention has been lavished in recent years on socio-economic and political aspects of health policies pursued by Western colonial powers in the nineteenth and early twentieth centuries in Africa and India. In the wake of criticism of colonialism and imperialism, 'medical imperialism' has been blamed for applying a 'biomedical' model to the non-medical world, and hence imposing Western cultural values in the non-Western world. In this context there has been an exhaustive search for signs of ill intentions and ulterior motives and lack of concern for native populations and native eco-systems in the great crusades against especially malaria and sleeping sickness carried out by the generation of Victorian physician-naturalists and their immediate successors. In these debates, working medical scientists have come in for their share of criticism. Some commentators have attacked those allegedly engaged in narrow-minded pursuit of pure science to the exclusion of attempts to improve sanitation and other public health measures, at the same time referring to public health as the 'handmaiden' to European medicine in a joint role as 'tools of empire'.[1]

There can be little doubt that on the political level such criticism is well justified, and that to the Colonial Office and the India Office, as to Belgian, French, and German authorities in the Congo and elsewhere, the health of their officers on the spot, and above all the economic consequences of ill health in Europeans and their native labourers, played a major role in decision making and formation of policies. As with Bismarcks' public health and welfare reforms in Germany in the 1880s, the driving forces were to be found, nationally and internationally, in politics and economics rather than in altruistic concern with individual human problems. But to adopt uncritically Ross's alleged observation that the empire had done more for tropical medicine than tropical medicine for the Empire would seem an over-simplification; in fact, Chernin has pointed out that Ross contradicted himself on this point with another 'favourite quip'.[2] In any case such a remark fails to take into account the sustained and often inspired hard work, clinically and scientifically, of many pioneers in the face of difficulties and disasters, and also the fact that epidemiology and constructive health policies, including rational preventive measures, could begin to be developed only when individual disease agents, both bacteria and the larger parasites, were known and the *modus vivendi* and the life-cycle of each were understood. This chapter sets out to concentrate less on politics and more on the achievements in clinical and pure science in this area prior to World War 1, many of which involved staff members and potential associates of both the London and Liverpool Schools.

When Patrick Manson, recently qualified, set out on the path which was to lead to China and Hong Kong, and eventually back to Britain and the founding of the LSTM[3] he was, like many a fellow Scot in the nineteenth century, motivated as much by lack of opportunities at home as by a taste for adventure. In his case, other driving factors were a degree of intellectual and scientific curiosity, and also a genuine concern for his patients, suffering from diseases of little known aetiology and doubtful prognosis. With no alternative but to learn from his mistakes as well as from occasional successes, in the absence of prior formal instruction, Manson's experiences in Amoy and Hong Kong became seminal for his belief in the need for specialist education in tropical medicine. This belief was strongly expressed in his passionate appeal for specialist teaching in his introductory lecture at St. George's in 1897. Five years later, these views were repeated and given practical expression in the lecture inaugurating the LSTM in October, 1899. In the 1897 lecture, he graphically described his abject helplessness when first confronted with unfamiliar diseases in his Chinese patients: on more than one occasion had he confused beriberi with dropsy. Nor did he spare himself when expressing his feelings of guilt when patients died following wrong diagnoses and treatment. Another puzzle involved frequently seen cases of elephantiasis and other manifestations of filariasis.[4] On home leave in 1875 he learned of Lewis's observations of microfilariae; when he returned to Amoy the following year, he had armed himself with a microscope.[5]

The rapid rise of medical bacteriology in the 1870s and 1880s in the hands of Pasteur and of Koch, and their respective schools, can be regarded as a corollary of experiences in parasitology earlier in the century. Worms and protozoa, larger than bacteria, could be seen sometimes with the naked eye, sometimes in primitive microscopes. The *acarus* mite and its causal relationship to scabies had been known since the late eighteenth century, and served as a point of reference for theories of the existence of other, 'infinitely small', invisible, disease causing organisms.[6]

In the Seamen's Hospital Ship *Dreadnought*, George Busk had found giant intestinal flukes (*Distoma crassum, Distoma Buskii,* now *Fasciolopsis buski*) in the duodenum of an Indian patient who had died there in 1843; by 1860, Theodor Bilharz (1825–62) had described eggs and adult forms of two species of *Schistosoma* in patients in Egypt.[7] Casimir–Joseph Davaine (1812–82), soon to turn his attention to anthrax, published the first edition of his textbook of parasitology in 1860. Microfilariae of filariasis and elephantiasis were observed in the 1860s by Jean–Nicolas Demarquay (1814–75) in Cuba and, independently, by Otto Wucherer (1820–73) in Bahia, Brazil, and later by Timothy Richard Lewis (1841–86) in Calcutta. The adult nematode was found, following a deliberate search, by Joseph Bancroft (1836–94) in Australia. Later established as species of *Wuchereria* and *Brugia*, it was under the name of *Filaria sanguinis hominis*, suggested by Busk when commenting on Lewis's paper of 1871, that the microfilariae of *Wuchereria* were studied by Manson in Amoy in the later 1870s.[8]

FILARIASIS

When Manson returned to Amoy with his new microscope in 1876, he had no difficulty in finding microfilariae in the blood of patients. But he was not satisfied with mere observation. The sheer numbers – hundreds of thousands – of larvae which might be present in one patient, led Manson to speculate on the possibility of their escaping to mature elsewhere before entering another human host. As for the path of transmission, he considered the possible role as vectors of a number of blood-sucking insects. In August, 1877, he began experimenting with mosquitoes fed on the microfilariae-containing blood of his Chinese gardener. Fortuitously,[9] he had made the right choice: painstaking daily examination of the stomach contents of mosquitoes, which had sucked the gardener's blood, revealed that '... the haematozoon which entered the mosquito a simple, structureless animal, left it, after passing through a number of highly interesting metamorphoses, much increased in size, possessing an alimentary canal, and being otherwise suited for an independent existence'.[10]

This was the discovery which first made Manson's scientific reputation both at home and abroad. His conclusion was not flawless. With little knowledge of the general natural history of the mosquito, he was unaware of its wide geographical distribution and of its ability to bite more than once in its lifetime: he erroneously concluded that after development in the mosquito gut the filariae escaped into water, and from there into new human hosts. Nevertheless it was his seminal discovery of mosquito transmission of filariae which was to lead directly to Ross's proof of mosquito transmission of the *Plasmodium* of malaria, and indirectly to all the subsequent work on malaria at the London and Liverpool Schools. Today that work promises to continue into a second century; not because of any failings in experimental methods, but because of the complexity of the problems of malaria and of the changing patterns of behaviour of the parasites and their vectors notably their ability to develop resistance to antimalarials and to DDT, respectively.[11]

When in the 1890s Manson, with characteristic pragmatism and generosity, guided Ross in his pioneering work on the malaria parasites and their transmission, the study of filariae and other helminths infesting man remained of absorbing interest to himself. Once his School was established, helminthological problems continued to play a considerable part in both clinical work at the hospital, and in the teaching and research of the School. Manson's seminal study of the mosquito transmission of *Filaria sanguinis hominis* (now *Wuchereria bancrofti*) was confirmed and extended in exemplary collaboration between Joseph Bancroft's son Thomas (1860–1933) in Australia, and Manson in London, and in experiments carried out by George Low at Manson's instigation in June, 1900.[12] These experiments finally established the way in which the filarial larvae passed through the salivary glands of the mosquito into its proboscis, ready to enter a new human host at the next bite. The young Low had completed his course after entering the School as one of the second intake of students in January, 1900; by then, he had already been working on the fate of *Filaria* larvae in *Culex fatigans* under Manson for more than two years.[13] His results were published in the *British Medical Journal* in June, 1900; a month later, Low left for Italy to take part in the School's first epidemiological malaria experiment. On July 19th, 1900, Low, Sambon, the Italian artist Enrico Terzi, and a servant, took up residence in a custom-built, mosquito-proof hut in the Roman Campagna. Three months later, having emerged from the hut only in the daytime, and remained free from malaria, they had proved an important epidemiological point.[14]

GUINEA WORM DISEASE

With the appointment of Robert Leiper as the School's helminthologist in 1905, Manson lost no time in introducing him to his own abiding interest in the transmission of filarial worms in man. Shortly after his arrival at the School, the young Leiper found himself at Accra on the African Gold Coast, learning on the job in the study of the perennial problems of the life-cycle of the Guinea worm *Dracunculus medinensis (Filaria medinensis)*. Manson had a long-standing interest in the Guinea worm, among the largest of the helminthic parasites of man. Calcified remains of the worm have been identified in a Egyptian mummy, and its very size – the adult female, found in prominent ulcers in the lower limbs of patients reaches a length of 1 metre – has earned it early appearances in the literature of antiquity, from the *Ebers Papyrus* to the Bible.[15]

At Accra in 1905 Leiper was able to complete the studies, prematurely ended, by A.P.Fedchenko (1844–73). Fedchenko in 1870 had implicated the crustacean *Cyclops* as intermediate host for developing larvae of *D.medinensis,* but was uncertain about the ultimate step in the path of transmission: the transfer of the embryo from *Cyclops* to man, and the final differentiation there of male and female worms. Leiper demonstrated that the acidity of gastric juice would kill the *Cyclops* without affecting the Guinea worm larvae, which were able to complete their development inside the human host. Following up this research, Leiper could finally describe the smaller male Guinea worm, found at autopsy, after a 6 months' interval, in a monkey fed on bananas containing infected *Cyclops*.[16] It was Leiper's definitive description of the life-cycle of the Guinea worm which finally brought control, and even prevention, of dracontiasis (dracunculiasis) within the realm of possibility. It also launched him in his career as an authority on parasitology and, as such, the teacher who above all was to inherit the mantle of Manson in influence on research and, on another level, as the personality guiding the School's further destiny when its concerns began to change from tropical medicine only, towards a broader concept of global public health between the two world wars.

Two years before the outbreak of The Great War Leiper, again at Manson's suggestion, went in search of the vector of another filarial worm, *Loa loa,* the eyeworm causing Calabar swellings. Ever supportive and keen to further Leiper's studies in a field which had always held his own interest, Manson encouraged travel abroad, and Leiper was the recipient of a number of grants and scholarships available at the School for study in tropical areas. In late autumn 1912 he was again in West Africa, as Wandsworth Scholar, in pursuit of the eyeworm.[17] Primed by Manson as to the diurnal periodicity of *Loa loa,* Leiper in Calabar adopted the 'blunderbuss' method, feeding a number of different insect species on an infected soldier, but without satisfactory results. Only when he found, at a local mission station, a rescued slave girl with the parasite in her blood, was he able to implicate an 'orange fly' *(Chrysops* species). Active in the daytime, the fly could be shown to contain the filarial larvae in its tissues after biting the girl (neither patient consent, nor other questions of ethics, seem to have been raised). Further experiments confirmed the full development of the worm in the 'orange fly', and Leiper could announce his discovery to the School on Christmas day.[18] In the meantime, between 1905 and 1912, Leiper, representing the School's Helminthology Department, had been studying other parasitic worms giving cause for concern: trematodes with immensely complex life-cycles and unpleasant effects on humans and the larger apes; and nematodes with somewhat simpler lifestyles and no intermediate hosts, but equally distressing effects on their human hosts. The former were the three species of blood flukes responsible for schistosomiasis in different parts of the world; and the latter the two main species of hookworm, *Ancylostoma duodenale* and *Necator americanus*.

SCHISTOSOMIASIS (BILHARZIASIS)

First discovered and described by Theodor Bilharz (1825–62) in Egypt in 1851, the vesical blood fluke, *Schistosoma haematobium* prevalent in Africa and the Middle East, has also been known as *Bilharzia haematobia*, and the disease as bilharzia. Other pathogenic species are *Schistosoma mansoni*, in Africa, South America, and the Caribbean islands, and *S.japonica* in the Far East. The three species vary little in their natural habitat, although their respective snail intermediate hosts each belong to species of three different genera: *Bulinus, Biomphalaria,* and *Oncomelania*. Only *S.japonica* include rodents and a number of domestic animals in its list of definitive hosts in addition to humans and the larger apes.[19]

The differences in distribution and identity of intermediate hosts not unnaturally gave rise to contradictions and controversies in early studies of the disease and its aetiology, although not until decades after Bilharz's premature death, in Cairo, from a 'febrile illness'.

The unravelling of the *Schistosoma* life-cycle, and of the clinical features of the disease caused, occupied many able researchers in the later decades of the nineteenth century. European governments with colonial interests encouraged fieldwork in North Africa: Italy, France, Germany and Britain all sent special missions to Egypt both before and after the turn of the century.[20] At that time of troubled politics in Egypt, consequent on the Suez Canal controversy, France and Britain dominated the weak governments of Tewfik Pasha; disagreements over the methods to be used in the face of nationalist riots eventually left Britain in virtual sole control between 1882 and 1907. Nevertheless, it was the German Arthur Looss (1861-1923) who was appointed the first Professor of Parasitology and Biology in the Egyptian Government School of Medicine in 1896. He was a German professor of the old school who, having made the major discovery of hookworm penetration of intact skin, went on to hold intractable, but erroneous, views on almost every aspect of schistosomiasis. It was to Looss's department that R.T.Leiper came on study leave in 1906-7, and it was there that his interests in the diseases caused by hookworms and schistosomes were kindled. Both were subjects which, in different ways, were to influence life at the London School in years to come.

The School's connection with the study of schistosomiasis began in 1902 when, at the Albert Dock Hospital, Patrick Manson examined a patient recently returned from fifteen years in the West Indies. Presenting with anaemia and a number of vague aches and pains, this patient did not, as Manson had expected, suffer from hookworm disease: ova in his stools were identified as schistosome eggs rather than hookworm eggs, and none was found in the patient's urine. Manson also noted that the spine on the eggs was 'placed laterally'. His results were to lead to a polarisation of German and British perceptions when, in the following year, he aired the possibility of the existence of two species of *Bilharzia*, one with lateral-spined ova depositing eggs in the rectum only, the other 'haunting the bladder and rectum indifferently'.[21] L.W.Sambon, lecturer at Manson's School, took up the subject. He proposed the names of *S.mansoni* and *S.haematobia* for the respective species, and was immediately subjected to what Grove has called a 'vitriolic blast' from Arthur Looss, whose rigidly held inaccurate views also included the theory of direct infection and the absence of any vector.[22] It was in such an atmosphere of acrimonious international controversy that Leiper in 1913 returned to the study of schistosomiasis.

When he first had encountered the problem on his early visit to Looss in Egypt, Leiper had felt that the problems of schistosomiasis, and the complex questions concerning individual species of schistosomes and their respective eggs, possible vectors, and overall life-cycles, could be more easily studied in the Far East where the disease occurs naturally in animals. Hence he was disappointed to learn, just before leaving England, that Japanese workers had described the reproductive stages of *S.japonicum* in snails, and had been able to infect mice experimentally by immersing them in the water of rice fields where the disease was endemic.[23]

However, much could still be learnt from, and possibly added to, the Japanese results, and Leiper set out on the journey. He did not go alone; his travelling companion was one E.L.Atkinson (1882–1928). Atkinson was the young surgeon who had been left in charge of the base camp when Scott and the rest of his companions set out on the final fatal dash to the South Pole in January, 1912. It was Atkinson who assumed the melancholy duty of organising the search party to bring back the bodies of his lost companions; it was Atkinson who found Scott's diary. Back in London later in 1912, he worked in Leiper's department at the School on his collection of worms from Antarctica, naming new species for his dead colleagues – e.g. scotti, wilsoni, oatsei, etc. The resulting papers were published with Leiper as senior author. Atkinson may have resented this; the relationship between the two men was never an easy one, and did not improve during their travels. Atkinson, a disciplined product of public school and St.Thomas's Hospital Medical School, sobered by his experiences in Antarctica, found it difficult to adjust to Leiper's spiky Scottish temperament and his autocratic ways within the department. Relations did not improve *en route* to the Far East. In a letter to a friend, Atkinson described Leiper as 'too damnable for words', and accused him of hampering their work by his lack of tact in dealing with local populations. On the other hand, Atkinson's own temper was frayed by Chinese attitudes, and he also complained that ' ... we were met by the most crass ignorance and suspicion'. There was clearly an impasse on several levels.[24]

The difficult situation between Leiper and Atkinson was an early indication of problems to come in the department. On the whole on friendly terms with his immediate staff and students, Leiper was not regarded as an easy colleague by his peers. During his long career, and especially in his later established position within the LSHTM, his pronounced scientific ego and often abrasive style in dealing with professional matters were repeatedly responsible for friction at administrative level, notably in a tussle over the appointment of an acting dean in 1943, when G.S.Parkinson resigned after only two years to become Director of the Public Health Commission to the Allied Military Government in North Africa. This episode will be analysed in a later chapter.

In spite of their personal differences, Leiper and Atkinson obtained valuable results during their time in the Far East. By July, 1914, they had confirmed the Japanese results; but only after a dash to Japan to collect the right species of snail, having failed in their efforts to infect any species native to the lower Yangtze Valley. With the international situation rapidly worsening, it was clearly time to return to London. Leiper and

Atkinson embarked on the voyage home accompanied by a number of mice which had been exposed to infected water. Only one mouse survived the long and rough journey back to the London School. That sole survivor, when examined, was found to contain adult male and female schistosomes. In this respect, the mission to the far East, on the eve of war in Europe, had been a success.[25]

The outbreak of war in Europe in August, 1914, which was so radically to alter the map of Europe and the balance of political power, had indirect effects on the study of schistosomiasis in Egypt. Large numbers of British troops were stationed there, and the dangers of contracting schistosomiasis were well understood in the RAMC. A Bilharzia Mission was established, under the command of Leiper. His staff included the protozoologist J.Gordon Thomson (1878–1937), recently arrived from Liverpool to take up a lectureship at the London School; and Leiper's own trusted technician, William McDonald (1895–1941).[26] Working space for the mission was found in the parasitological laboratory of the Cairo Medical School, vacated by the departure of Looss in November, 1914. Looss had never abandoned his theory of direct transmission of what he considered a single disease; Leiper, since his early visit to Looss's laboratories, had developed very different ideas. Working from a village with a virtual 100 per cent infection rate with *S.haematobium*, Leiper and his staff systematically examined numerous species of Egyptian snails, selecting those producing typical cercariae. During the first half of 1915, they solved the main outstanding problems of the life-cycles of the African schistosomes. In a Cairo crowded with wounded from Gallipoli, and later back in London, the study of about fifty species of Egyptian snails showed that as many as half of them harboured various types of cercariae, many of them of bilharzial origin. To conclude the study, Leiper was able to identify snail vectors for both African species, and to demonstrate the full cycle of development of the parasites in the snails.[27]

HOOKWORM DISEASE (ANCHYLOSTOMIASIS)

The work on schistosomiasis may have been the culmination of Leiper's achievements in the studies of life-cycles; but he had many strings to his bow. His work on hookworm, already mentioned in the previous chapter, was of a different character: the life-cycle of the hookworm is relatively simple, and there is no intermediate host. Yet the implications of its study were such that it was to influence the development of public health education, and public health policies, on both sides of the Atlantic during the first quarter of the twentieth century, and beyond. It had long been a problem in many parts of the world when, in 1909, John D.Rockefeller (1839–1937), on the advice of Frederick Gates (1853–1929), decided to offer financial support to the hookworm campaign envisaged by Charles W.Stiles (1867–1941) in the southern United States.[28]

The resulting Rockefeller sponsored Sanitary Commission was established in 1909, and within a period of four years it had achieved a measure of control of the debilitating disease in the southern United States.[29] In 1913, the Rockefeller philanthropic activities were incorporated as the Rockefeller Foundation, and in the same year its International Health Board was established under the able directorship of Wickliffe Rose (1862–1931). It was at this point that American and British interests joined forces in an effort to control hookworm over a range far beyond the narrow area delimited by the southern United States. The decision to do so was to influence not only future policies for disease control on a global scale, but also the development of Manson's School, and the disciplines with which it was to be associated in the twentieth century.

The problems of hookworm infestation in poor working populations were not unknown to the School's helminthologists well before 1913. Egypt, although not declared a British protectorate until the outbreak of war in 1914, was effectively controlled by British consuls general in the early years of the century; and British and other European physicians and surgeons played a not inconsiderable role in the work of the Egyptian Government Medical School in Cairo. One of them was Fleming Mant Sandwith (1853–1918).

Sandwith had spent twenty years in Egypt when in 1904 he returned to England to work at the Hospital for Tropical Diseases at the Albert Dock, and to lecture at Manson's School there.[30] During the Egyptian years he had been associated with Arthur Looss, before the later controversies, at a time when Looss was justly respected for his discovery that infective hookworm larvae penetrate intact skin. When Sandwith arrived at the Albert Dock, shortly to be joined by Robert Leiper as helminthologist, he was armed with more than cursory knowledge of hookworm disease in Egypt, and had published several papers on the subject.[31] It was the expertise of Leiper and of Sandwith which attracted Wickliffe Rose when in 1913, as director of the newly established International Health Board (IHB), he began a fact-finding tour with a visit to London. He conveniently arrived in time for the 17th International Congress of Medicine, and lost no time in making contact with members of the tropical section, and especially with Leiper and Sandwith, acknowledged experts on hookworm disease. In their presence, lecturing on the work of the Sanitary Commission, Rose offered, on behalf of the IHB, to assist Britain in fighting hookworm disease in countries of the British Empire. Afterwards Rose confided with some satisfaction to his diary that Sandwith had congratulated him on having made more headway 'in one evening than we have been able to ... at all'. When Rose set out on a more extensive tour at the beginning of 1914, he took Sandwith with him as adviser in Egypt and Ceylon.[32] It was the beginning of a cooperation, on a semi-official level, which was to have important consequences for the London School in the years following the end of the Great War.

When Sandwith first began working on hookworm disease in Egypt before the turn of the century, he pointed out that a disease described in the medical papyrus, found by George Ebers at Thebes in 1872 and dating back to more than a millennium BC, has been thought by scholars to be possibly identical with anchylostomiasis. The characteristic anaemia, highly debilitating and eventually fatal when left untreated, was reported from South America and the West Indies in the late seventeenth and early eighteenth centuries. In Europe the disease was first observed among miners early in the nineteenth century, and Angelo Dubini (1813–1902) in Milan described the worm in 1843.[33] From the late 1870s, the disease was widely reported in Italy, and in mining communities throughout Europe; but it was the outbreak among workers on the St.Gotthardt tunnel in 1880 which concentrated the minds of medical scientists and clinicians on the disease.[34] The early contributions by Leiper and by Sandwith had been primarily concerned with differentiation between the 'European' *(Anchylostoma duodenale)* and the 'American' *(Necator americanus)* species of hookworm, and the pathway of infestation. In their cooperation with the Rockefeller Foundation it was the epidemiology, and the control of the disease in the field, which became paramount issues. This emphasis was to shape the approach to the wider issues with which the IHB and the LSHTM were to be concerned during the period between the wars.

RIVER BLINDNESS (ONCHOCERCIASIS)

Manson's position as an authority on filariae and microfilariae was established well before the development of plans for a school of tropical medicine. As such, he was brought into contact, albeit only fleetingly in the early 1890s, with a parasite whose full importance would become apparent only slowly in the minds of those concerned with tropical health around the world, and especially in Africa and South America.

The parasite first named as *Filaria volvulxus* by either Rudolf Leuckart (1822-98) or Patrick Manson, and eventually established as *Onchocerca volvulus*,[35] had been described by an Irish naval surgeon on the Gold Coast in 1874, as the cause of a dermatological complaint known locally as 'craw-craw'. The surgeon, one John O'Neill (1848-1913), had degrees in medicine and surgery from Queen's College, Cork, and was of a studious bent. He also possessed a microscope. Examining the skin of patients, he found 'a filaria which I believe to be the immediate cause of the complaint'.[36]

Similar observations, though not necessarily of identical microfilariae, were made in Brazil by Silva Araujo at the same time. Only much later were O'Neill's observations resurrected and related to the considerable volume of literature which had meanwhile accumulated on the filariae and microfilariae of what had become known as *Onchocerca volvulus*, the convoluted filaria of river blindness. Even that definition was long in doubt: complex clinical features and pathology caused confusion, as did international controversy regarding possible specific differences between causative filariae in Africa and South America, respectively, and their development in blackflies of the genus *Simulium* as intermediate hosts. Further difficulties of definition arose over differences in clinical features on presentation, since the incidence of the blindness referred to in the common name varies widely in infected individuals from different geographical locations.[37] Even within its range, distribution patterns of the disease vary. In northern Ghana, for example, it was estimated in the 1950s that about 3 per cent of the population were totally blind from onchocerciasis; in the 1970s the WHO estimated that out of 10 per cent infected in a 10 million population in the region of the Volta Basin, 70,000 individuals must be regarded as 'economically blind'.

The study of onchocerciasis, and consequent policies aimed at eradication, or at least control, of the disease, has involved French, German, and British teams for much of the twentieth century. After World War II, the international efforts were coordinated and directed by the WHO in collaboration with the Food and Agriculture Organization, the United Nations Development Programme and the World Bank. In all of these activities both before and after 1945, names connected with the London and Liverpool Schools stand out. The later history will be discussed in Chapter 12.

Filariasis and filariae had been in the forefront of Manson's clinical and research interests throughout his career. With Leiper established as head of the School's helminthology department after 1905, the study of filarial worms was assured a bright future. However, in the early years of the School's existence, and of tropical medicine as an established medical specialty, certain other tropical diseases were perceived as greater immediate threats, more deserving of concerted national and international action. Thus the Malaria Commission, jointly sponsored by the Royal Society and the Colonial Office, predated the openings of both the London and Liverpool Schools. In the United States, the turn of the century also marked milestones in the knowledge and understanding, and hence the ability to control, mosquito-borne disease; but there, by force of immediate circumstances in Cuba and in Panama, the focus was primarily on yellow fever, although malaria also played a part. The heroic experiments of Walter Reed (1851-1902) and his associates confirmed the identity of the agent as a 'filterable virus', and provided evidence for the long suspected transmission of the disease by the mosquito vector, following Ross's work on malaria.[38] At the same time, the practical epidemiological efforts of William C.Gorgas (1854-1920) facilitated control in Cuba and on the Panamanian Isthmus, enabling US teams to succeed in building the Panama Canal where a few years earlier France had failed in the face of appalling statistics of morbidity and mortality. Only later was yellow fever in Africa and in South America to take its place among major concerns for European and American researchers, largely under the aegis of the Rockefeller Commission.[39] In the early years of the twentieth century it was African sleeping sickness which in addition to malaria commanded the better part of the attention of parasitologists.

SLEEPING SICKNESS (TRYPANOSOMIASIS)

In Britain at the turn of the century, prime targets of concern were sleeping sickness and malaria in colonies and dependencies in Africa, and on the Indian subcontinent. When in 1901 medical missionaries in Uganda, notably the brothers Albert (1870-1951) and John (1871-1946) Cook reported beginnings of an epidemic of sleeping sickness, the Royal Society in London responded with a commission and an expedition to investigate the disease. It has been suggested – although this is a controversial and frequently disputed hypothesis – that the slowly developing, but lethal, form of sleeping sickness, caused by *Trypanosoma gambiense*, was first brought east from Gambia with participants in

PREVENTION AND CURE

Stanley's later expeditions in the 1870s and 1880s. Certainly the opening up of East Africa to trade around the turn of the century was a not unimportant factor in an accelerating and alarming spread of the disease in Uganda.[40]

The first of successive Sleeping Sickness Commissions to work in Uganda in the initial decade of the twentieth century arrived in Entebbe in the summer of 1902. Its composition of three, somewhat ill-assorted, members reflected the choice of Manson. George Low, his erstwhile assistant in filaria research, had demonstrated the true function of the mosquito vector – and the error of Manson's initial views – by finding embryos of *Wuchereria bancrofti* in the proboscis of infected mosquitoes. The fact that they were thus ready to transmit the disease in the very act of biting showed the different pathway of this filaria from that of the Guinea worm, *Filaria medinensis*.[41] Now Manson wanted Low to study the possible role of another filaria, *Filaria perstans*, which had been found in the blood of patients with sleeping sickness. Aldo Castellani was chosen from among student volunteers at the School to join the expedition as its bacteriologist. They were both under thirty when they left for Africa. The third commission member, Cuthbert Christy (1864–1932), can best be described as a medical adventurer. On his return from Uganda in early 1903 he joined the Liverpool School as lecturer for a very short period indeed; thirty years later he was killed by a rhinoceros in that other stronghold of sleeping sickness, the Belgian Congo. He was an able field naturalist with tropical experience and an uncertain temper, whose chief contribution appears to have been the collection of useful epidemiological information during long solitary marches.[42]

Of the original three members of the first Royal Society Commission, it was Castellani who was to leave a permanent mark on research into the disease. While Low left after having established that *Filaria perstans* was merely a harmless concomitant, and Christy travelled widely in search of epidemiological knowledge, Castellani was hard at work in the makeshift huts hastily erected to serve as hospital wards for a growing number of patients, and as his laboratory. Observing clinical cases and examining post-mortem material, he found and cultivated a streptococcus from the heart blood of a number of patients. With his bacteriological training and 'research style', he suspected that this might be the causal organism until, in November 1902, he found trypanosomes in the cerebrospinal fluid of another patient. Unwilling to abandon his theory of streptococcus involvement, he wavered in his attitude to the presence of trypanosomes until, the following March, David Bruce and D.N.Nabarro arrived as new members of the Commission (Low and

Christy had returned to England at the beginning of 1903). With the arrival of Bruce, the scene was set for the long drawn out and painful controversy over priority in recognising trypanosomes as causal organisms in sleeping sickness, which was to rumble on for a very long time, to nobody's credit.

David Bruce (1855-1931) had been in pursuit of animal trypanosomes since 1894, although these protozoa were not linked to disease in man until J.E.Dutton's (1875-1905) observations in 1901. The presence of parasitic trypanosomes had first been recorded in the blood of trout as early as 1841, by Gabriel Valentin in Berne. Shortly afterwards, others noted similar organisms in frogs, and in 1843 David Gruby (1810-98), the distinguished albeit eccentric microscopist, described and named *Trypanosoma sanguinis* in a paper delivered at the *Académie des Sciences* in Paris. Gruby, a successful practising physician, compared his findings to contemporary observations of filariae in the blood stream. The healthy appearance of the frogs which harboured the parasites convinced him that they were not pathogenic, a conclusion also reached by Timothy Lewis (1841-86) thirty-five years later, concerning motile parasites found by him in rats in Bombay.[43]

To these early observers, the trypanosomes were no more than zoological curiosities. Not until 1880 was a connection established to animal disease. In that year Griffith Evans (1835-1935), a veterinary officer then serving in the Punjab, noticed parasites which were similar to those described by Lewis from the blood of rats, in horses and mules dying of surra.[44] From then on, attempts were made to discover possible ways of transmission. In his report, Evans had mentioned that native tradition blamed spread of surra on blood-sucking species of gadflies (tabanids). At the turn of the century, Leonard Rogers (1868-1962) confirmed this as the path of transmission, although the process is strictly mechanical, and the trypanosomes do not develop within the fly.[45] This discovery belongs to Rogers's early years in the Indian Medical Service (IMS), when he willingly turned his hand to the control of prevailing epizootics, rinderpest as well as surra. It predated his later absorption in the fevers of man, and in the political problems of the founding of the Calcutta School of Tropical Medicine, and even more his eventual return in 1920 to London, where he was to join in the work at the Hospital for Tropical Diseases, and to lecture at the School.[46]

By the time Rogers's paper on surra was published, David Bruce had demonstrated the role of tsetse flies as carriers of the trypanosomes of nagana, a fatal disease of cattle in the Natal tsetse-fly belt. Bruce became involved in work on this animal disease when in 1894, as a surgeon-major in the RAMC, he was switched from a post at Netley to field service in South Africa. Sir Walter Hely-Hutchinson, Governor of Natal and Zululand, who had known Bruce in Malta and admired his work on Malta fever, contrived to have him seconded to Natal to investigate nagana. 'Nagana', a Zulu word for 'in low or depressed spirits', was a cattle disease occurring in an area of Zululand defined by the presence of tsetse-flies. In the course of investigations between 1894 and 1897, Bruce was able to establish first that nagana was identical with the 'fly-disease' described since the 1830s by hunters, explorers, and missionaries – it figured prominently in the writings of David Livingstone (1813–73) and of his associate, John Kirk (1832–1922). From their travels along the Zambesi River between 1858 and 1863, Kirk wrote to Joseph Hooker of a 'constant sleepiness which acts very injuriously on Europeans, but of which they become insensible after some time'.[47] Bruce's main achievement in Natal in the 1890s was to demonstrate conclusively the role of the tsetse-fly as vector of nagana, transmitting the causative trypanosome from wild game to domestic cattle although he did not at first fully understand the developmental cycle of the trypanosome within the fly. In all his fieldwork, Bruce was ably supported by his wife, one of many spirited women who at that time, denied a university education of their own, found satisfaction in dedicated service as assistants to their husbands. By all accounts, Lady Bruce was not only an able fieldworker, but a charmer who was universally beloved by all who met her, whereas her husband most certainly was not.[48]

The story of the discovery of the aetiology of sleeping sickness in man is exciting on a scientific level; on a personal and political level, it was among the more complex of priority disputes, and does in no way serve to improve the images of any of the strong personalities involved, neither the men on the spot, nor the warring factions in London, i.e. what one not entirely disinterested observer has called ' … top-hatted, bewhiskered characters living in the smoky air of Victorian London'.[49] According to this commentator, the main culprit in London was Ray Lankester (1847–1929), using every opportunity for intrigue to favour the cause of Bruce, for the glory of the RAMC, and to the detriment of Castellani. On the other hand, this source also shows signs of having been influenced to no small extent by conversations with Castellani, and by reports from disgruntled members of the Church Missionary Society. The most objective account is probably the most recent, by Sir John Boyd, who has carefully examined the available sources. The perceptions of the men in the field, of their work and results at the time, were given in their individual papers read to the meeting of the British Medical Association in August, 1904.[50]

However undignified the squabbles between the individual members remained, the main objective of the Royal Society Commission had been reached by late 1903 with the conclusion that 'sleeping sickness is, in short, a human tsetse-fly disease', and that the trypanosome agent was transmitted by the bite of the fly *Glossina palpalis*. With the aetiology of sleeping sickness established, the original members of the commission left Uganda; but many questions remained to be solved concerning the epidemiology of the disease, and especially policies for its control. The Royal Society continued to support the activities of subsequent investigators in Uganda through its sleeping sickness subcommittees of its Tropical Disease Committee, of which Bruce remained the one permanent member in an otherwise changing composition.[51]

The British authorities were not alone in their concern over the threat of sleeping sickness in Africa; Belgian, French and German possessions in the Congo and elsewhere in the tsetse-fly belt in East and Central Africa were similarly afflicted. In October, 1906 a French expedition went to Brazzaville to study the disease; and by the summer of 1907, representatives of the interested parties met in London to consider joint international efforts for control. Only one concrete result was achieved: the establishment of a central bureau to collate and offer information on current research and control measures. It began work as The Sleeping Sickness Bureau in London, on Royal Society premises, in June, 1908, under the direction of A.W.G.Bagshawe (1871–1950). Bagshawe had recently returned from the Uganda expedition which had attempted to check spread of the disease by moving whole populations to tsetse-fly free areas. The first issues of the *Sleeping Sickness Bulletin* appeared in October, 1908. It soon became evident that sleeping sickness was not the only disease in urgent need of attention; in 1911 the *Kala Azar Bulletin* was published, and the following year the Bureau moved to the Imperial Institute, widening its scope to emerge as the Tropical Diseases Bureau and publishing the *Tropical Diseases Bulletin*. From 1914 onwards the Bureau, maintaining a comprehensive international sphere of interests, emphasised a growing awareness of sanitation as a necessary factor in control of disease in tropical latitudes by publishing also a monthly *Bulletin of Hygiene*. In 1920 the Bureau moved again, to share the new premises of the London School and its Hospital in Endsleigh Gardens. Five years later it underwent a final change of title to the Bureau of Hygiene and Tropical Diseases. Shortly afterwards, the Bureau moved with the School into its new buildings in Keppel Street, where it has remained, as part, and yet not a part, of the School and its library, until final severance in March, 1993, when after personal and practical difficulties, and problems of logistics, the Bureau left Keppel Street to join the group of Commonwealth Agricultural Bureaux International (CABI) at Wallingford.[52]

In spite of all the activity surrounding the subject of sleeping sickness, in the field in Uganda and elsewhere, and in London in the Bureau and in Royal Society sub-committees on pathology and therapy, little progress was made in control of the disease before the outbreak of war in 1914. By then, it was certainly evident that one stumbling block was the scant knowledge of the natural history of the vector. The pressing need was for practitioners of medical entomology, a discipline only just beginning to evolve at Manson's School, to study the habits of the tsetse-fly in Africa. In 1910 G.D.H.Carpenter (1882–1953) arrived in Uganda, fresh from a course at the School and selected by the Colonial Office, to do just that. For the next ten years he was to pursue the tsetse-fly, on infected islands in Lake Victoria, studying relative densities of the flies in different areas, their life-spans, and the possibility of destroying their larvae. He also paid attention to their feeding habits, examining the stomach contents of wild flies for mammalian and non-mammalian blood.[53]

Carpenter's studies on deserted islands in Lake Victoria followed a major attempt to control, if not eradicate, the disease in Uganda by moving whole populations away from areas with infected flies, in the hope that in the absence of human hosts the infection would die out, and hence allow the return of the temporarily displaced population. The attempt failed; but the fact that it was made at all should be kept in mind in prevailing discussions of the complex interactions of the 'evils' of the politics and economics of colonialism on the one hand, and the development of tropical (colonial) medicine on the other, as a 'positive' counterbalance. Certainly the latter development did serve to bring a measure of help with prevailing endemic and epidemic diseases, and to some extent opened the road to public health movements in previously neglected areas. Unfortunately, in the case of the trypanosomiases in particular, the relentless progress of agricultural development and advancing 'civilisation' disturbed existing delicate ecological patterns, often with disastrous results in Africa's tsetse-fly belts.[54] It will be seen below that some complex ecological problems were appreciated at an early date.

It had been in response to the obvious need for further knowledge of the behaviour and habits of the infecting flies that Carpenter had carried out his long and arduous researches on the islands of Lake Victoria. At the same time, further discoveries concerning the strains of trypanosomes and the species of vectors of importance in human diseases were made back in England, by J.W.W.Stephens and H.B.Fantham at the Liverpool School of Tropical Medicine, and by Bruce in Nyasaland.[55] Their results raised more questions than they answered, and also presented the unwelcome problem of whether or not to deracinate certain species of wild animals, which were suspected of harbouring the trypanosome of nagana, in case it could also cause human sleeping sickness. This spectre of an expensive and ethically dubious policy of wild game destruction was avoided by the report of a committee appointed by the Colonial Office. In May, 1914, this committee stated its preference for the option of destruction of tsetse-flies and evacuation of inhabitants from threatened areas rather than the 'hasty and imperfectly considered action of a drastic character, such as an attempt to effect a general destruction of wild animals ... not justified by the evidence ...'.[56]

In spite of all the intense activity of fieldworkers in Uganda, and of observations of clinical cases back in London and in Liverpool, there was to be little real progress in the control of sleeping sickness in Africa until the development of therapeutic drugs in the 1920s, and of chemoprophylaxis in the later 1940s. Difficulties arose over differences in infectivity of the different strains and forms of *Trypanosoma brucei (T.b.brucei, T.b.rhodesiense and T.b.gambiense)* for man and animals, and the differences in feeding habits of various species of tsetse-flies *(Glossina palpalis, G.morbitans, G.pallipides, G.fuscipes,* and *G.tachanoides,* the two latter species known as 'riverine tsetse'). The complex interrelationships between the various strains of trypanosomes and species of tsetse-flies have been discussed at length in the literature on human and animal trypanosomiasis for the better part of the twentieth century. It has been suggested that outbreaks of trypanosomiasis during this time could have been caused by a clash between opposing ecosystems, i.e. the 'natural' one of bush, wild animals and tsetse-flies, and the 'artificial' one of man, domestic animals and cultivated land.[57] It is a problem which is still far from solved. Later attempts at control, and the School's involvement in their theoretical background and practical execution will be discussed in a later chapter.

MALARIA

Among the diseases which acted as catalysts for the development of the new medical specialty of 'tropical medicine' towards the end of the nineteenth century, malaria occupied a central position. The case of malaria is perhaps unique in the succession of hopes, apparent successes, and reversals, for attempts at its control, from the early work of Manson and of Ross, via the optimism of eradication attempts in the 1950s and the 1960s, to the dispiriting resurgence in the 1970s, and the most recent burgeoning hopes for new 'tools for control'. The story of the road to some measure of control of malaria has involved the London and Liverpool Schools and their staffs at every turn, and looks set to continue to do so for a long time to come.[58]

Speculation concerning the origins of malaria covers all periods of human history, and it has been suggested that species of *Plasmodium* affecting man may have been evolving with man in Africa already in the neolithic period.[59] Comparison of the extent of distribution of malaria and of sleeping sickness is an instructive indication of the importance of the natural history of a vector for the range of spread of a disease. The speed of breeding and adaptability of the *Anopheles* mosquito has ensured a wide distribution of malaria, where the reproductive parsimony of the female tsetse-fly, which produces only one living larva at a time, and a total of only a dozen larvae in a lifetime, has helped to limit the range of sleeping sickness to narrow bands of riverine and rain forest areas in Africa.

From the Hippocratic writings and Thucydides's account of the siege of Syracuse, the dangers of fevers in marshy areas have been part and parcel of history's warnings to armies and civilians alike. The introduction of the bark of South American *Cinchona* species ('Peruvian fever tree') as a remedy in the seventeenth century was a first, empirical, step towards a method of controlling 'agues'. The bark's main active alkaloids, quinine and cinchonine, were isolated as early as 1820 in France.[60] The story of nineteenth-century attempts to collect and propagate *Cinchona* trees in order to meet the growing demands of therapy based on the bark, is as exciting as all stories of the great plant collectors of the period. Sadly, Charles Ledger (1818–1905) and his gallant servant in Peru, Manuel Incra Macrami, had scant reward for great enterprise and hard work, which in the end benefited only Dutch planters in Java. It is an unhappy reminder that the authorities in Victoria's Britain failed to exploit native talent, i.e. Ledger's discovery of a new species, *Cinchona ledgeriana*, as miserably as did later generations when they let the British discovery of penicillin slip from their grasp to commercial development overseas.[61]

Charles Ledger's *Cinchona* variety was found to produce considerably more quinine than the older known varieties; once Dutch production was firmly established in the 1870s, it became easier to satisfy world demand for therapy. At the same time, nascent scientific tropical medicine was moving closer to an answer to the question of the aetiology of malaria. It has been claimed that as early as 1717 Giovanni Maria Lancisi (1655–1720) suggested the possibility of mosquito transmission of malaria, although other interpretations are possible in the context of his times and the metaphors then used for putative disease-carrying microorganisms.[62] More rational formulation of ideas on disease carrying arthropods began to emerge in the second half of the nineteenth century. Manson's discovery of the development of microfilariae in blood-sucking female *Culex* mosquitoes was published in 1877. This seminal paper spawned speculation on possible transmission of other diseases by other insects, not all of them species of mosquito. Carlos Findlay (1833–1915) suggested *Stegomyia (Culex)* mosquitoes as possible carriers of yellow fever in Cuba in 1881. Albert F.A.King (1841–1914) followed suit with malaria in 1883, the year after the discovery of the malaria parasite by Alphonse Laveran (1845–1922).[63]

Having observed and described the metamorphosis of microfilariae into infective larvae within the mosquito, Manson continued to prefer to believe that they escaped from dead mosquitoes into water, and were then ingested by man, rather than inoculated with the bite of live mosquitoes. He still believed this when, in 1894, he began to draw comparisons between his own filaria results and some of the structures observed by Laveran in malaria blood. Then, the following year, he was visited in London by Ronald Ross on home leave from the IMS. Having obtained the DPH during an earlier leave, Ross had recently become interested in the problems of malaria and its control in India, but had so far had scant regard for Laveran's observations. His attitude changed when Manson showed him stained blood-films of malaria parasites. Under Manson's influence, Ross became an enthusiastic hunter of malaria parasites, and fired with ambition to solve the problems of malaria transmission in the light of the mosquito theory outlined to him by Manson.[64] For two years he laboured at every opportunity at his microscope, in the face of appalling climatic conditions on the subcontinent, and suffering periodic and highly frustrating interruptions by other IMS duties. In August, 1897, his perseverance was finally rewarded. On August 20th (henceforth 'Mosquito Day' to Ross), he dissected an *Anopheles* mosquito earlier fed on malaria blood; in the wall of the insect's gut, he found cysts containing the characteristic pigment seen in erythrocytes of malaria patients. Before he could amplify these promising results, Ross suffered another frustrating interruption: an order to report for duty a thousand miles away, in a malaria free locality.

Not until five months later, in February, 1898, was it made possible for Ross to return to work in Calcutta. It was now the 'healthy season', and malaria cases were difficult to find; but meanwhile advances had been made with bird malaria in the United States, and the faithful Manson kept Ross informed. As a result, Ross was able to follow the development of the cysts in the gut wall of mosquitoes fed on caged, infected sparrows and larks. By May, 1898, he could submit a full and detailed report explaining the transmission of malaria from bird to bird, and describing the development of the parasite in the mosquito until released through the proboscis of the biting mosquito into the next host.[65] Less than a year later, Giovanni Battista Grassi (1854-1925), collaborating with Amico Bignami (1862-1929) and Giuseppe Bastianelli (1862-1959) confirmed an identical cycle for three parasites of human malaria (*Plasmodium* species) in species of *Anopheles* mosquitoes. Grassi had earlier, between 1890 and 1892, described two parasites of avian malaria.[66]

The results of Ross and Grassi were obtained before the opening of the London and Liverpool Schools, but only just; and malaria was still very much a focus of interest in the early years of the new century. The London School and the Rome team led by Grassi collaborated in experiments designed to throw light on the epidemiology of the disease, and to establish beyond doubt the role of its vector. Mosquitoes infected by feeding on malaria patients in Rome were sent to London, where they were allowed in turn to feed on volunteers, one Manson's son, another his laboratory assistant. Requiring more complex arrangements was the experiment organised by Manson in the Roman Campagna, where George Low, Sambon, the Italian artist Enzio Terzi, and a servant, lived for three months in a mosquito-proof hut from dusk to dawn, emerging only in the daytime. Under these conditions they remained unaffected by malaria, in an area where the disease was rife among the unprotected population. It was triumphant proof of the precise timing of the biting of the mosquito vector.[67]

The fragility of an early spirit of cooperation and determination to pool resources in the face of the threat of malaria, and the equally fragile nature of personal relationships nationally and internationally, are demonstrated in a surviving letter from George Low, then in the West

Indies, to Manson. It is dated St. Lucia, December 14th, 1901, barely two years after the opening of the London and Liverpool schools, and a year before Ross received the Nobel Prize for 'his work on malaria, by which he has shown how it enters the organism and thereby has laid the foundation for successful research on this disease and methods of combating it'. The contents of the letter also offer a depressingly clear indication that the lack of warmth between the two schools dates to no small extent from the Liverpool School's association, however truncated, with Ronald Ross; and that the latter's determination to be seen as the sole instigator of an epidemiological approach to the problems of malaria led him to activities little short of ill-intentioned intrigue. It does not detract from the importance of his early results and his pioneering work in epidemiological modelling; but it does raise questions about the received perception of Ross's disinterested concern for local communities and public health matters, as opposed to Manson's narrower clinical and research interests.

In December, 1901, Low's letter to Manson was a *cri de coeur*. He was reporting on his own work in St. Lucia, where malaria and yellow fever were taking their toll. On arrival, he had been briefed by his local contact, Gray, who had received a letter from Ross asking for information concerning the local malaria situation. Low went on to tell Manson:

> Ross then said he would incorporate this in his report and would send a man to St. Lucia to destroy mosquitoes (*a thing I have been slaving at and doing for the last six months*). I did not think Ross would leave this part of the world alone for long as he knows that I representing the London School was out here and I see through his little game perfectly. He would send someone out, boom the thing up in a big report and pose as the pioneer of mosquito destruction in the West Indies, just as in a report of his (I saw in Gray's house) he poses as the saviour of West Africa and gives the Italians and others no credit. [authors' italics]

Low then suggests that Manson might put a diplomatic note in the medical journals and even the 'day papers', hurry a so far neglected paper by Low and Gray into print, emphasising their ongoing work on mosquito destruction. Having outlined the text for such a communication, he continues:

> I think that this should about represent the matter and get the kudoss [*sic*] for the London School of Tropical Medicine. I hate

advertising myself in any way but I think after the hard work I have gone through it is only right that the London School which I represent should get the credit; and that *Ross and the Liverpool people should not calmly step in and snatch up the work done....* Well to pass to more pleasant topics than scientific jealousy, I arrived ... .[68] [authors' italics]

It had all begun more amicably when the first of the Royal Society's commissions on malaria was established in late 1898, and when the first 'Report to the Malaria Committee of the Royal Society' arrived in London in February, 1899. It was C.W.Daniels's account of his visit to Ross, to be shown the methods used and the results obtained in the studies on bird malaria. Ross gave demonstrations to Daniels in Calcutta in late December, 1898, and early January, 1899. A total of eight Reports were published between July, 1900, and October, 1903. The three main investigators, Daniels (1862–1927), J.W.W.Stephens (1865–1946), and S.R.Christophers (1873–1978) travelled widely in India and West Africa, mapping the distribution of *Anopheles* species serving as vectors, and studying their morphology and the development of the *Plasmodium* parasites in the vector.[69]

Stephens and Christophers were appointed directly by the Royal Society, whereas Daniels, as a member of the Colonial Medical Service, represented the Colonial Office. His last contribution to the Report, on *Anopheles* and on blackwater fever in British Central Africa, was printed in 1901, after he had returned to London in 1900 for a brief period as superintendent at Manson's School, as successor to D.C.Rees (cf. Chap.1). Stephens and Christophers continued their studies on the endemicity and epidemiology of the disease, focusing on the geographical distribution of the vector, and on conditions particularly favourable to the spread of malaria, e.g. in the camps housing families of the labourers employed in the construction of the growing network of railways in both India and Africa. The very title of one early paper by Stephens and Christophers bears witness to an objectivity which today would certainly require more sensitive handling. 'The segregation of Europeans' is in no way a racist document; it is a careful analysis of age-related acquisition of immunity to malaria, showing a high degree of asymptomatic endemicity in native children, followed by absence of infection in adults. Writing in the autumn of 1900, Stephens and Christophers were able to compare their results obtained on the Gold Coast with those of Robert Koch from Dutch New Guinea, published earlier in the same year.[70] On the other hand, the segregation policy was even at that time, in the heyday of colonial rule, when plague precautions in South Africa gave rise to legal justification for the removal of Africans from the slums of Cape Town to special 'clean' isolation camps outside the city, viewed with reservations in some quarters. In August, 1904, Stephens wrote defensively in the *Journal of Tropical Medicine:*

> On general sanitary grounds there can be no doubt that were the Europeans to segregate themselves away from Native dwellings, it would be advisable, so far as the Europeans were concerned. Some, however, regard this mode of dealing with the question as *unjust, impolitical &c, and academical;* apart, however, from sentimentality, segregation has much to recommend it. [authors' italics].[71]

Daniels's last contribution to the Reports, on *Anopheles* and on blackwater fever in British Central Africa, was printed in 1901, when he was already back in London. Stephens and Christophers continued to work for the Malaria Commission until 1902. At the end of this period Stephens was appointed Walter Myers Lecturer in Tropical Medicine at Liverpool, beginning a long association with that School. Ten years later he succeeded Ross as Alfred Jones Professor of Tropical Medicine. He remained heavily involved in malaria work, both in Liverpool and during the School's many expeditions and activities at the Freetown laboratory, funded by a bequest in Alfred Jones's will in 1913.[72] Christophers on the other hand, eager for the opportunities for research into tropical diseases found in India, entered the IMS at the conclusion of the Malaria Commission investigations.

Like many of the great names in the early years, Christophers went straight into tropical medicine with no special training, learning on the job. His talents were obvious, and he was soon involved, with S.P. James (1870–1946), in the not entirely successful attempts to control a malaria outbreak at Mian Mir in the Punjab. It was an episode which caused a clash between, on the one hand, Christophers and James, who questioned the efficacy of mosquito control as a means of reducing the incidence of malaria, and, on the other Ross, who in return criticised their report and their methods. The ensuing bitter dispute, with more emphasis on the differences between the strong and unyielding personalities involved than on scientific fact, was to cloud malaria research and attempts at control in India for several decades.[73] Shortly afterwards, Christophers went to Madras as director of a new institute of preventive medicine. During four years there, and for many years subsequently, his main interests lay in the study of malaria and blackwater fever. Accounts of his distinguished work in India, in the field, and coordinating surveys on behalf of the Central Malaria Bureau at the Research Institute at Kasauli, leave vivid impressions of his scientific flair as much as of his human qualities, his concern in equal measure for troops in campaigns in India and Iraq, and for native children. In the survey work in particular, his personal charm, and his ability to talk through any problems with self-effacing tact and understanding of others' point of view, were invaluable. Disinterested observers have commented on his abundant humanity, integrity, and generosity of spirit, compared to some of his contemporaries, who regarded themselves as very much part of the colonial establishment, and acted accordingly.[74]

Only when he retired from the IMS in 1931 did Christophers join the LSHTM as Professor of Malaria Studies in the University of London. He was one of the great pioneers in the field. By dint of longevity, his working life covered a period which saw a shift from the much maligned 'colonial', 'imperial', medical policies, to policies implemented by newly independent states both in Africa and on the Indian subcontinent. By temperament he was ideally suited to preside over the changes brought about in scientific, epidemiological research attitudes, which accompanied the sometimes violent political adjustments. Unfortunately, the more extreme examples of politically inspired violent activities have interfered, and are interfering, with later attempts to implement policies designed to help developing nations. Such attempts, together with the later achievements by Christophers and colleagues in and out of the LSHTM, will be considered in a subsequent chapter. The period until the end of World War I, when Manson's School began a near decade of transformation into the new LSHTM, was characterised by much steady work rather than any one remarkable advance, along the frontiers of the fight against malaria. The same could be said for another 'fever' which had, for the better part of the nineteenth century, been considered a type of malarial fever.

KALA-AZAR

Since the early days of research on fevers in India, difficulties in differential diagnosis had been exacerbated by patients' tendency to describe any illness as 'fever', regardless of any symptoms felt or observed. Such difficulties had been, in particular, associated with the disease which since the 1880s had been referred to as kala-azar, and been regarded as a form of malarial fever, in Sanitary Reports in Assam. In 1896 the young Leonard Rogers, who had established his credentials with a study of interactions between local ecology and pathogenesis in malaria, was posted to Assam to investigate the nature and spread of kala-azar in the district.[75] Six years earlier the prevailing ideas of the disease as a type of 'relapsing malarial fever' had been challenged by one G.M.Giles in a report from Assam. Giles suggested that the main symptom of kala-azar was not fever, but anaemia; anaemia caused by infestation with hookworm. His theory was refuted, when others found no difference in the level of hookworm infection between kala-azar patients and healthy controls. Now Rogers, after a year's meticulous work, was able to demonstrate the difference between the blood picture in anaemias caused by, one the one hand, anchylostomiasis, and on the other, kala-azar and malaria. In the case of the latter two diseases, the blood changes were identical. Rogers concluded that kala-azar was caused by a particularly virulent 'super-malarial' germ.[76] Not long afterwards, W.B.Leishman (1865–1926), and also C.Donovan, both using the new Romanovsky stain perfected by Leishman, were able to demonstrate the presence of a hitherto unknown parasite, named *Leishmania donovani* by Ross in 1903.[77] In spite of identification of the parasite, the question of a possible vector was to remain open for a number of years.

In the summer of 1914, just before the outbreak of war and the ensuing disruptions to research work and international exchanges of knowledge, Bassett-Smith, now a Fleet-Surgeon RN, reviewed the progress made since Leishman's identification of the parasite. In the intervening years, kala-azar had been observed around the Mediterranean littoral. Italian workers, studying leishmania infections in dogs, had implicated the dog-flea in dog-to-dog transmission. Although blood-sucking insects were high on the list of suspected vectors, the identity of the species responsible for transmission of leishmania was still undecided. In 1914, mosquitoes, fleas, and tabanid flies in South America, were all considered possible agents of transfer from host to host. It was only following epidemiological studies in the 1930s, which showed a correlation between the distribution of certain sandflies (*Phlebotomus argentipes*), and kala-azar in India, that sandflies were finally recognised as the vectors in kala-azar, and in the cutaneous form of leishmaniasis.[78]

NOTES

[1] David Arnold (ed), *Imperial Medicine and Indigenous Societies,* Manchester University Press, 1988;
Roy MacLeod and Milton Lewis (eds), *Disease, Medicine and Empire. Perspectives on western medicine and the experience of European expansion,* London and New York, Routledge, 1988.

[2] Eli Chernin, 'The early British and American journals of tropical medicine and hygiene: an informal survey', *Med.Hist.,* 1992, *36:*70–83, pp.74–5;
for Bismarck's reforms see
Paul Weindling, *Health, race and German politics between national unification and Nazism 1870–1945,* Cambridge University Press, 1989.

[3] P.H.Manson-Bahr and A.Alcock, *The life and work of Sir Patrick Manson,* London etc., Cassell and Co., [1927];
P.Manson-Bahr, *Manson: the father of tropical medicine,* London and Edinburgh, Thomas Nelson and Sons, Ltd., 1962;
P.Manson's Amoy Journal, etc., LSHTM Archives.

[4] Patrick Manson, 'The necessity for special education in tropical medicine', *The Lancet,* 1897, *ii*:842–5.

[5] David Grove, *A history of human helminthology,* Wallingford, CAB International, 1990, p.606.

[6] L.Wilkinson, *Animals and Disease,* Cambridge University Press, 1992, p.45 and p.139.

[7] T.Bilharz, 'Distomum haematobium und sein Verhältniss zu gewissen pathologischen Veränderungen der menschlichen Harnorgane', *Wiener med.Wschr.,* 1856, *6*:49–65.

[8] C.Davaine, *Traité des entozoaires et des maladies vermineuses de l'homme et des animaux domestiques,* Paris, J.B.Ballière; J.Théodoridès, *Un grand médecin et biologiste Casimir-Joseph Davaine (1812–82),* Analecta medico-historica, 4, Oxford, Pergamon Press, 1968, pp.160–6;
Grove, op.cit note 5, pp.597–613;
T.R.Lewis papers, LSHTM MSS FB: D4.

[9] Grove, p.606.

[10] P.Manson, 'Further observations of *Filaria sanguinis hominis*', China Imperial Maritime Customs. Medical Reports for the half-year ended 30th September 1877, 14th issue, 1878, pp.1–26, p.10;
P.Manson, 'On the development of *Filaria sanguinis hominis* and of the mosquito considered as a nurse', *J.Linnean Soc. (Zoology),* 1878, *14:*304–11;
Eli Chernin, 'Sir Patrick Manson's studies on the transmission and

biology of filariasis' *Rev.infect.dis.*, 1983, *5*:148–66.

[11] D.Bradley, 'Malaria-whence and whither'?, *in:* G.A.T.Targett (ed), *Malaria. Waiting for the Vaccine,* Chichester etc., John Wiley & Sons, 1991.

J.D.Gillett, 'Forlorn hope for a malaria vaccine'?, *Nature* 1990, *348*:494.

[12] G.C.Low, 'A recent observation on *Filaria nocturna* in *culex:* probable mode of infection in man', *Br.med.J.,* 1900, *i:*1456–7.
Similar observations were made almost simultaneously, and independently, by James in Travancore, S.P.James, 'On the metamorphosis of the *Filaria sanguinis hominis* in the mosquito', *ibid.* 1900, *ii:*533–7.

[13] LSTM School Register, vol.1;

N.H.F.[Neil Hamilton Fairley], 'George Carmichael Low', *Trans.R.Soc.Trop.Med.Hyg.* 1952, *46*:571–3;

G.C.Cook, 'George Carmichael Low FRCP: twelfth President of the Society and underrated pioneer of tropical medicine', *ibid.,* 1993, *87*:355–60.

A full scale biography of Low by G.C.Cook is currently under preparation and nearing completion.

[14] Cf. Chapter 1, note 46, and note 67 below.

[15] Grove, op.cit note 5, pp. 693–719.

[16] R.T.Leiper. 'The etiology and prophylaxis of dracontiasis', *Br.med.J.,* 1907. *i:*129–32;

idem, Report of the helminthologist, LSTM, for the year ending April 30th, 1913; abstract in *Trop.Dis.Bull.* 1913, *2:*195–6.

[17] P.Manson-Bahr, *History of the School of Tropical Medicine in London*, London, H.K.Lewis, 1956: 'Diary', p.276.

[18] P.C.C.Garnham, 'Robert Thompson Leiper', *Biogr.Mem.Fell.Roy.Soc.,* 1970, *16:*385–404, p.394.

[19] Grove, op.cit., chapters 8,9 and 10; pp.187–295.

[20] *ibid.,* pp.195–200.

[21] P.Manson. 'Report on a case of *Bilharzia* from the West Indies', *Br.med.J.,* 1902, *ii:*1894–5;

idem, Tropical Diseases, 3rd ed., London, Cassell & Co., 1903, and 4th ed. 1907, p.661.

[22] L.W.Sambon, 'Remarks on *Schistosomum mansoni'*, *J.Trop.Med.Hyg*, 1907, *10:*303–4;

R.T.Leiper. 'On the relation between the terminal-spined and lateral-spined eggs of *Bilharzia'*, *Br.med.J.,* 1916, *i:*411.

[23] K.Mayairi and M.Suzuki, 'On the development of *Schistosoma japonicum'* (in Japanese), Tokyo Iji Shinsi no.1836, 1913, pp.1–5. Cited

by Grove, op.cit., pp.270-2, who described their work, and that of others, and ensuing priority disputes.

[24] G.S.Nelson, 'A milestone on the road to the discovery of the life-cycles of the human schistosomes', *Am.J.Trop.Med.Hyg.*, 1977, *26:*1093-1100; John Ford, 'Edward Leicester Atkinson', *St.Thomas's Hosp.Gaz.*, 1985 (Summer): 64-7.

R.T.Leiper and E.L.Atkinson. 'Helminths of the British Antarctic Expedition 1910-1913', *Proc.Zool.Soc.Lond.* 1915:222-6.

[25] R.T.Leiper, Report on an expedition to China to study the nematode infections in man. Unpublished report to the Colonial Office, 15 January 1915; abstract in *Trop.Dis.Bull.*, 1915, *6:*295-6;

R.T.Leiper and E.L.Atkinson, 'Observations on the spread of Asiatic schistosomiasis', *Br.med.J.*, 1915, *i:*201-3.

[26] Manson-Bahr, op.cit. note 17, pp.219-21, and 245-6.

[27] R.T.Leiper, 'Report on the results of the *Bilharzia* Mission in Egypt, 1915', *J.RAMC*, 1915, *25:*1-55; 147-92; 253-67; 1916, *27:*171-90; 1918, *30:*235-60.

Trop.Dis.Bull. 1916, *8:*610.

[28] P.J.Hotez and D.I.Pritchard, 'Hookworm Infection', *Sci.Amer.*, June 1995, pp.42-8;

John Ettling, *The germ of laziness. Rockefeller philanthropy and public health in the New South*, Cambridge, Mass., Harvard University Press, 1981; Chapter 4: 'Philanthropy for the ages'.

[29] *ibid.,* Chapter 8: 'Henceforth thy field is the world: from Sanitary Commission to the Rockefeller Foundation'.

[30] Manson-Bahr, op.cit. note 17, 'Diary', pp.271-2, for 1904-5; LSTM, 'Syllabus of Lectures' for 1907, pp.16-17;

'F.M.Sandwith', *The Lancet,* 1918, *i:*347-8;

'Fleming Mant Sandwith', *Trans.R.Soc.Trop.Med.Hyg.*, 1917-18, *11:*232-6.

[31] Grove, op.cit., pp.507-12;

papers by Sandwith in *The Lancet, Br.med.J.* and *J.Trop.Med.* between 1894 and 1904.

[32] J.Ettling, op.cit note 28, pp.189-190, identifies the quotation as 'from the journal kept by Rose on his trip to England', in the Rockefeller Archives;

'The Dinner', *J.Trop.Med.Hyg.*, 1913, *15:*294-6;

R.Acheson and P.Poole, 'The London School of Hygiene and Tropical Medicine: a child of many parents', *Med.Hist.*, 1991, *35:*385-408.

[33] F.M.Sandwith, 'Observations on four hundred cases of anchylostomiasis', *The Lancet,* 1894, *i:*1362-8;

Angelo Dubini, 'Nuovo verme intestinal umano (*Agchylostoma duodenale*) constituente un sesto genere dei nematoidea proprii dell 'uomo', *Annali universali di medicina,* 1843, *106:*5–13; cited by Grove, translated *in:* B.H.Kean, K.E.Mott, and A.J.Russell, *Tropical medicine and parasitology. Classic investigations,* Ithaca, Cornell University Press, 1978.

[34] E.Perroncito, 'Observations helminthologiques et recherches expérimentelles sur la maladie des ouvriers du Saint–Gothard' *C.r.hebdom.des sèances Acad.Sci.,* 1880, *90:*1373–5; idem, *La malattia dei minatori dal S.Gottardo al Sempione,* Torino, Carlo Pasta, 1910; R.Peduzzi and J.C.Piffaretti, '*Ancylostoma duodenale* and the Saint Gothard anaemia', *Br.med.J.,* 1983, *ii:*1942–5.

[35] Grove, op.cit., pp.662–4.

[36] John O'Neill, 'On the presence of a filaria in "craw-craw"', *The Lancet,* 1875, *i:*265–6.

[37] Grove, op.cit., pp.673–7; K.David Patterson, 'Onchocerciasis', *The Cambridge History of Human Disease,* K.F.Kiple (ed), Cambridge University Press, 1993, pp.895–7, p.895.

[38] Francois Delaporte, *The history of yellow fever. An essay on the birth of tropical medicine,* Cambridge, Mass. and London, M.I.T.Press, 1991.

[39] John M.Gibson, *Physician to the world. The life of General William C.Gorgas,* Tuscaloosa and London, University of Alabama Press, 1989; J.R.Busvine, *Disease Transmission by Insects,* Berlin etc., Springer-Verlag, 1993.

[40] Because of the controversies surrounding the participants in the expeditions, and their results, the literature on the subject both by contemporary observers and by later commentators is copious. See for example:
C.A.Wiggins, 'Early days in British East Africa and Uganda', *E.Afr.Med.J.,* 1960, *37:*699–708;
J.N.P.Davies, 'The cause of sleeping-sickness', parts 1 and 2, *ibid.,* 1962, *39:*81–99, and 145–60.
W.D.Foster, *A history of parasitology,* Edinburgh and London, E.&S.Livingstone, 1965, pp.115–37;
On Albert Cook, Wellcome CAMC, pp/COO;
W.D.Foster, *The Church Missionary Society and modern medicine in Uganda: the life of Sir Albert Cook, KCMG, 1870–1951,* [Prestbury], the author, 1978.

[41] Cf. notes 12 and 13 above on G.C.Low.

[42] 'Cuthbert Christy', *The Lancet,* 1932, *i:*1284; also op.cit. Davies,

pp.89-90; Wiggins, p.704, and Foster, p.125.

G.C.Cook, 'Correspondence from Dr.George Carmichael Low to Dr.Patrick Manson during the first Ugandan sleeping sickness expedition', *J.Med.Biogr.*, 1993, *1:*215-29, p.217.

[43] D.Gruby, 'Recherches et observations sur une nouvelle espèce d'hématozoaire, *Trypanosoma sanguinis'*, *C.r.hebd.séanc.Acad.Sci.*, 1843, *17:*1134-6;

T.R.Lewis, *In Memoriam. Physiological and pathological researches,* London, 1888, p.611;

W.D.Foster, op.cit. pp.115-17;

J.E.Dutton, 'Preliminary note upon a trypanosome occurring in the blood of a man', *Thompson Yates Lab.Reports,* 1902, *4:* 455-69.

[44] Griffith Evans, 'On a horse disease in India known as surra, probably due to a haematozoon', *Vet.J.*, 1881, *13:*1-10; 82-8; 180-200; 326-33; 'Dr.Griffith Evans. The professions's centenarian, *Vet.Rec.*, 1935, *15:*890-4;

'The postulates of Griffith Evans MD, MRCVS (1835-1935), and the specificity of disease', *in: De novis inventis,* Amsterdam, Holland University Press, 1984, pp.[81]-93.

[45] Leonard Rogers, 'Note on the role of the horse fly in the transmission of *tyrpanosoma* infection' *Br.med.J.* 1904, *ii:*1454.

[46] Helen Power, 'Major-General Sir Leonard Rogers (FRS): Tropical Medicine in the Indian Medical Service', Ph.D.thesis, University of London, 1993;

Manson-Bahr, op.cit. note 17, 'Diary', p.283;

LSHTM, 'Diary of lectures in the Ordinary Course', *in: Prospectus* of the School, from 1922 onwards;

on Rogers appointment, SHSMB *16,* p.264;

also Leonard Rogers papers, LSHTM MSS, FB: D3.

[47] D.P., 'Sir John Kirk, 1832-1922', *Proc.R.Soc.B,* 1923, *94:*xi-xxx; p.xiii.

[48] D.Bruce, Croonian Lecture on 'trypanosomes causing disease in man and domestic animals in Central Africa', *The Lancet*, 1915, *i:*1323;

D.Bruce, *Further report on the tsetse-fly disease, or nagana, in Zululand,* London, Harrison & Sons, 1897;

W.D.Foster, op.cit. note 40, pp.118-23;

John J.McKelvey, *Man against tsetse,* Ithaca, Cornell University Press, 1973, pp.64-75;

A.J.Duggan, 'Bruce and the African trypanosomes', *Am.J.Trop.Med.Hyg.*, 1977, *26:*1080-3;

G.C.Cook, 'Sir David Bruce's elucidation of the aetiology of *nagana* -

exactly one hundred years ago', *Trans.Roy.Soc.Trop.Med.Hyg.*, 1994, *88:*257-8;
Basil J.S.Grogono, 'Sir David and Lady Bruce. Part I: a superb combination in the elucidation and prevention of devastating diseases', *J.Med.Biogr.*, 1995, *3:*79-83;
idem., 'Sir David and Lady Bruce. Part II: further adventures and triumphs', *ibid.*, 1995, *3:*125-32.
[49] Davies, op.cit. note 40, part 1, p.82
[50] Sir John Boyd, 'Sleeping sickness. The Castellani-Bruce controversy', *Not.Rec.R.Soc.*, 1973, *28:*93-110;
D.Bruce, 'Trypanosomiasis', *J.Trop.Med.*, 1904, *6:*250;
D.Nabarro, 'Remarks on trypanosomiasis', *ibid.;*
C.Christy, J.E.Dutton and J.L.Todd, 'Human trypanosomiasis and its relation to Congo sleeping sickness', *ibid.*, pp.250-1.
[51] The Royal Society, Minutes of the Tropical Diseases Committee and its Sleeping Sickness Sub-Committees, 476/Lxr1.b.15/CMB 50; 477/Lxr1.b.16/CMB 51; 479/Lxr1.b.18/CMB 53.
[52] Manson-Bahr, op.cit. note 17, pp.106-9;
C.M.Clark and J.M.Macintosh, *The School and the Site*, London, H.K.Lewis, 1954, (LSHTM Memoir no.9), pp.75-6;
Mary Gibson, 'Vale BHTD', *The Chariot, LSHTM Newsletter,* March, 1993, p.11;
LSHTM *Research Report* 1992, p.86.
[53] G.D.H.Carpenter, *A naturalist on Lake Victoria,* London, T.Fisher Unwin, 1920;
Carpenter obituaries, *The Lancet*, 1953, *i:*300-1; *Br.med.J.*,1953, *1:*406-7; Royal Society Reports of the Sleeping Sickness Commission for 1912, 1913 and 1919;
Foster, op.cit. note 40, pp.130-1.
[54] Maryinez Lyons, 'Sleeping sickness, colonial medicine and imperialism: some connections in the Belgian Congo', *in: Disease, medicine and empire, [op.cit. note i;]* 'Sleeping Sickness epidemics and public health in the Belgian Congo', *in: Imperial medicine and indigenous societies*, op.cit. note 1; *The colonial disease: a social history of sleeping sickness in Northern Zaire,* Cambridge University Press, 1992.
[55] J.W.W.Stephens and H.B.Fantham, 'On the peculiar morphology of a trypanosome from a case of sleeping sickness and the possibility of its being a new species (*T.rhodiense)*', *Proc.Roy.Soc.*, 1910, *83:*28-36;
idem, 'Further measurements of *Trypanosoma rhodiense* and *T.gambiense', Ann.Trop.Med.Parasit.*, 1913, *7:*27-39;
D.Bruce, 'Trypanosomes causing disease in man and domestic animals in

Central Africa', *Br.med.J.*, 1915. *i:*1073–8.
[56] Foster, op.cit. note 40, pp.132–3.
[57] J.Ford, *The role of trypanosomiases in African ecology. A study of the tsetse fly problem,* Oxford University Press, 1971.
[58] G.A.T.Targett (ed), *Malaria,* op.cit. note 11;
S.C.Oaks et al. (eds), *Malaria. Obstacles and opportunities,* Institute of Medicine Report, Washington DC., National Academy Press, 1991.
[59] A.J.Knell (ed) for the Wellcome Trust, *Malaria,* Oxford University Press, 1991, p.3.
[60] J.Pelletier et J.Caventou, 'Recherches chimiques sur les quinquinas', *Ann.Chim.Phys.,* 1820, *15:*289–318; 337–61.
[61] Gabriele Gramaccia, *The life of Charles Ledger (1818–1905): alpacas and quinine,* Basingstoke, Macmillan, 1988.
[62] W.C.Gorgas and F.H.Garrison. 'Ronald Ross and the prevention of malarial fever', *Sci.monthly,* 1916, *3:*133–50, p.135;
L.Wilkinson, 'Rinderpest and mainstream infectious disease concepts in the eighteenth century', *Med.Hist.,* 1984, *28:*129–50, pp.138–9.
[63] F.Delaporte, op.cit. note 38.
[64] G.H.F.N.[Nuttall], 'Sir Ronald Ross 1857–32', *Obit.Not.Fell.Roy.Soc.* 1932–5, *1:*108–14;
Mary E.Gibson, Introduction to *A catalogue of the Ross Archives,* LSHTM, 1983.
[65] Ronald Ross, 'Report on the cultivation of *Proteosoma Labbe* in grey mosquitoes', Calcutta, Office of the Superintendent of Government Printing, 1898;
Announcement by Manson to the BMA annual meeting, July, 1898, *Br.med.J.,* 1898, *ii:*849–53;
for a full account of Ross's papers see M.E.Gibson's Catalogue, as above.
[66] G.C., 'Giovanni Battista Grassi', *Trans.R.Soc.Trop.Med.Hyg.,* 1954, *48:*369–72.
[67] Grassi telegraphed from Rome: '... perfect health experiments ... I salute Manson who first formulated mosquito malarial theory'; LSHTM MSS FC: D2.
[68] CMAC, WTI/RST, F.30.
[69] C.W.Daniels, 'On the transmission of *Proteosoma* to birds by the mosquito: a report to the Malaria Committee of the Royal Society', *Reports to the Malaria Committee of the Royal Society,* I, 1899–1900, published 6 July, 1900, pp.1–76.
Further reports II–VIII, August 1900–October, 1903.
[70] J.W.W.Stephens and S.R.Christophers, 'The segregation of Europeans', *Reports to the Malaria Committee of the Royal Society,* 3rd series,

December 1900, pp.21-4.

[71] J.W.W.Stephens, 'The prophylaxis of malaria', *J.Trop.Med.*, 1904, 6:253-5, p.254;
for such developments in South Africa, see Molly Preston Sutphen, 'Imperial hygiene in Calcutta, Cape Town and Hong Kong: the early career of Sir William John Ritchie Simpson (1855-1931), Ph.D. thesis, Yale University, 1995.

[72] [J.W.W.Stephens, W.Yorke, B.Blacklock], *Liverpool School of Tropical Medicine. Historical Record 1898-1920*, Liverpool University Press, 1920, pp.56-7, 59.

[73] S.P.James and S.R.Christophers, 'The success of mosquito destruction operations', *J.Trop.Med.*, 1904, 6:255;
R.Ross, 'The anti-malarial experiment at Mian Mir, Punjab, India', *ibid;*
M.Watson, 'The lesson of Mian Mir', *J.Trop.Med.Hyg.*, 1931, 34:183-9;
W.F.Bynum, 'An experiment that failed: malaria control at Mian Mir', *Parassitologia*, 1994, 36:107-20.

[74] H.E.Shortt and P.C.C.Garnham, 'Sir (Samuel) Rickard Christophers', *Biogr.Mem.Fell.R.Soc.* 1979, 25:179-207;
'A tribute to Sir Rickard Christophers on his 100th birthday', *Trans.R.Soc.Trop.Med.Hyg.*, 1973, 67:729-54.

[75] Helen Power, op.cit. note 46.

[76] L.Rogers, *Report of an investigation of the epidemic of malarial fever in Assam, or Kala Azar*, Shillong, Assam Secretariat Printing Office, 1897;
'Kala Azar', *Br.med.J.*, 1897, i:1434-5.

[77] W.B.Leishman, 'On the possibility of the occurrence of trypanosomiasis in India', *Br.med.J.*, 1903, i:1252-4:
C.Donovan, 'On the possibility of the occurrence of trypanosomiasis in India', *ibid.*, 1903, ii:79;
R.Ross, 'Further notes on Leishman's bodies', *Br.med.J.*, 1903, ii:1401.

[78] M.J.Allison, 'Leishmaniasis', *in:* K.F.Kiple (ed), *The Cambridge World History of Human Disease*, pp. 832-4;
'Kala-azar and allied conditions', *Br.med.J.*, 1914, ii:394-5.

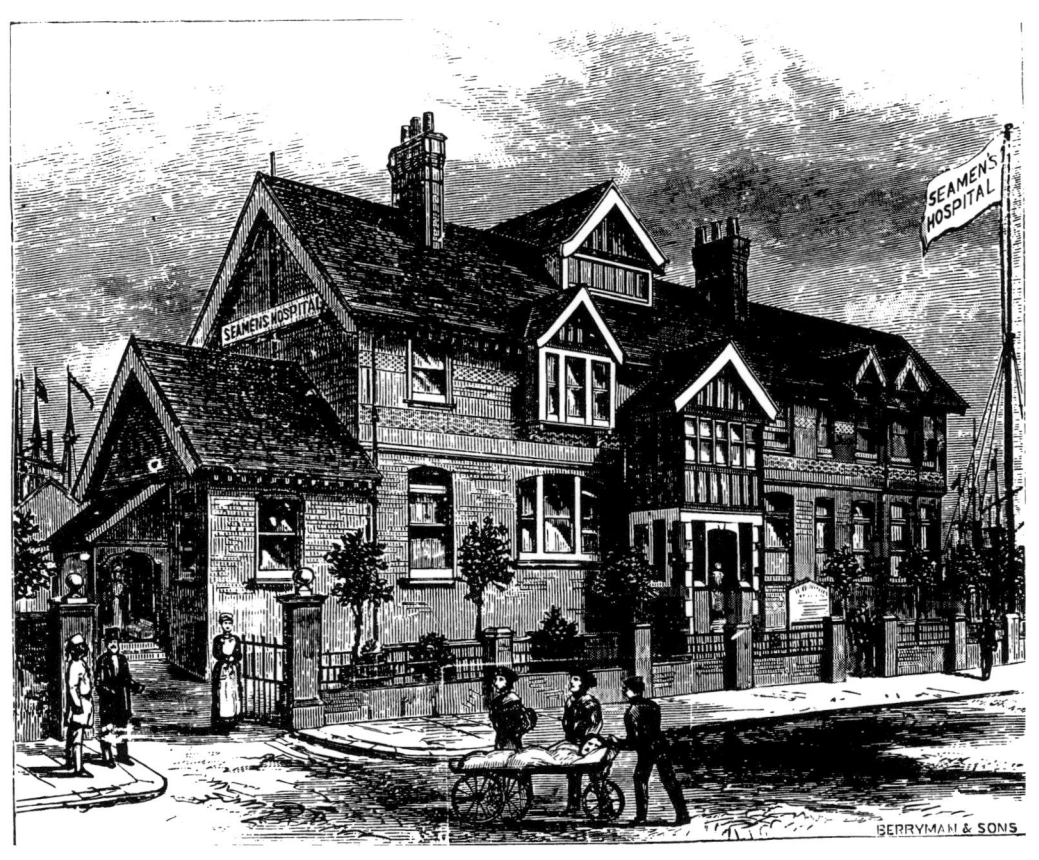

Fig.1 The Albert Dock Branch Hospital, opened in 1890, where it all began in 1899.
(Courtesy Wellcome Institute Library, London)

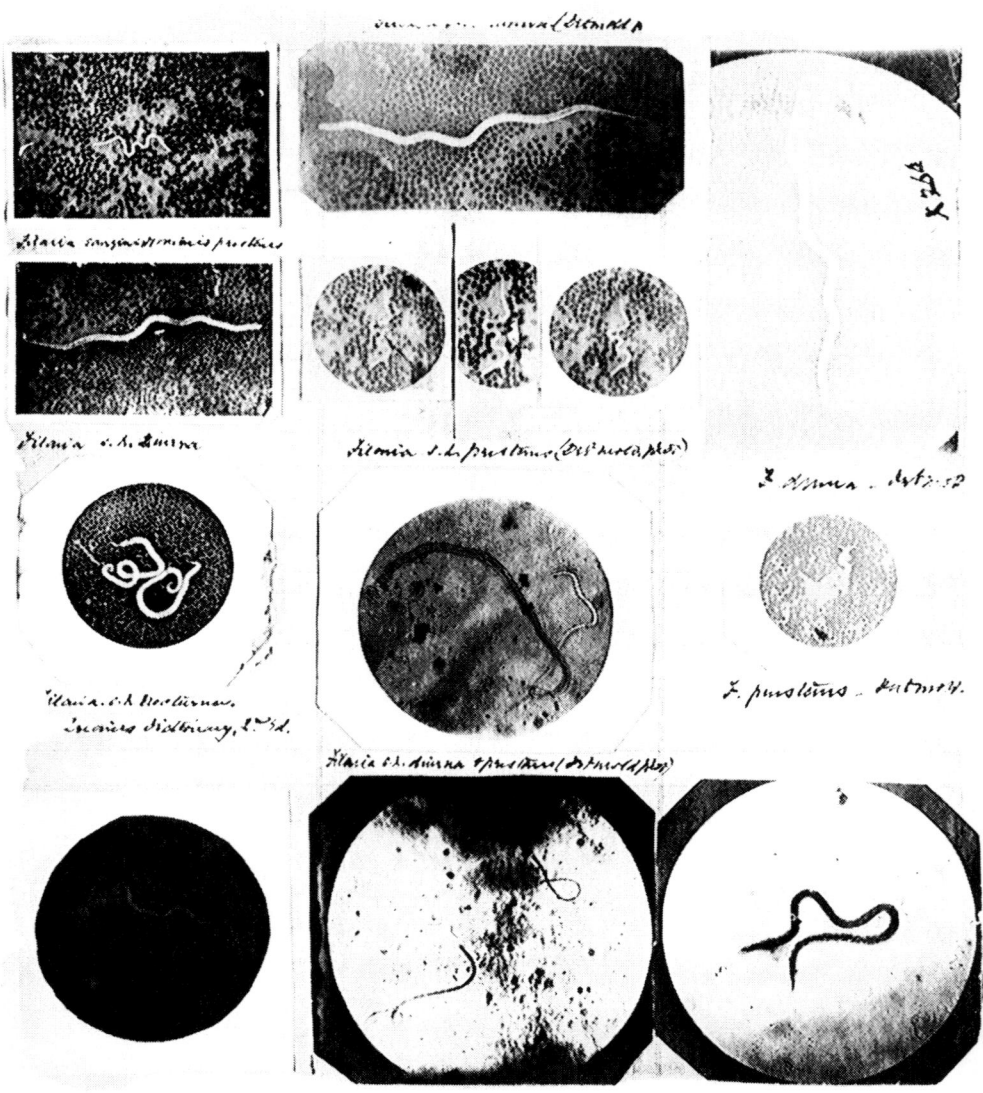

Fig.2 Manson's photomicrographs of *Filaria* species (1890s).
(Wellcome Institute Library, CMAC)

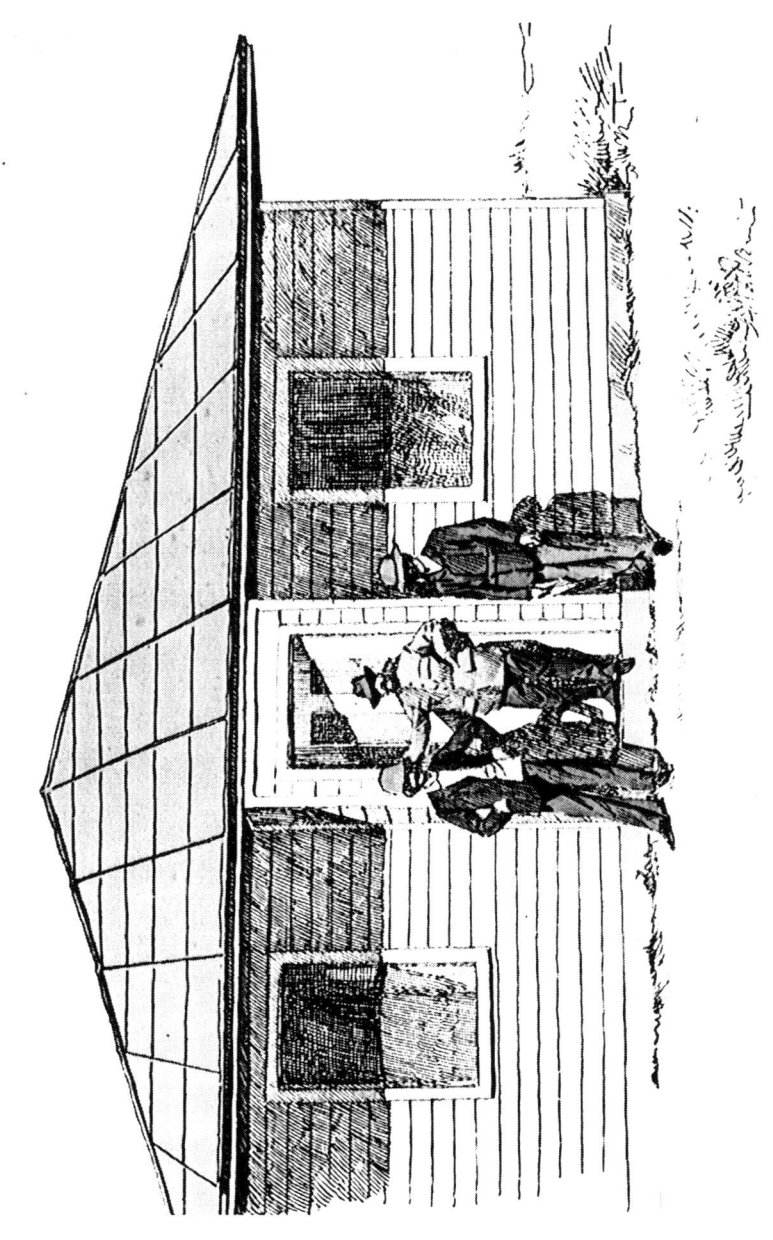

Fig.4 The mosquito-proof 'Humphrey's Hut' at Ostia in the Roman Campagna, 1900.
(Wellcome Institute Library, CMAC)

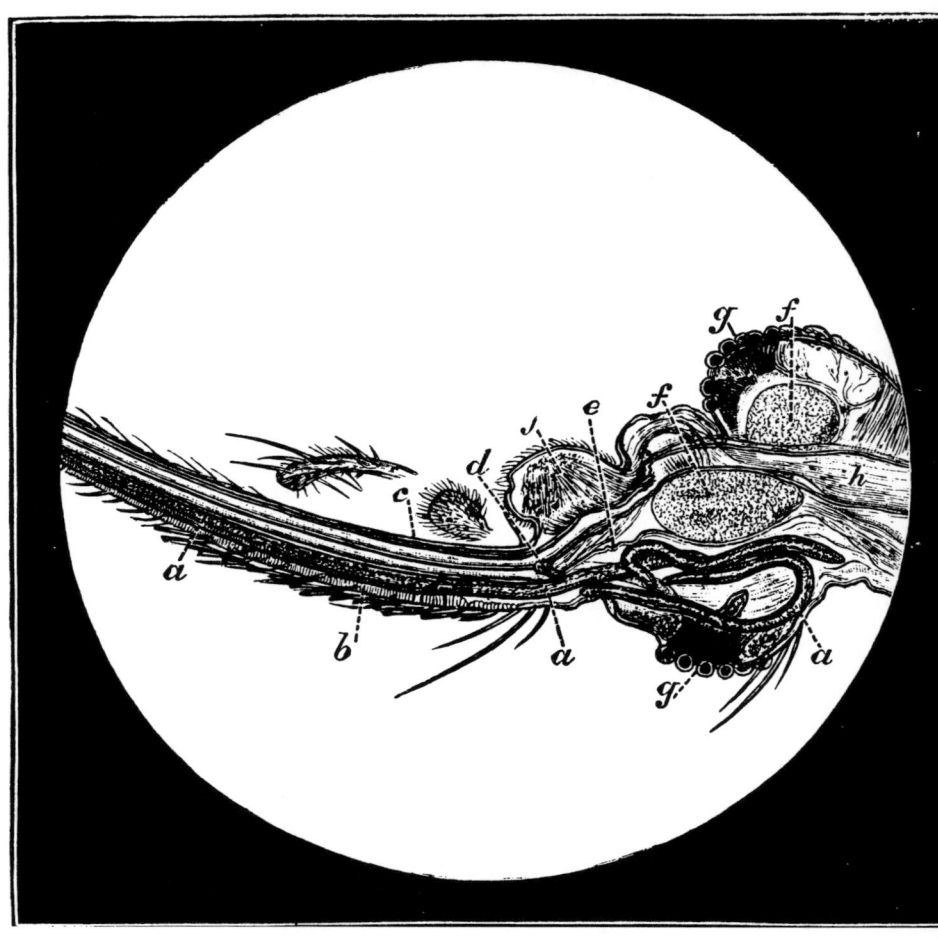

Fig.3 *Filaria nocturna* in head and proboscis of mosquito. From Manson's *Tropical Diseases*, 1900.
(Wellcome Institute Library)

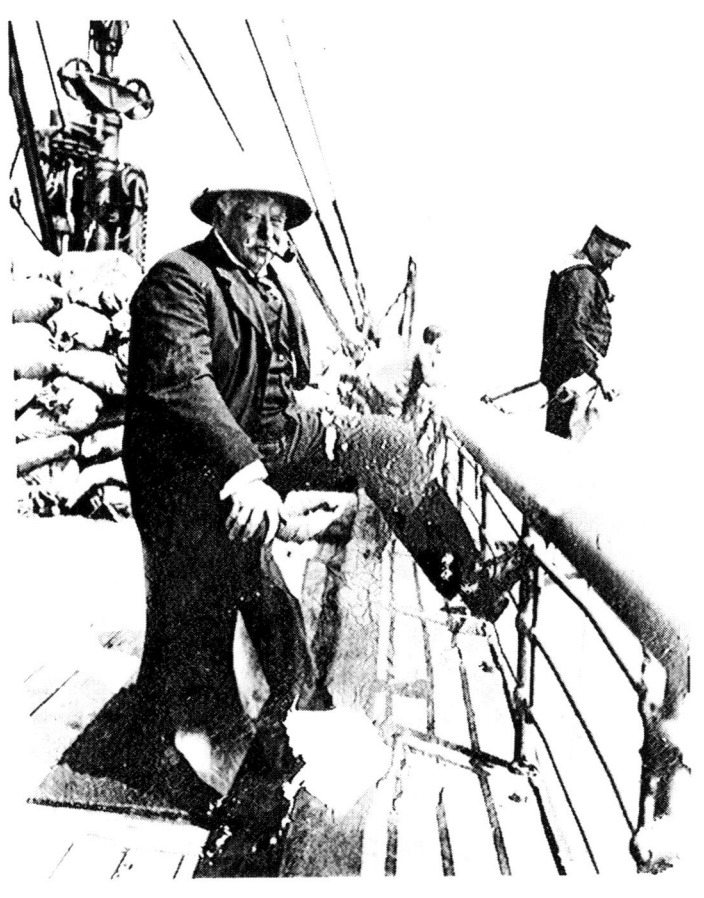

Fig.5 Patrick Manson on board the 'Union Castle' bound for Cape Town, June 1913, having retired in 1912.
(Wellcome Institute Library, CMAC)

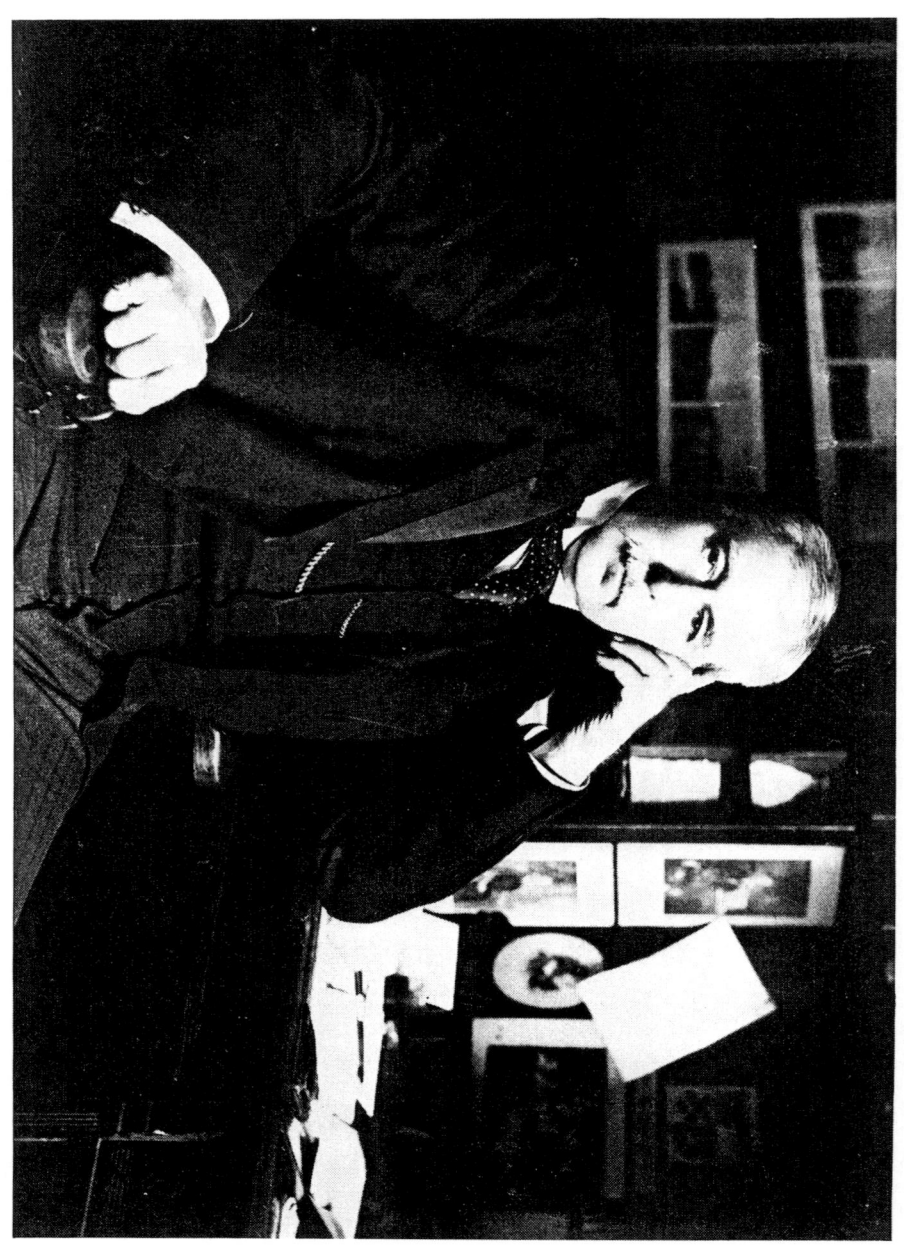

Fig.6　Manson at his desk in London.
(Wellcome Institute Library, CMAC)

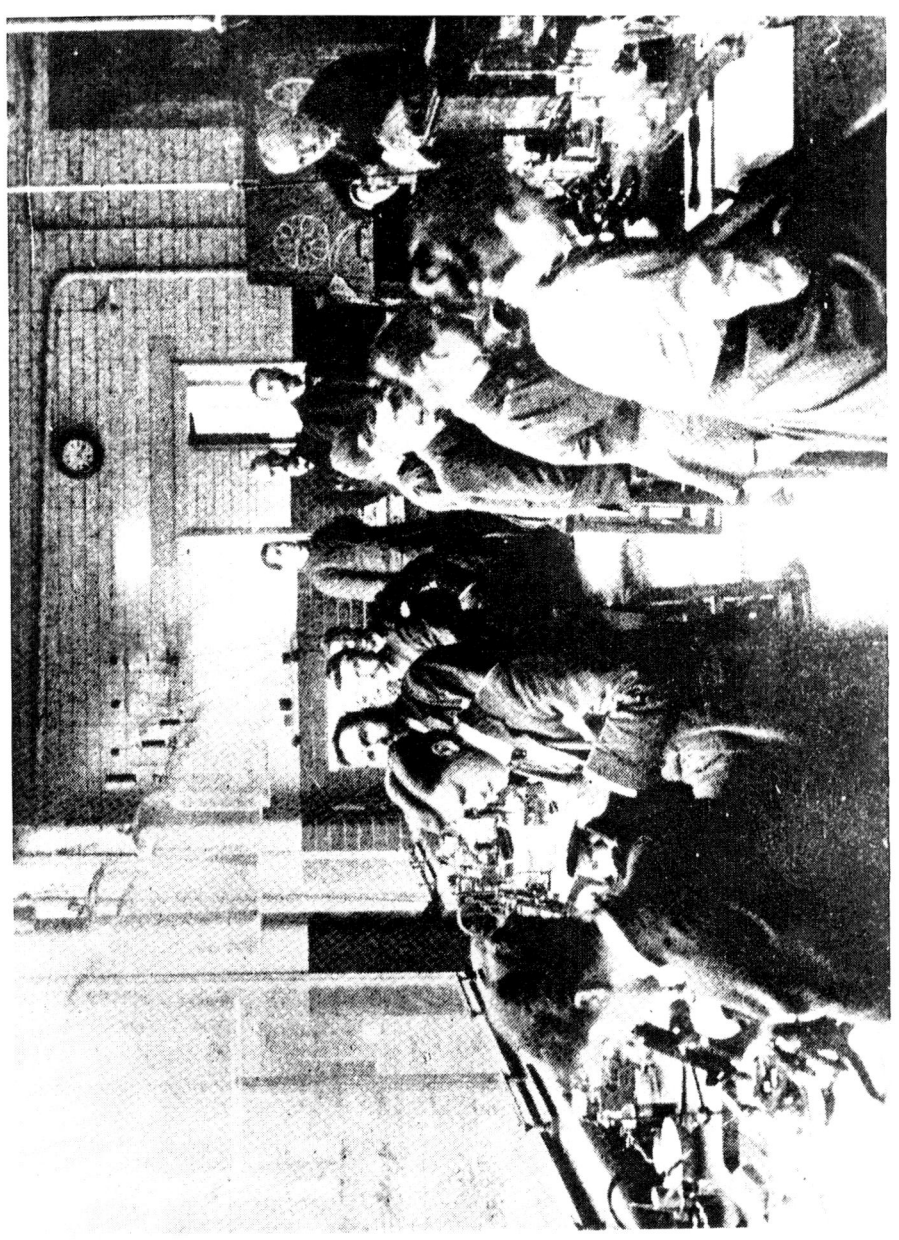

Fig.7 Class at their microscopes at the turn of the century: women medical missionaries in foreground, Manson in front of blackboard. (Wellcome Institute Library, CMAC)

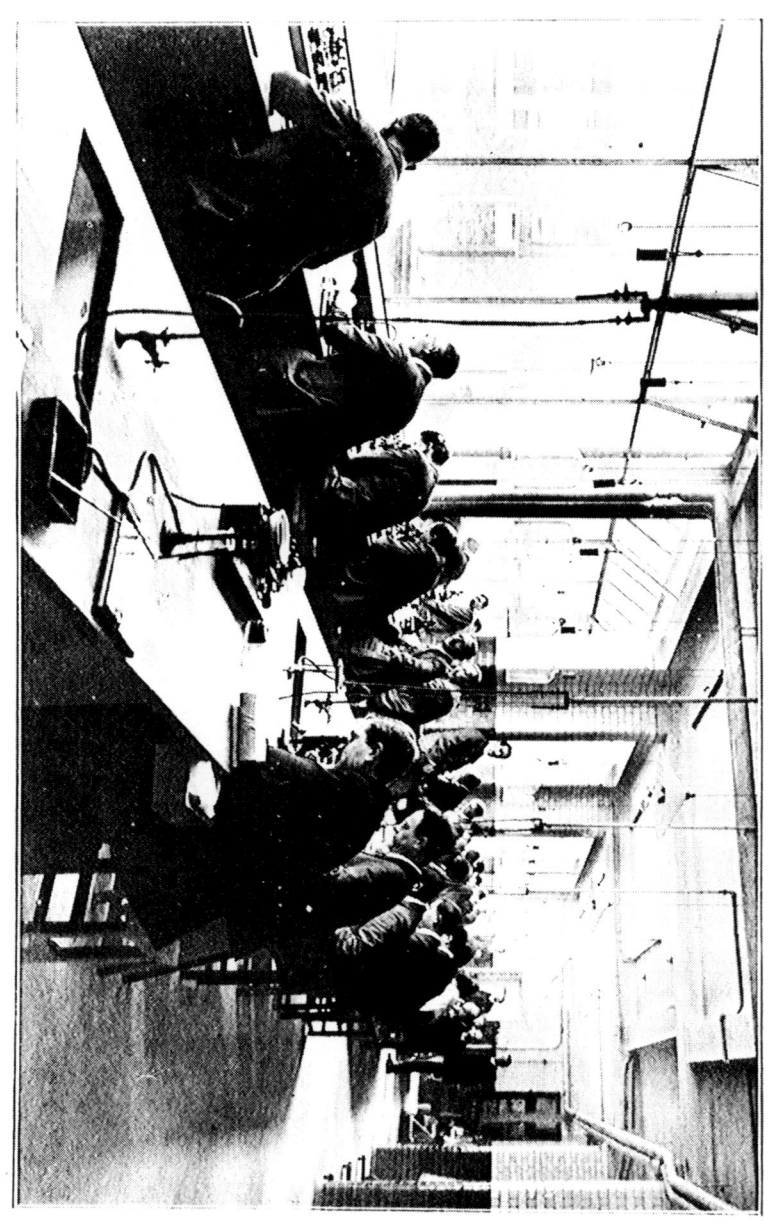

Fig.8 The new laboratories at the Albert Dock, 1910.
(Wellcome Institute Library, CMAC)

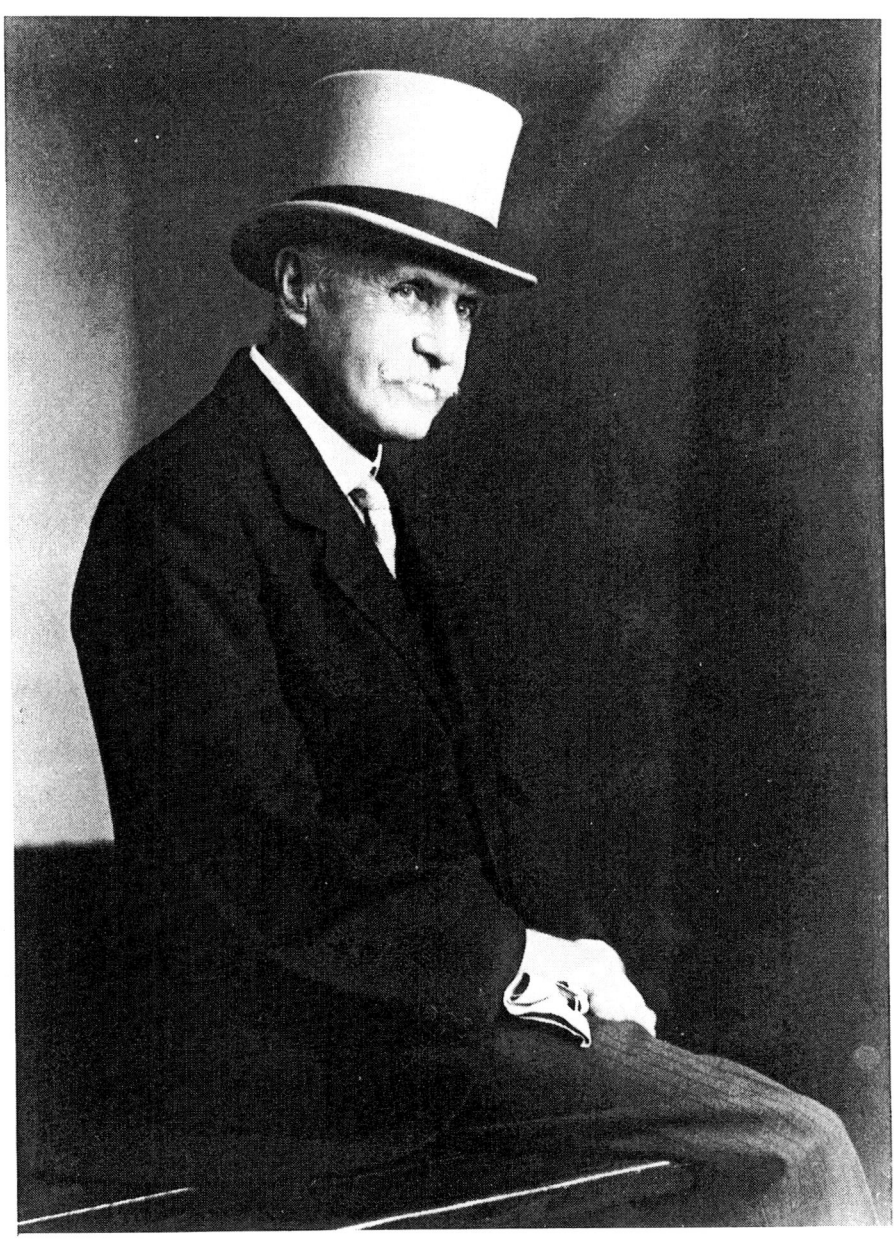

Fig.9 Sir James Michelli (1853-1935), Secretary of the Seamen's Hospital Society and of Manson's School.
(Wellcome Institute Library, CMAC)

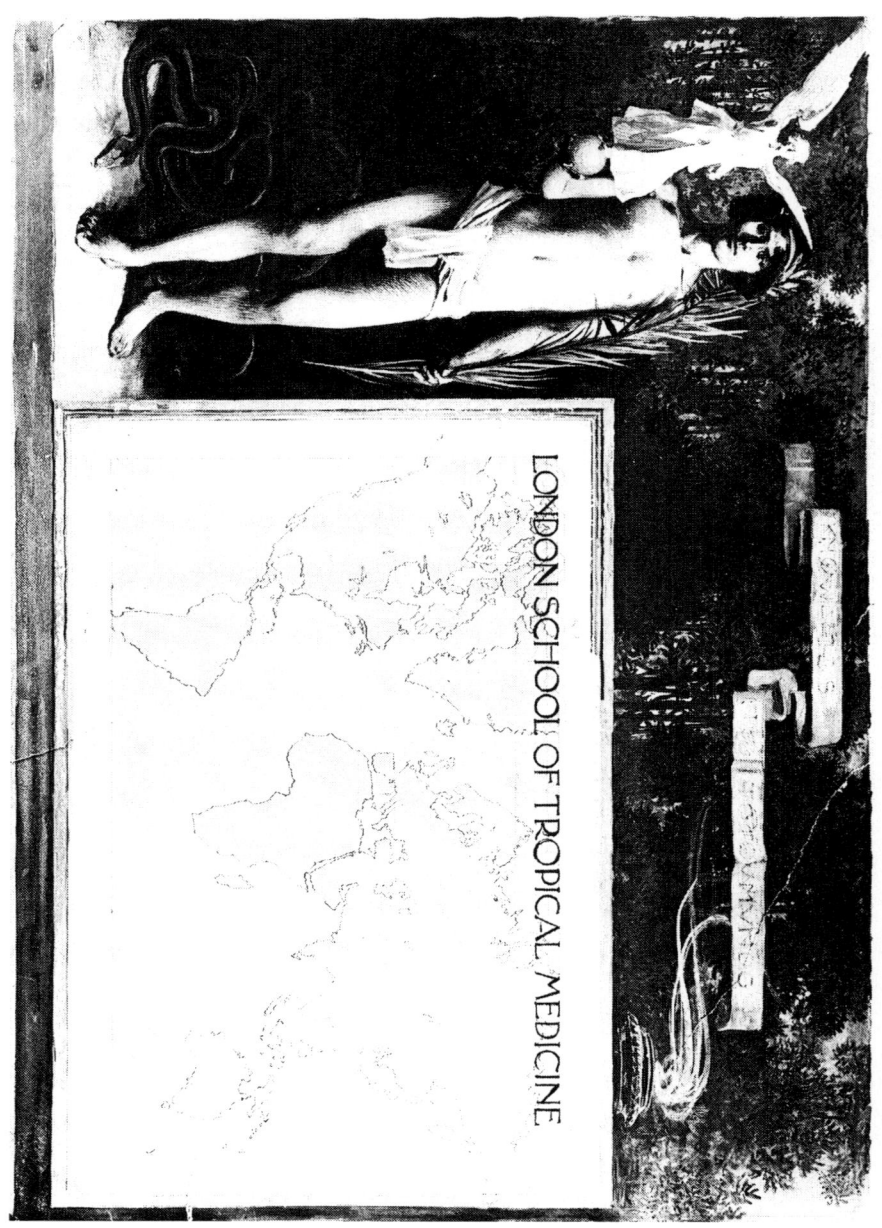

Fig.10 The original Diploma (abandoned 1924) awarded to students on completion of course.
(Wellcome Institute Library)

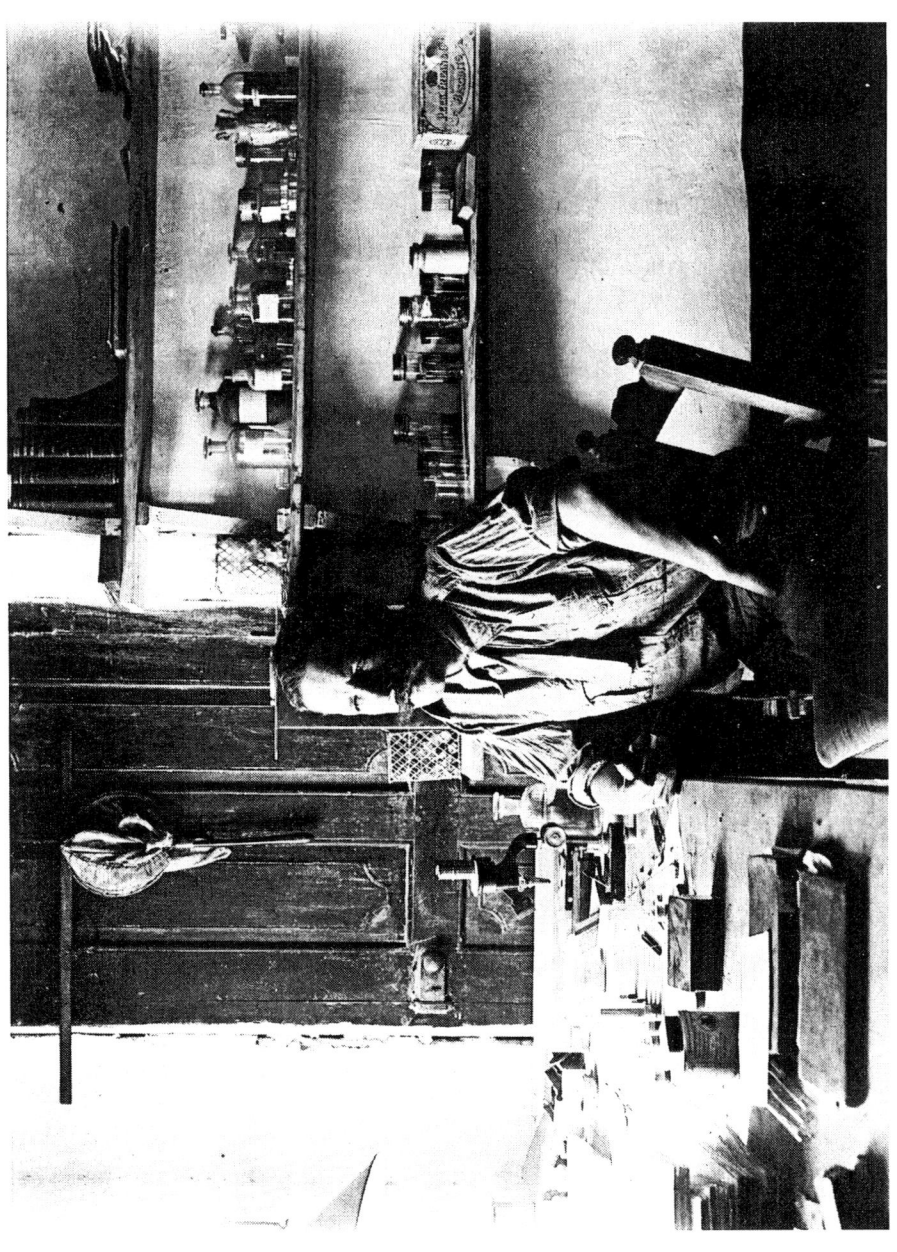

Fig.11 S.R.Christophers in his laboratory on board the *Elphinstone* during the Mesopotamia campaign, c.1916.
(Wellcome Institute Library, CMAC)

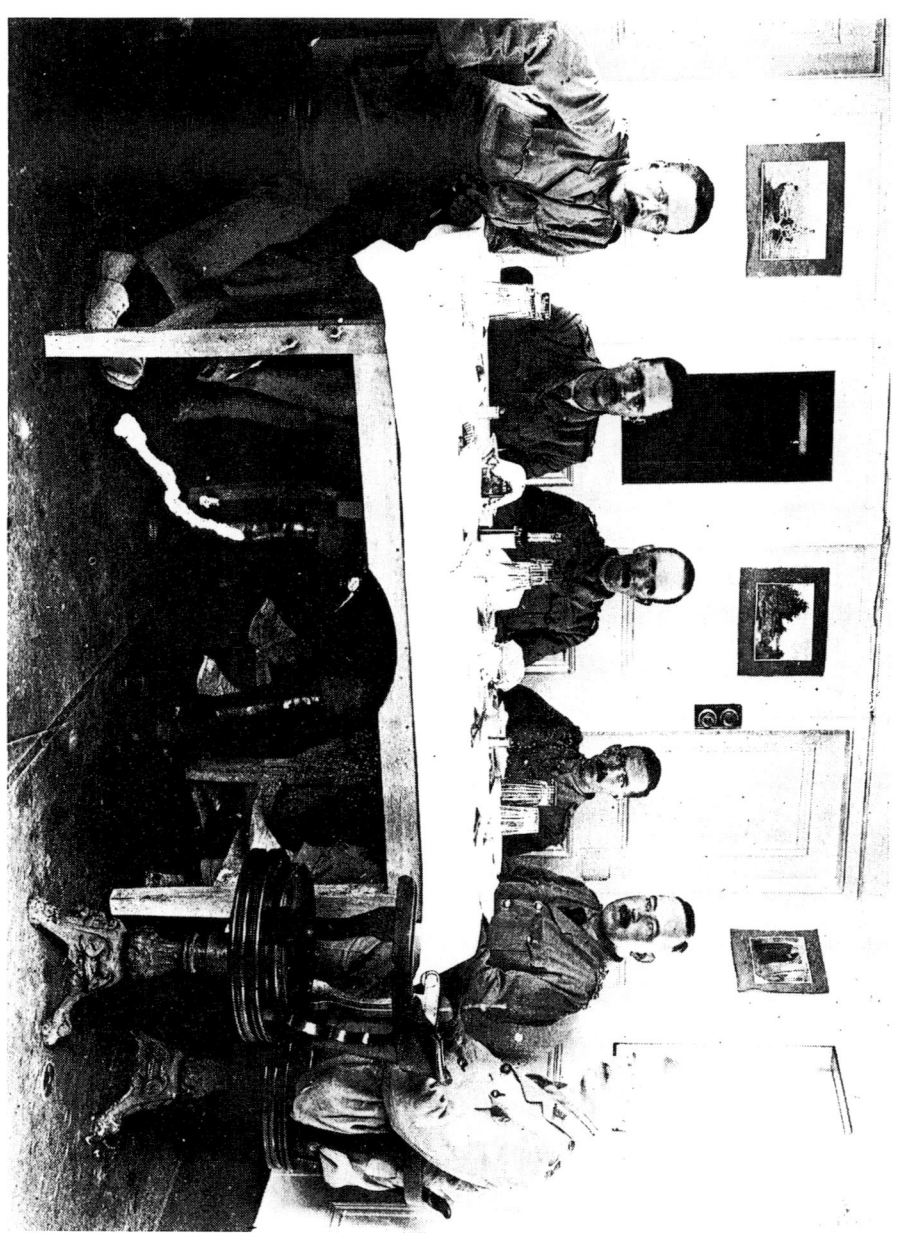

Fig.12 Sunday lunch on board the *Elphinstone* during the Mesopotamia campaign: Christophers at extreme left, Shortt 3rd from right.
(Wellcome Institute Library, CMAC)

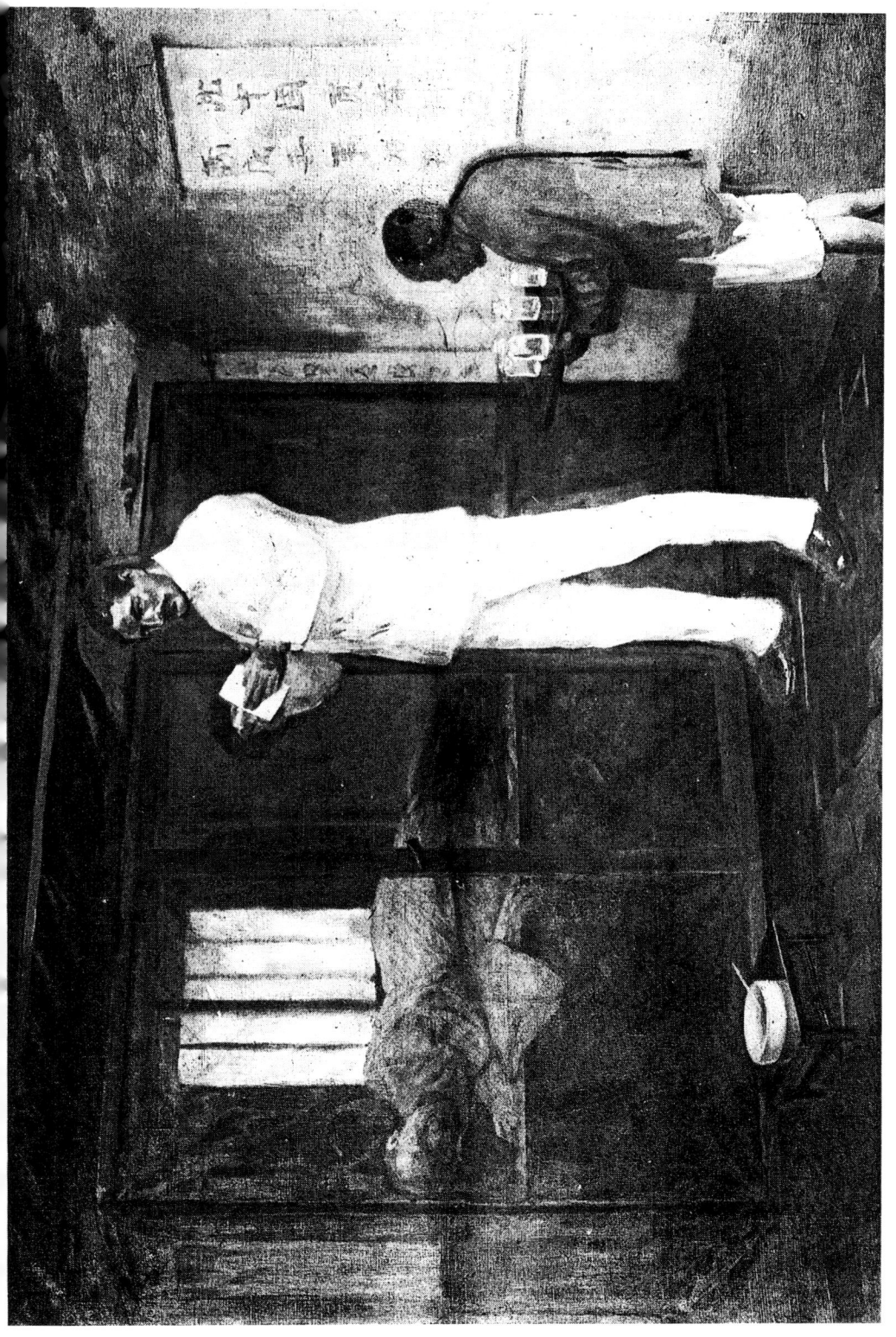

Fig. 13. Oil painting by Ernest Board: Manson, the Chinese gardener, and experiments on filariasis.
(Wellcome Institute Library, Iconographic Coll.)

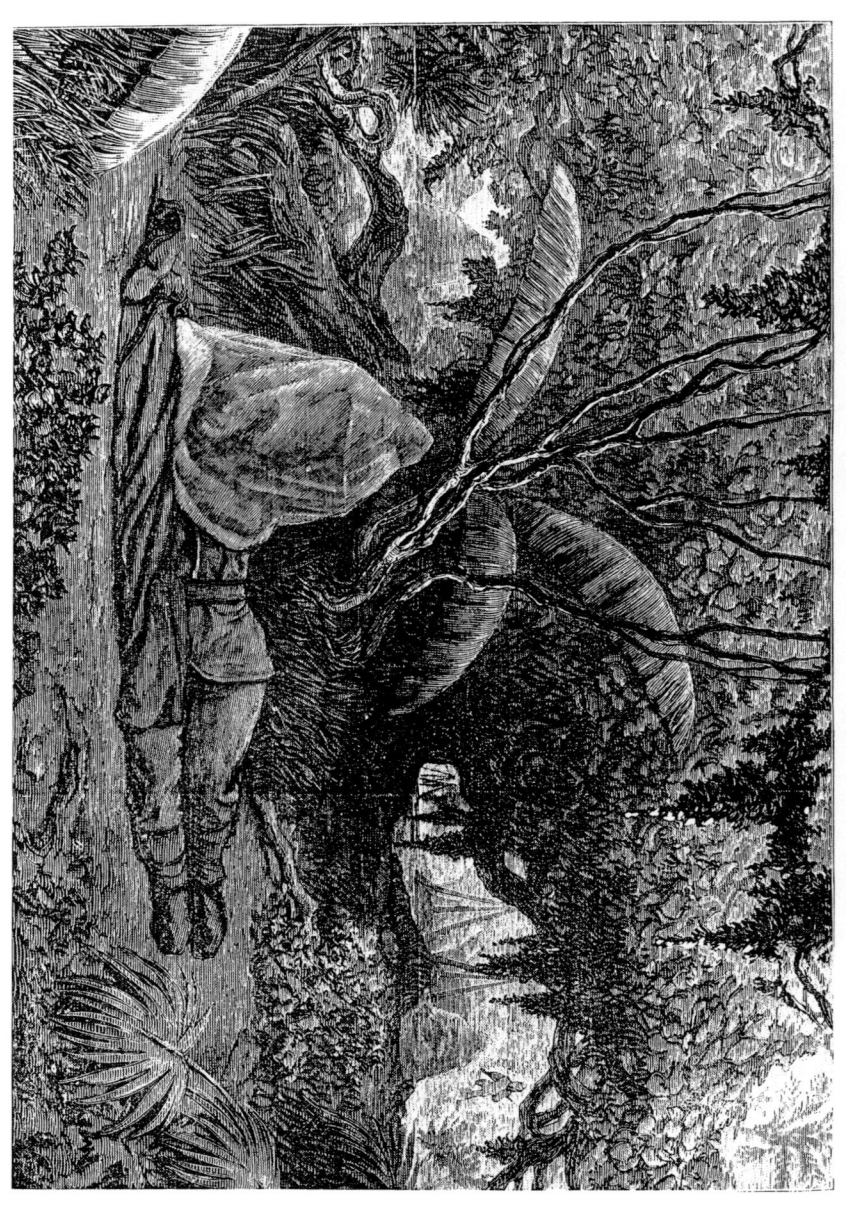

Fig.14. 'Mosquito curtain for the soldier's rest', c.1873. (Wellcome Institute Library Iconographic Coll.)

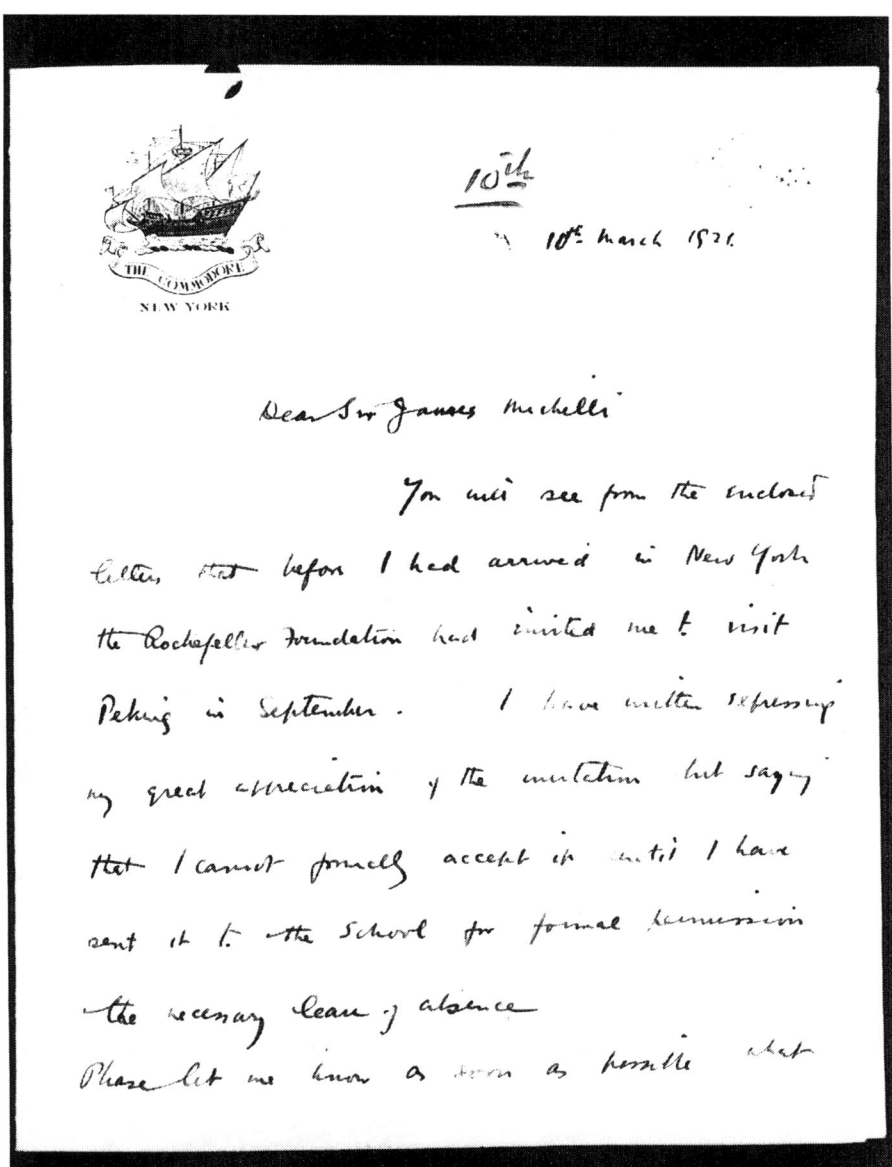

Fig.15 Letter from Leiper in New York to Michelli in London, keeping him informed of the situation *vis à vis* the Rockefeller Foundation. (LSHTM Archives, MSS FA:D3)

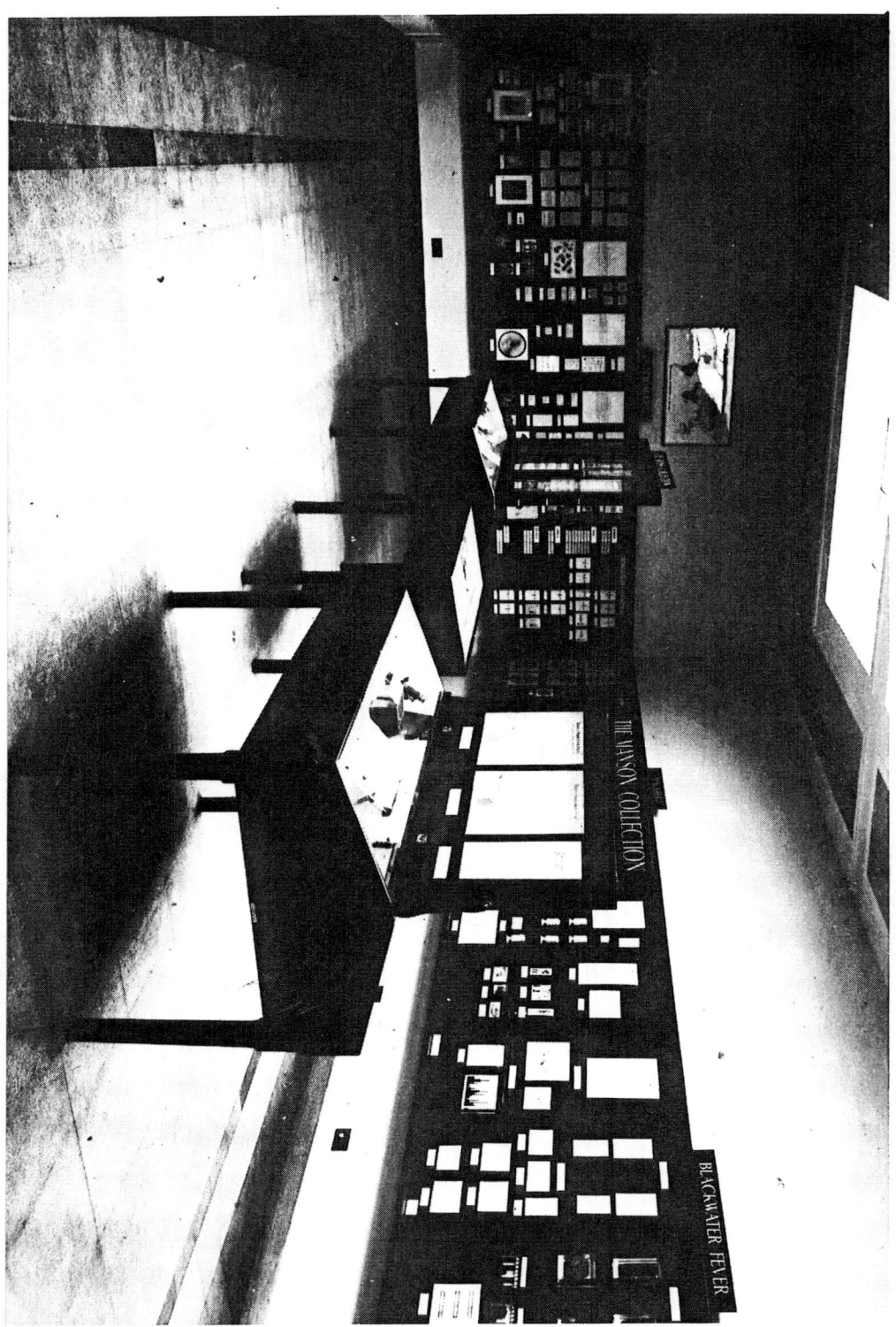

Fig.16 The School's Museum before the ravages of World War II.
(LSHTM Library collections)

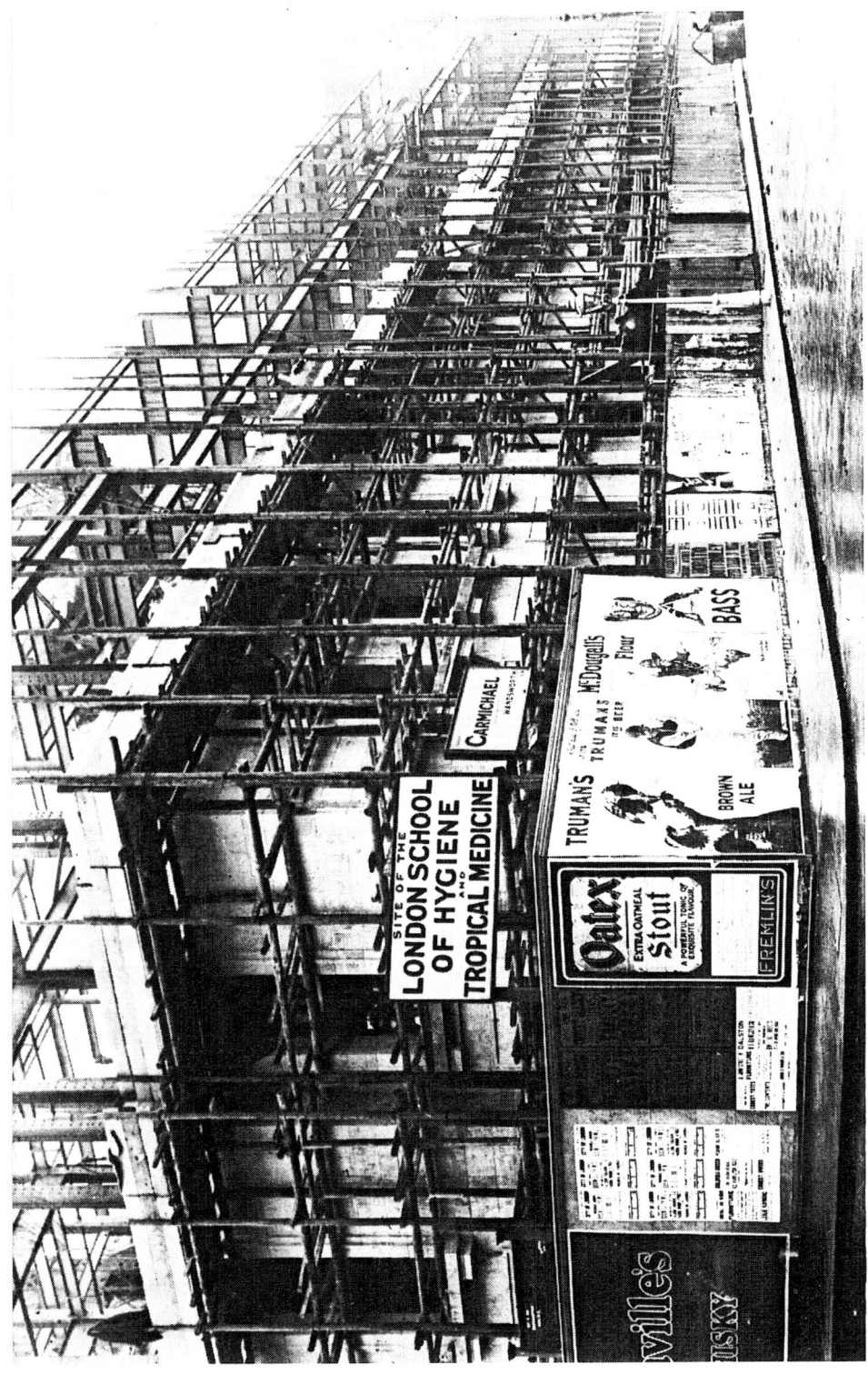

Fig.17 The Keppel Street building under construction in the 1920s. (LSHTM Library collections)

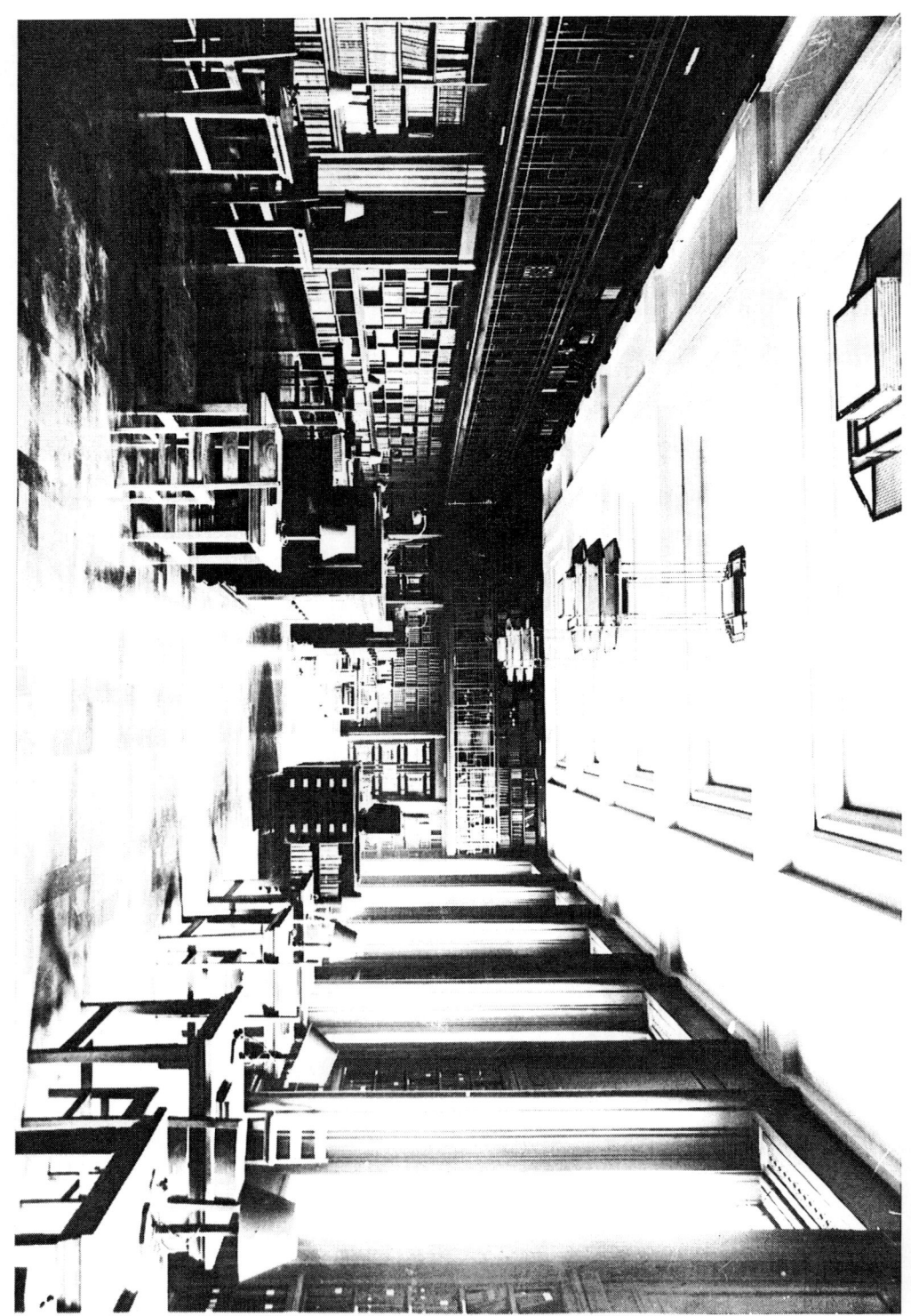

Fig.18 The School Library in the 1930s.
(LSHTM Library collections)

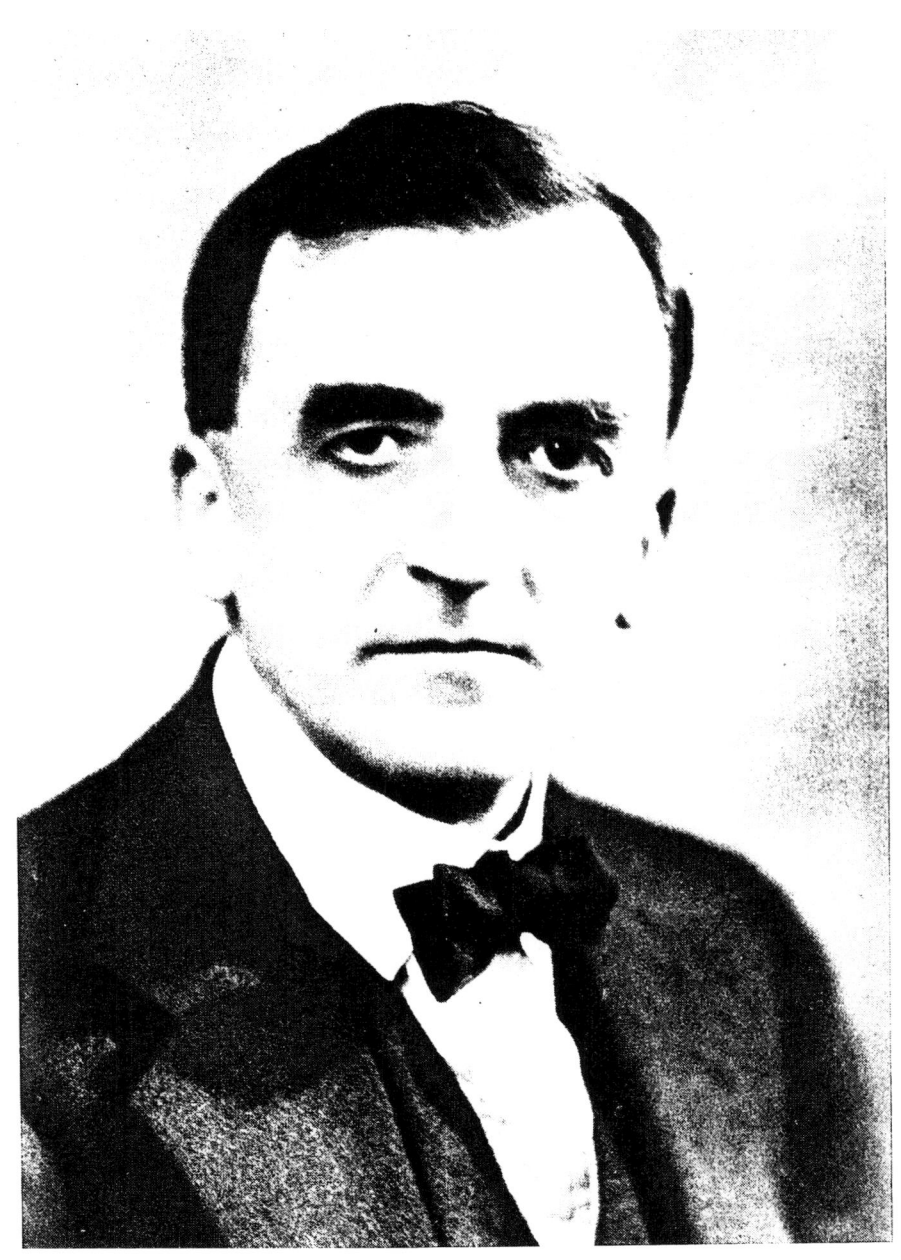

Fig.19 Major Greenwood (1880–1949). (LSHTM Board Room)

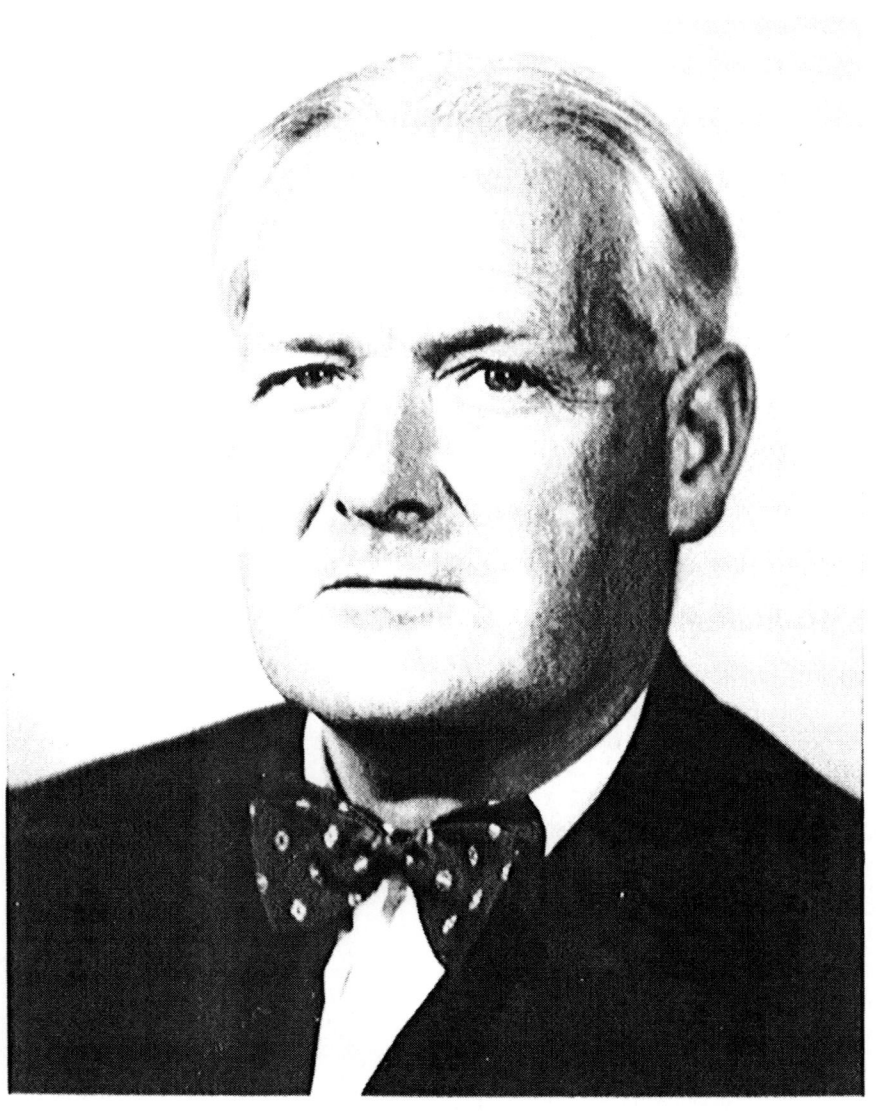

Fig.20 Sir Austin Bradford-Hill (1897–1991).
(LSHTM Board Room)

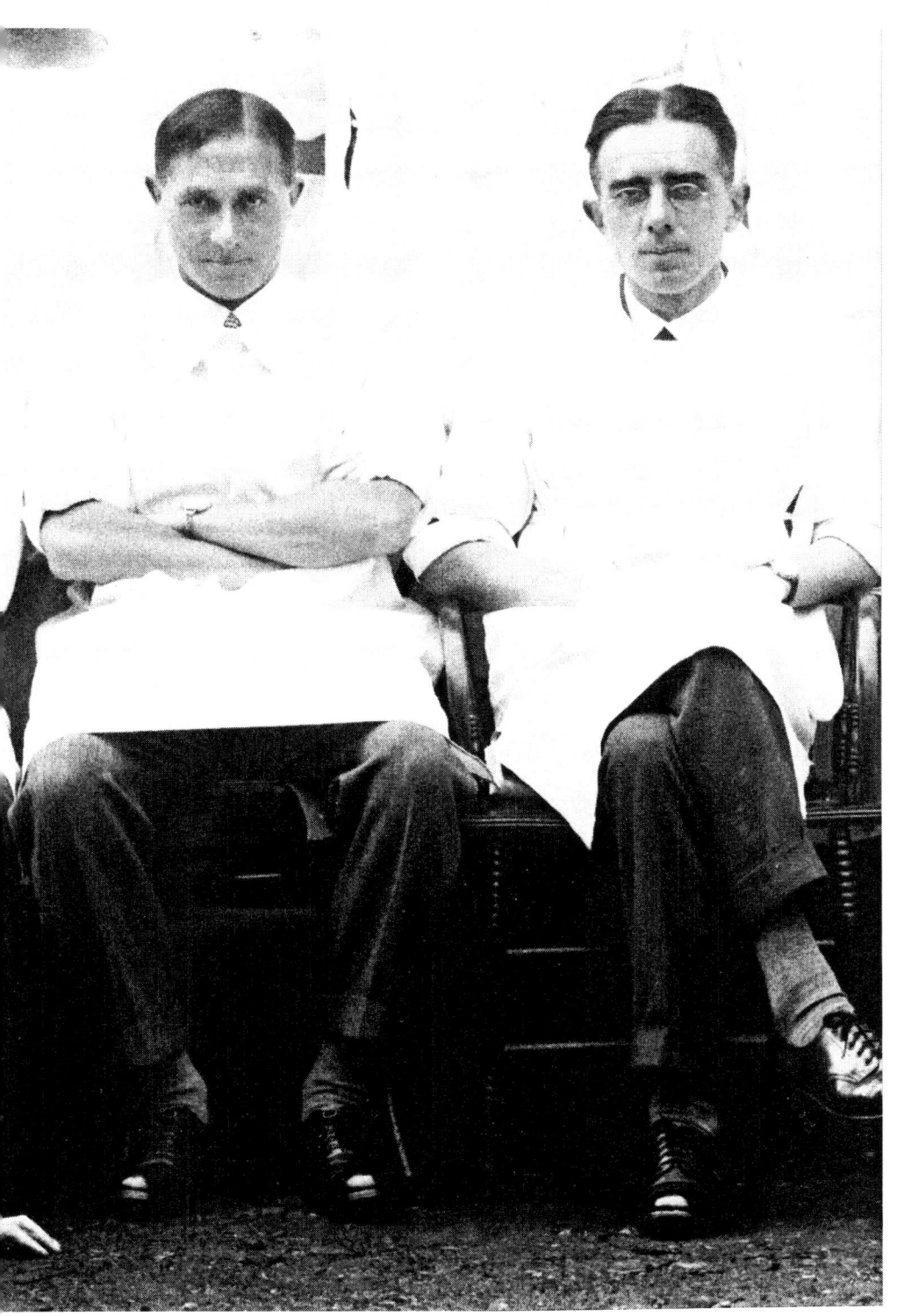

Fig.21 W.W.C.Topley and Forrest Fulton at the PHLS.
(Courtesy Prof.B.S.Drasar)

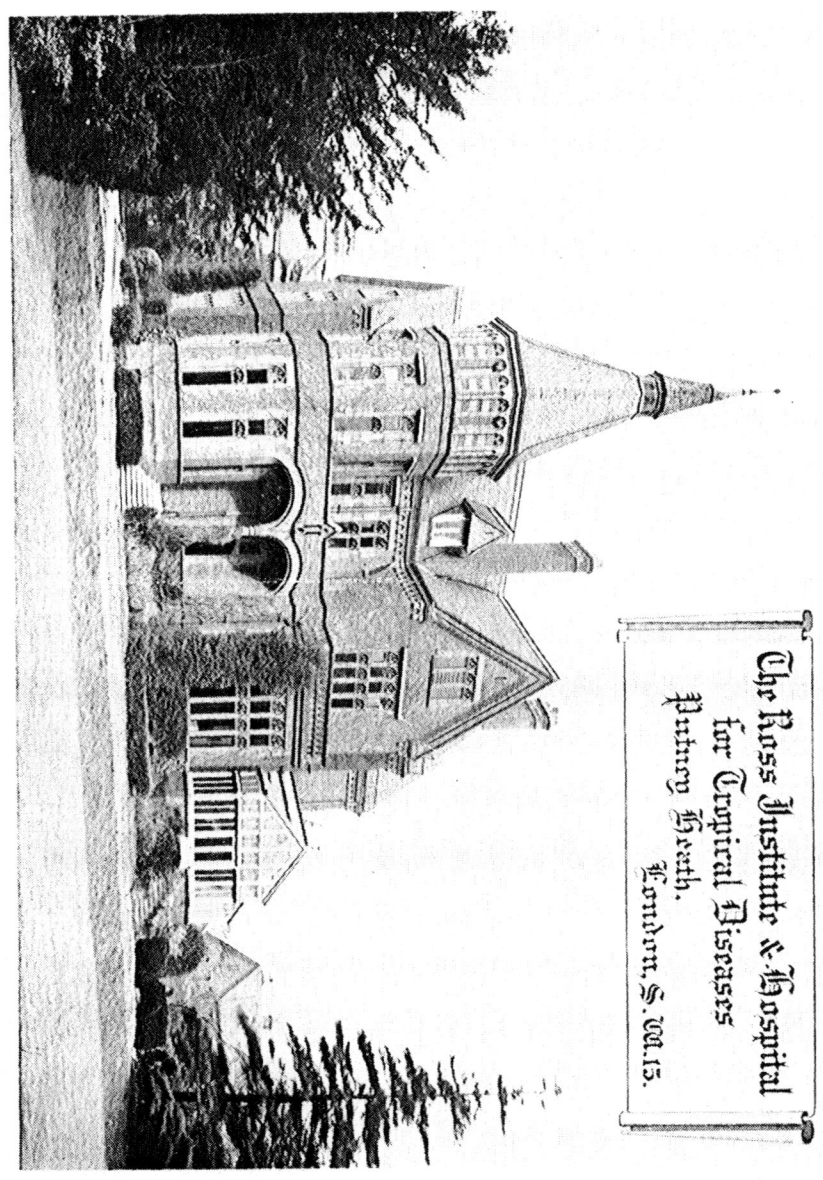

Fig.22 The Ross Institute at Putney in the late 1920s.
(Courtesy Prof.D.J.Bradley)

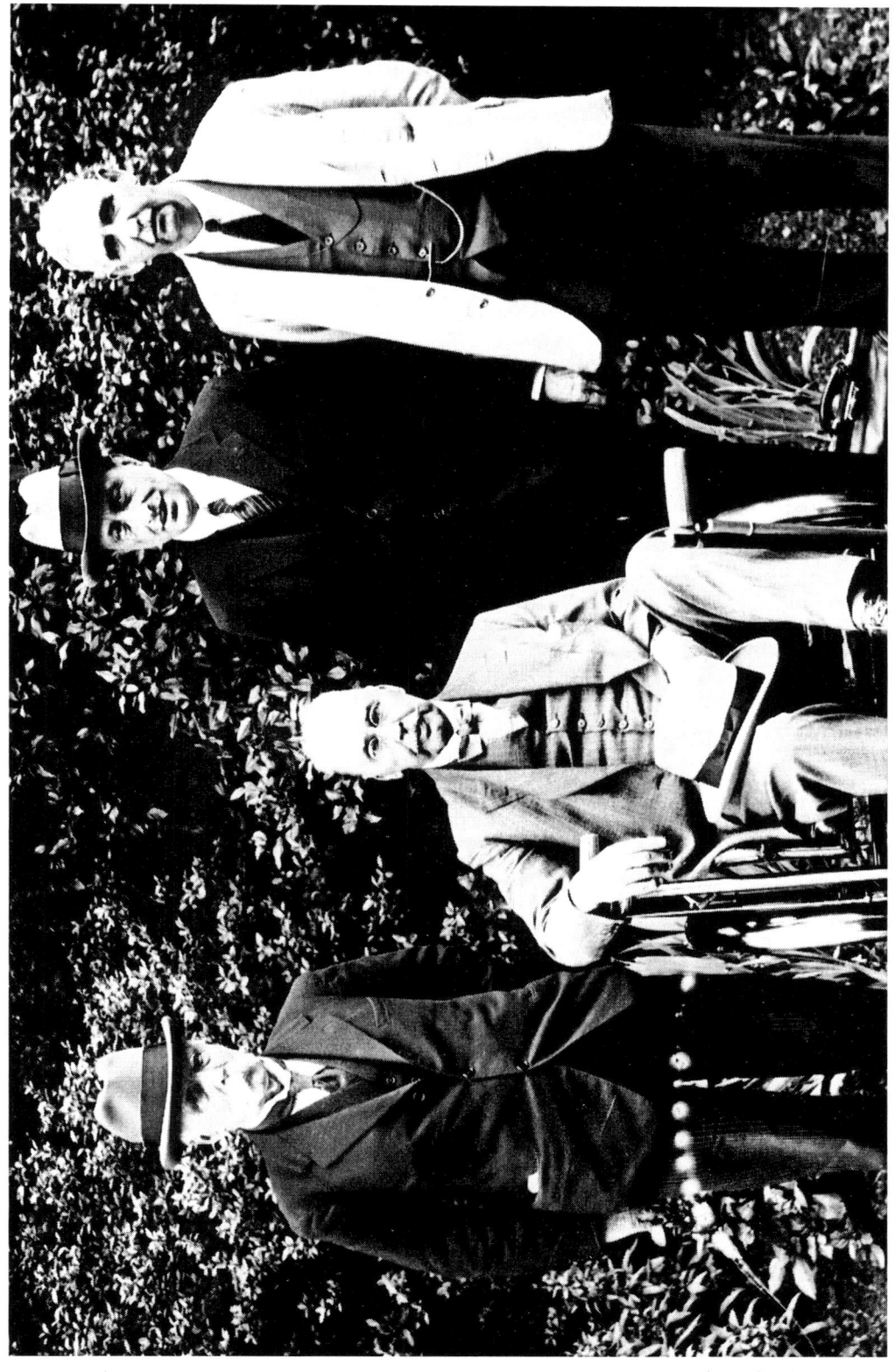

Fig.23 Heroes and villains of the Ross Institute and Hospitals in the grounds at Putney, l. to r.:, Sir William Simpson, Sir Ronald Ross. Aldo Castellani and Malcolm Watson, c.1930. (Courtesy Maty Gibson, LSHTM Library)

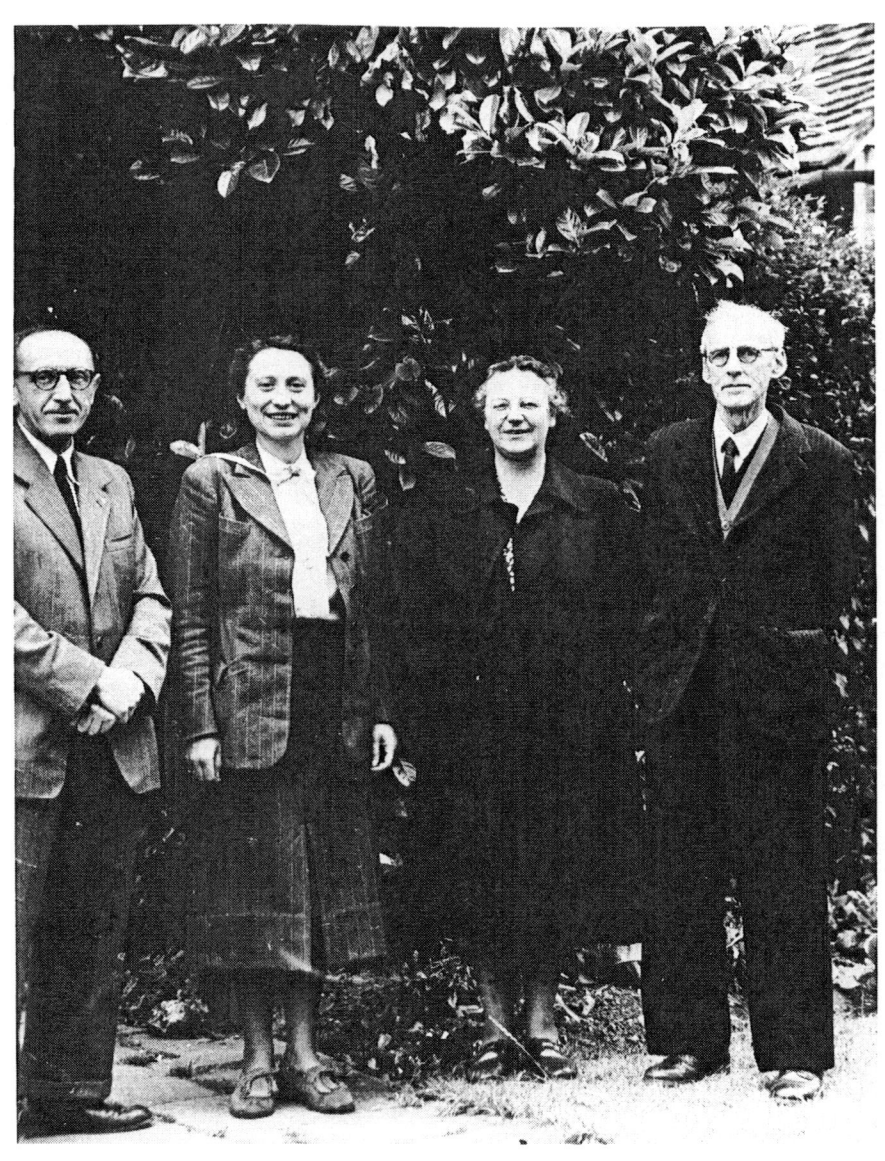

Fig.24 R.T.Leiper in later years with colleagues at Winches Farm, l.to.r. Dr.Oldham, Dr.Sheila Wilmot, Miss A.Walton). (LSHTM Library collections)

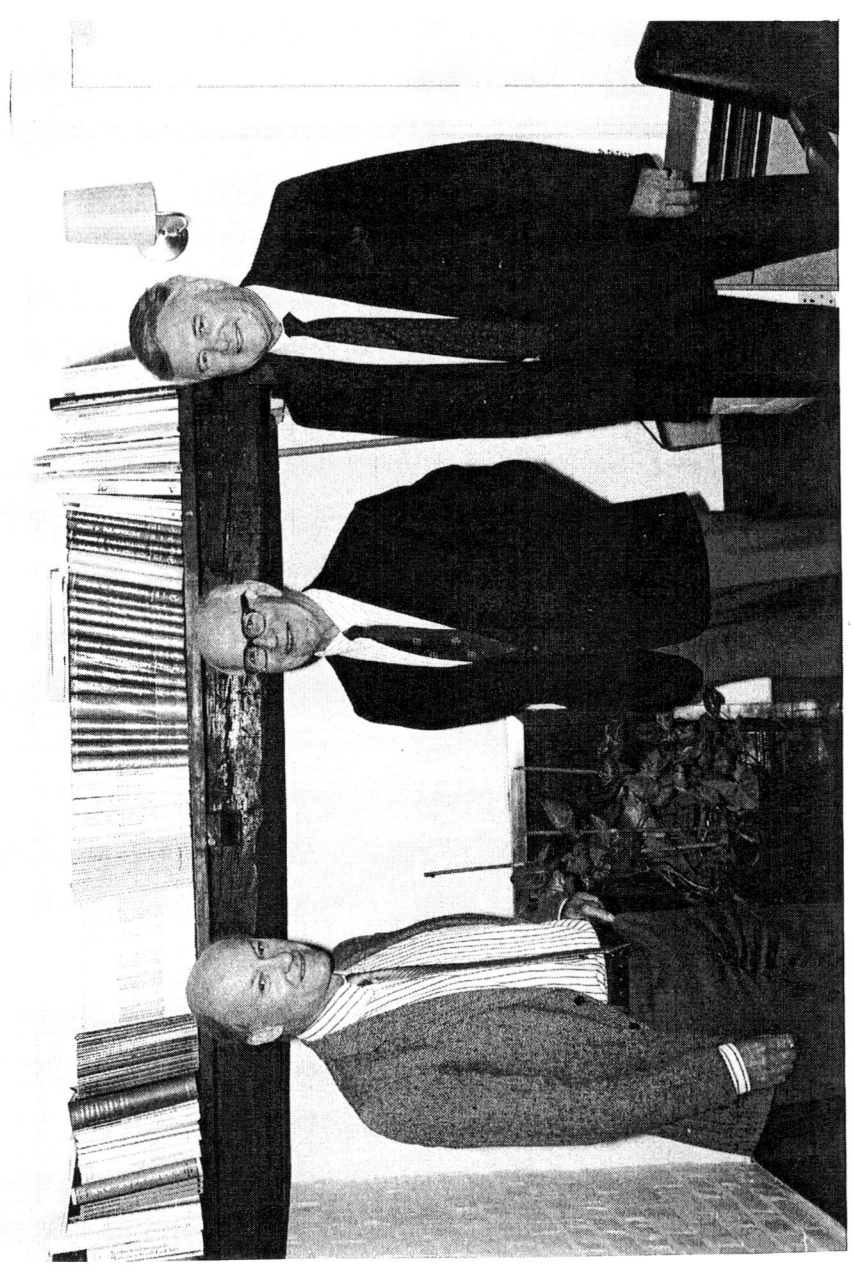

Fig.25 The second - and final - flowering of Winches Farm: Dr.R.L.Muller, Professor W.Peters, Professor and Sub-Dean G.Webbe in front of the restored 16th century fireplace in the Sub-Dean's office, 1991.
(Courtesy Professor Webbe)

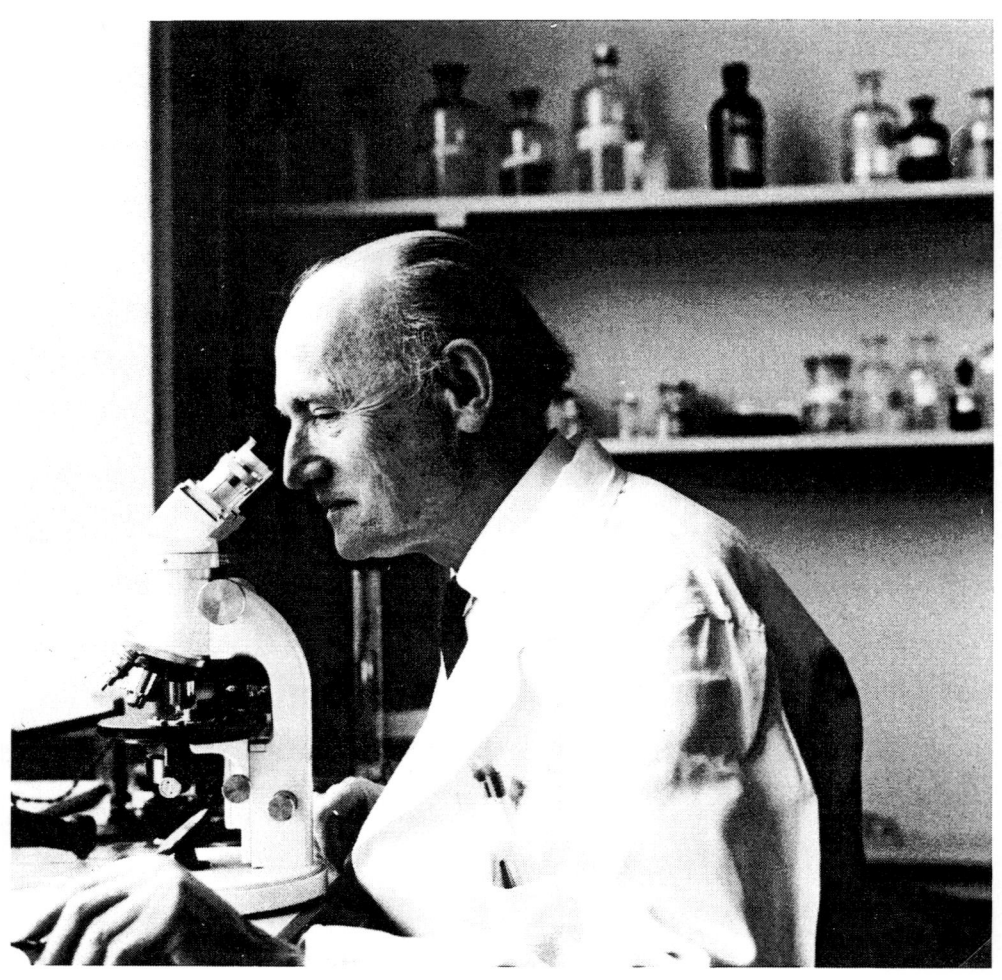

Fig.26 P.C.C.Garnham at the microscope in the 1960s.
(Wellcome Institute Library, CMAC)

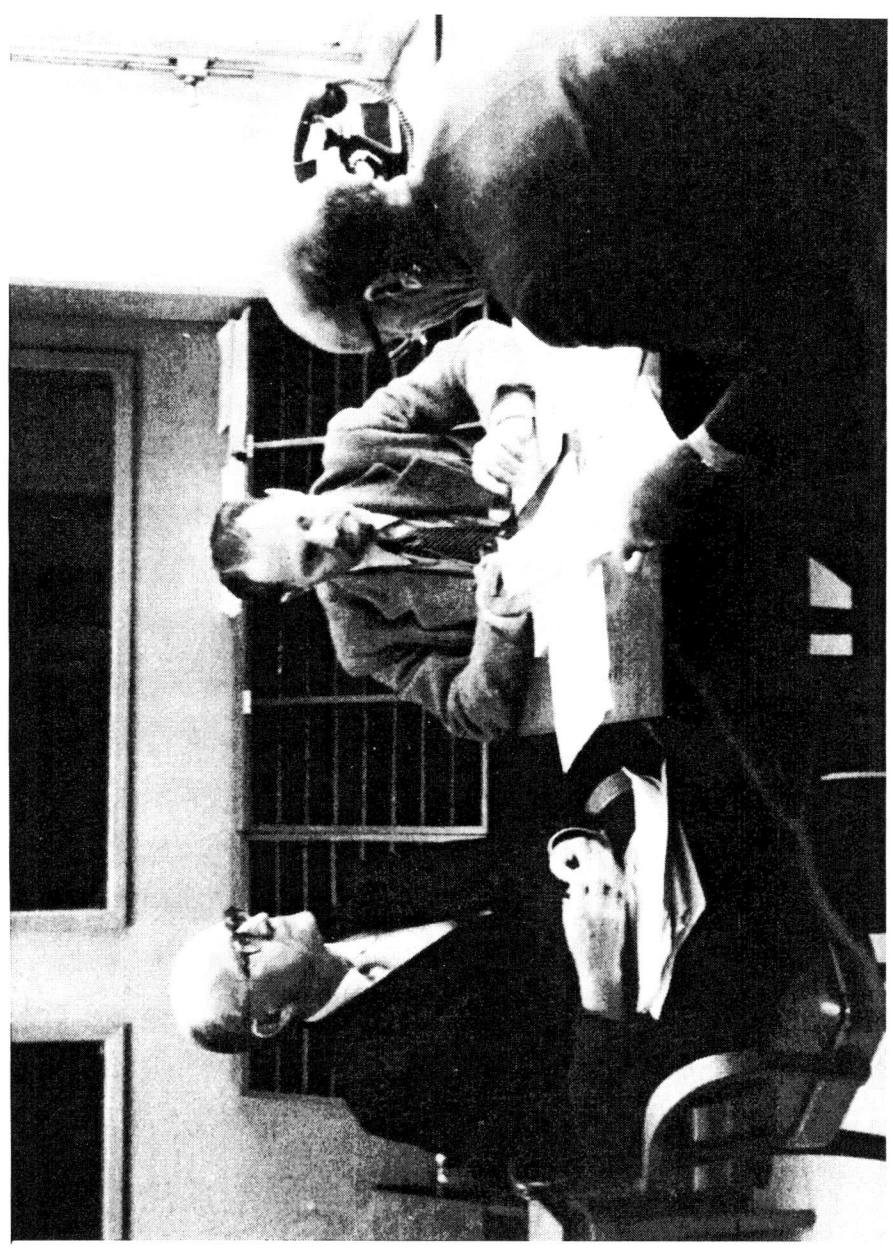

Fig.27 Keeping the peace: Bruce-Chwatt in his Geneva office, discussing WHO matters with P.C.C.Garnham (left, contemplating distant vistas), and George Macdonald.
(Wellcome Institute Library, CMAC)

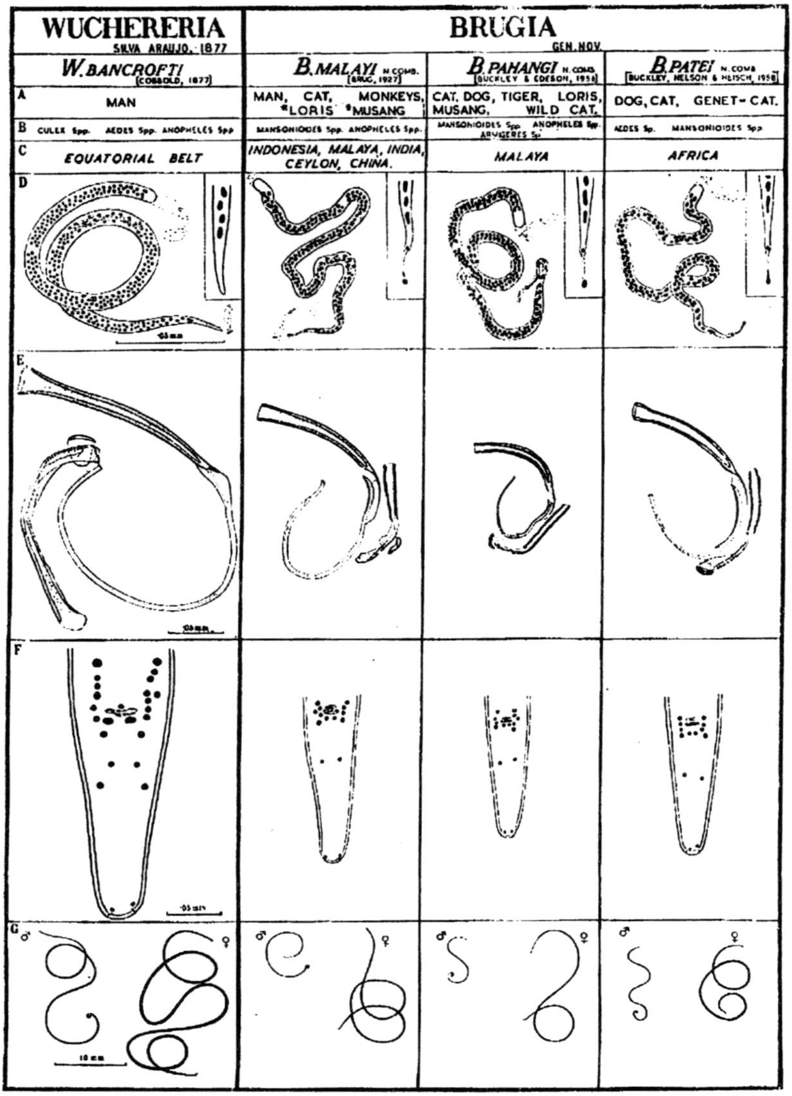

Fig.28   J.J.C.Buckley *et al.:* schematic separation of *Wuchereria* and *Brugia* species, 1956–8. *Ann.Trop.Med.Parasit.*, 1960, 54:75–7.

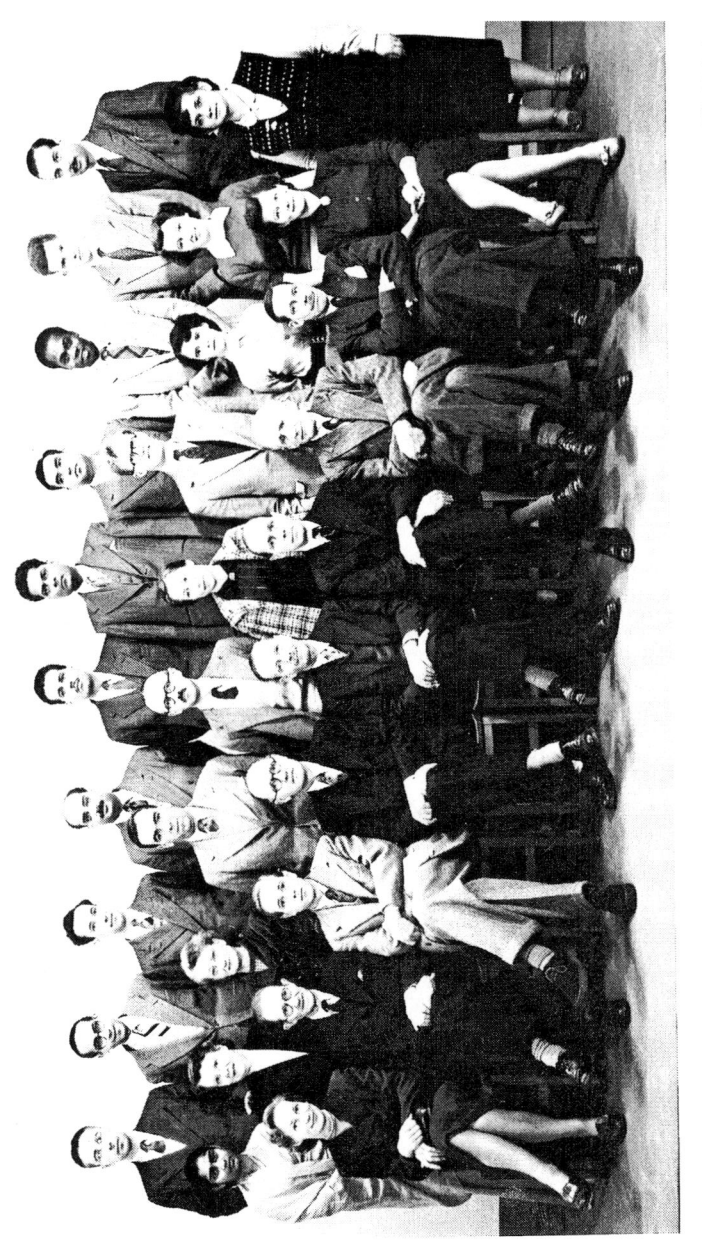

Fig.29 The Parasitology Department, LSHTM, 1952. Front row centre: Garnham, Shortt, Buckley.
(Wellcome Institute Library, CMAC)

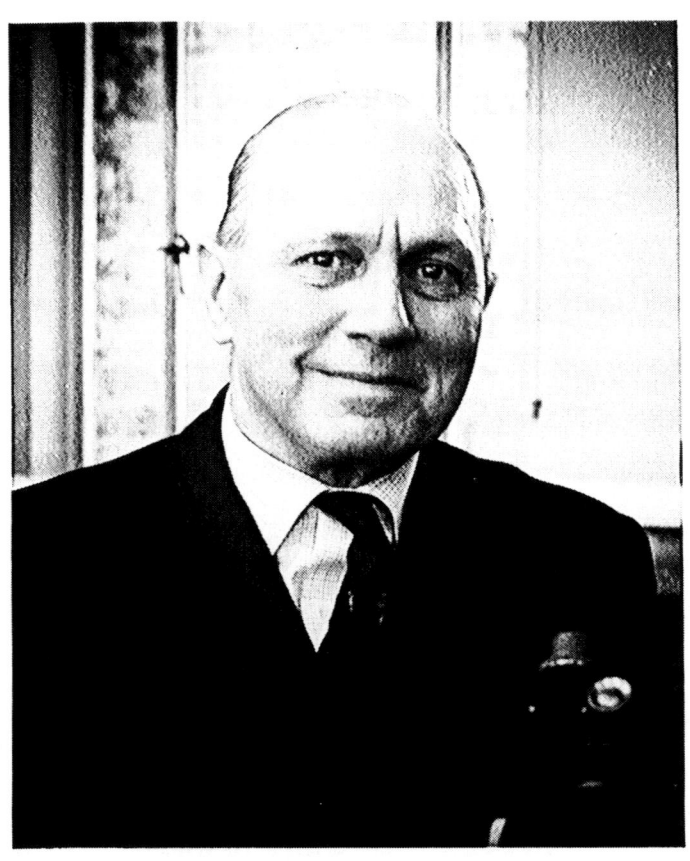

Fig.30   J.J.C.Buckley and microscope, 1960s.
(Courtesy Dr.D.Denham; now CMAC)

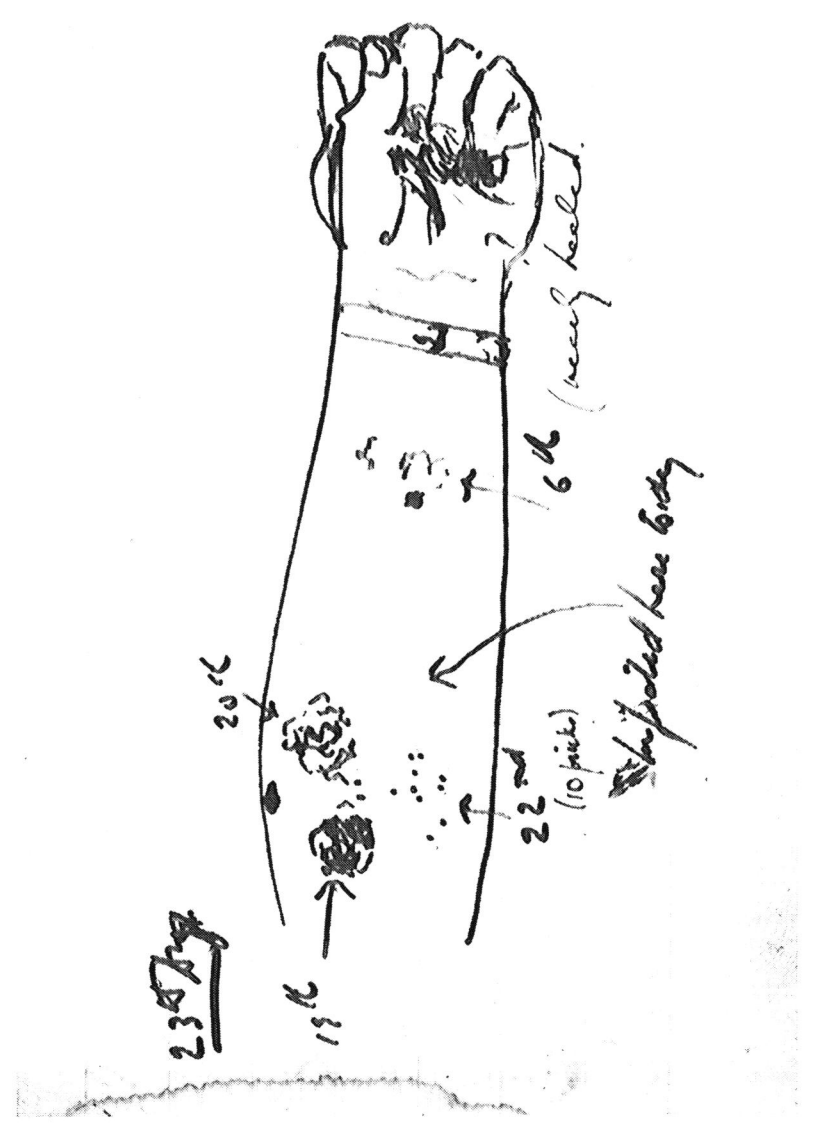

Fig.31 J.J.C.Buckley's sketch of self-experimentation on arm; Buckley notebook on hookworm (*Necator*) experiments, Caribbean Islands, April 1932.
(Courtesy Dr.D.Denham; now in Wellcome CMAC)

PLATE XII
BRICK-SHAPED PARTICLES SHOWN IN PHOTOGRAPHS
OF SKIN LESION SCRAPINGS FROM MISS ALGEO[1]

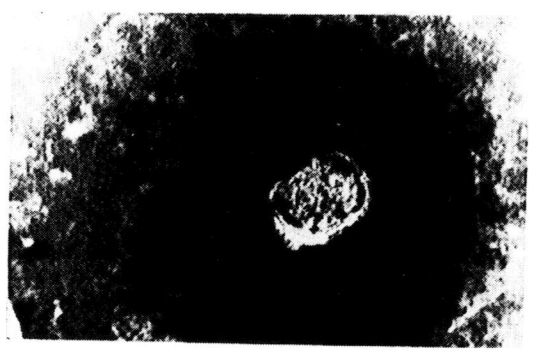

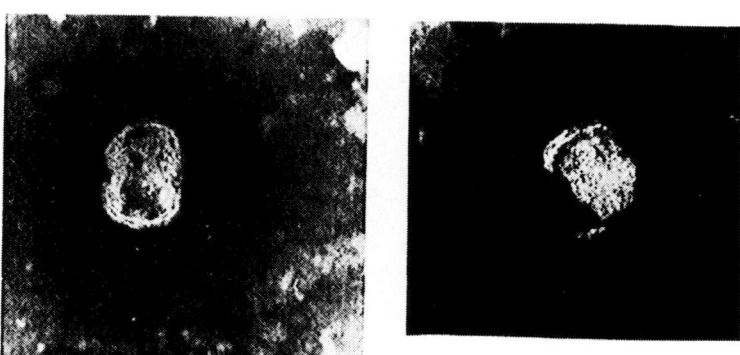

Fig.32 Three images of smallpox virus from 1973; and Ebola virus, 1978.
(Courtesy Dr.D.S.Ellis)

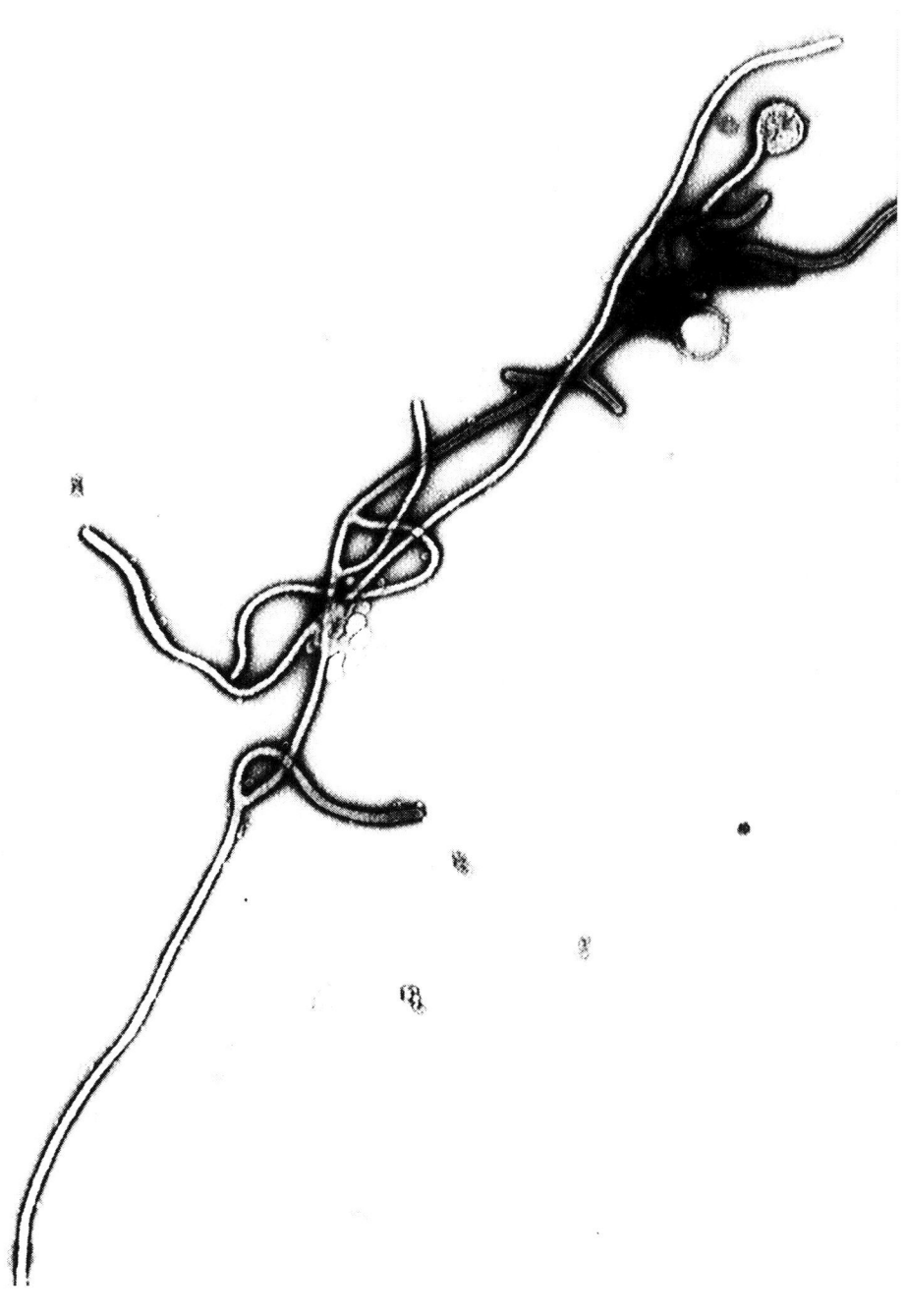

3

TRANSITION 1919–29: FROM TROPICAL MEDICINE TO GLOBAL PUBLIC HEALTH

The transformation of Manson's School at the Albert Dock to a central London institution concerned with teaching and research in not just tropical medicine, but in public health on a wider global scale, took place over a period of ten years, from 1919 to 1929, when, after an interlude in Endsleigh Gardens described below, the London School of Hygiene & Tropical Medicine opened in new buildings in Keppel Street, close to University College, University College Hospital and Medical School, and to the site where the Senate House of the University of London was to be built a few years later. The ten-year period can be neatly split in two: five years of synthesis of a number of ideas and plans put forward by interested individuals and official bodies on both sides of the Atlantic; and another five years of building on the site finally acquired in Bloomsbury, and simultaneous development of the infrastructure of teaching and research departments. The first new departments to be established and added to what had become designated the 'Tropical Division', in 1927, were the Division of Epidemiology and Vital Statistics under Major Greenwood, and the Division of Bacteriology and Immunology under W.W.C.Topley. At the same time, the Tropical Division was divided into two, one of Tropical Medicine and Hygiene under Balfour, and another of Medical Zoology under Leiper. It was the intention to group all teaching in six administrative divisions.[1] The burden of administering the changes and innovations fell to Andrew Balfour, who had been appointed Director in October, 1923.

The appointment of a director had been closely watched at the Rockefeller Foundation, the main benefactor of the new school. On October 19th, Victor Heiser informed F.F.Russell that Balfour was leading the field in the search for a director of the 'Health School'. A week later this was confirmed when Sir Arthur Robinson sent Russell a telegram: 'Transitional Executive Committee have to day appointed Dr.Andrew Balfour director school of hygiene'. Russell wrote a letter of congratulation to Balfour on the same day; Vincent, on behalf of the Foundation, followed suit on November 2nd.[2]

At first sight, these developments may appear to be a matter concerning just one school within the University of London; but they were more than that. They constituted only one aspect of a complex combination of a post-war review of medical education in Britain, of political changes giving rise to a Ministry of Health, and of a Rockefeller policy aimed at establishing a network of public health centres at strategic points throughout the world; centres intended to promote research and teaching of the gospel of comprehensive preventive medicine.

The extent of Rockefeller influence in shaping the structure and policies of the future LSHTM has been examined by Donald Fisher, in a wider context, and, more recently, by Acheson and Poole.[3] Both studies are based to a considerable degree on the material in the extensive and meticulously catalogued Rockefeller Archives at Tarrytown, New York. Acheson and Poole have covered much the same ground as Fisher, but claim to have interpreted it differently because of their additional scrutiny of the Vincent and Rose diaries and of the Senate Minutes of the University of London. On the other hand, they in turn have ignored sources closer to home, i.e. the Public Record Office and the LSHTM Archives, the latter with their Leiper letters, Michelli correspondence, and private messages between Leiper, Michelli, Vincent, and Rose; archives which are not as yet catalogued, and consequently much less easy of access. A number of these documents testify to the role Leiper had played, and continued to play, behind the scenes where planning was taking place.[4]

In the United States, Rockefeller philanthropy had been involved in support of changes in medical education and research since the turn of the century. Such changes were rooted in a reversal of a previous trend: the almost obligatory period of study spent in European research laboratories by any self-respecting American physician. The 1890s saw the beginnings of an erosion of the European stranglehold on teaching of scientific medicine, especially such rapidly developing disciplines as pathology, histology, and bacteriology. The Johns Hopkins Medical School had introduced research laboratories linked to clinical teaching, with William H. Welch (1850–1934) as professor of pathology, in 1893. At the same time, John D. Rockefeller (1839–1937) had shown his interest in support of higher education by generous funding, which had ensured the opening of the University of Chicago. By 1897, his financial adviser, the shrewd Baptist clergyman Frederick T. Gates (1853–1929), had been reading Osler's *The principles and practice of medicine,* and was aiming to convince Rockefeller of the potential advantages of medical philanthropy as an improver of a somewhat flawed image.[5]

Ten years later, a chance meeting between Gates and Charles W. Stiles (1867–1941), who was seeking sponsorship for an anti-hookworm campaign in the Southern United States, led to Rockefeller involvement in an escalating fight against the disease. It was a development which was in turn to lead directly to not only the Sanitary Commission and its determined campaign against the disease on United States territory; but also to a consolidation of Rockefeller philanthropic policies, with incorporation of the Rockefeller Foundation and its International Health Board (both in 1913), and, in 1916, the establishment of the Johns Hopkins School of Hygiene and Public Health. The supreme pioneer in scientific medical research in the United States, the Rockefeller Institute for Medical Research, opened in 1904.[6]

Already in 1913, towards the end of the hookworm campaign in the Southern States, transatlantic contacts had been made. Wickliffe Rose (1862–1931), who had no medical experience, but plenty of organisational talent, had been appointed Director of the International Health Board (IHB). Almost immediately he visited London, seeking experienced help from the hookworm experts at the LSTM, and from the politicians at the Colonial Office, with a view to widen the campaign internationally, and especially in British controlled territories.[7] The ultimate goal was to be an ambitious quest for global public health as not only an immediate benefit to humanity, but also as a social investment in the longer term. Disease everywhere was seen, in the words of Gates, as ' ... the main source of ... human ills, poverty, crime, ignorance, vice, inefficiency, hereditary taint, and many other evils'.[8] It was a sweeping indictment, which was echoed, albeit in less extreme terms, in London by the Medical Research Committee, in its last Annual Report before it became the Medical Research Council in 1919.

Initial contacts between the Rockefeller Foundation and London had been interrupted by the exigencies of the 1914–18 war. When Rose was able to return to the subject after the war, he found that a number of factors had strengthened his hand. The alarming pandemic of influenza in 1918–19, following war in Europe, had stretched health services everywhere, and emphasised the need for world-wide vigilance on the epidemiological front. In London, a Ministry of Health was created in June, 1919, with Christopher Addison (1869–1951) as Minister of Health. In April, 1921, he was replaced by Alfred Mond (1868–1930), with George Newman (1870–1948) continuing in his post as the Ministry's Chief Medical Officer.[9] At about the same time, William Osler (1849–1919), interested in developing medical specialties and especially in the new tropical medicine coming to the fore under the aegis of Manson and of Ross, and who had himself introduced a course in tropical diseases at Johns Hopkins in September 1899, had been spearheading a campaign for Government support to create a postgraduate medical school in London. Addison responded in January, 1921, by appointing a committee, chaired by the Earl of Athlone (1874–1957), to explore the possibilities for developments. By chance, this was the same month that saw a prolonged visit to University College, London, by Abraham Flexner (1866–1959), author of the two authoritative reports on medical education in the United States and Canada (1910), and in Europe (1912), and G.E. Vincent (1864–1941), President of the Rockefeller Foundation.[10]

Ostensibly, Flexner and Vincent were in London to inspect the workings of the 'unit' scheme introduced at University College, with University College Hospital and its Medical School, which had just received substantial support from the Foundation.[11] Inevitably, it was an opportunity not to be missed for contacts between the leading players in the complex developments involving University College, its Hospital and Medical School, members of the Athlone Committee – and Robert Leiper, playing for high stakes with regard to the future of the LSTM. For there can be little doubt that ever since the early contacts over the hookworm campaign in 1913, Leiper had nurtured hopes of involving the Rockefeller Foundation and the IHB in wider, but initially very tentative, plans for expansion of the modest LSTM and its research activities. His firmness of purpose in his correspondence with Michelli of the Seamen's Hospital Society, and with Vincent, Rose and Heiser, was no sudden development.

Leiper's confidence had been strengthened, and his hopes for the future of the School had been given new reality, when at the end of the war the Seamen's Hospital Society received a donation from the British Red Cross, which at the conclusion of hostilities found itself with a healthy surplus of funds. Sir Havelock Charles, Dean of the LSTM 1916–24, had suggested already in July, 1918, well before the armistice, the desirability of moving the School to a more central site in London.[12] Six months later, the war over, the Seamen's Hospital Society formally accepted the suggestion, and the former Endsleigh Palace Hotel at Euston, used as a hospital during the war, was acquired.[13] This was made possible by the Red Cross contribution. The Society noted 'with gratitude' in June, 1919, that the Red Cross was setting aside £15,000 for beds in the Hospital for Tropical Diseases, 'making a total of £45,000 for endowment'. A further £55,000 were earmarked for purchase of buildings, making 'a grand total of £100,000'. Lord Milner, at the Colonial Office, raised another £80,000, and by February, 1920, the former Endsleigh Garden Hotel had been refurbished, and could open as the new LSTM and Hospital for Tropical Diseases.[14] The tall building, still on the corner of what was Endsleigh Gardens and what is still Gordon Street, is now occupied by the University College Students' Union. In 1920, the ground floor housed general offices, the School's Board Room, and general laboratories; on the first floor were the museum and departments of tropical pathology and entomology; on the second floor helminthology and protozoology; on the third floor the Tropical Diseases Bureau; and the upper four floors were given over to the hospital (perhaps not the most practical arrangement), with staff quarters, waiting rooms, and private and general wards on separate floors, topped by operating theatre and dispensary.[15]

Soon after receipt of the Red Cross donation, in August, 1919, Leiper had informed Victor G. Heiser, Director, IHB for the East, of the promising developments. In reply, Heiser wrote of his hopes that ' ... the next step in Great Britain will be the establishment of a great school of hygiene and public health'.[16] This revealing remark accompanied a variety of information on hookworm disease: details of results from California, and experiments by Dr. Stiles with chemical destruction of hookworm larvae in latrines. Heiser also professed himself 'greatly interested' in the question of hookworm infestation in Cornwall mines. He concluded: 'Wickliffe Rose, our General Director, will arrive in London in the latter part of December'. On cue, three days before Christmas, 1919, Rose and Richard M. Pearce, newly appointed Director of the Foundation's Division of Medical Education, arrived in London to explore the possibilities for fulfilling Heiser's pious hopes.[17] Clearly the 'hookworm connection' had lasted far beyond the first friendly contacts and the fact-finding tour in 1913–14.

It was from the time of Rose's Christmas visit in 1919–20 that transatlantic contacts and ties began to grow, and that efforts and initiatives on both sides of the Atlantic began to coalesce. On their return to New York, Rose wrote in his Report of his hopes for future cooperation in the field of public health medicine between the now neighbouring institutions of the LSTM, the University College Medical School, about to adopt the 'unit-plan' for teaching and research, and the Wellcome Bureau of Scientific Research under Andrew Balfour (1873–1931), who three and a half years later, in October, 1923, became Director of the new London School of Hygiene and Tropical Medicine. Noting the close proximity of the three institutions, Rose's Report concluded that the nucleus for a future school of hygiene and public health could be found in the London School of Tropical Medicine and the existing Department of Hygiene at University College.[18]

Surviving correspondence between Leiper and Michelli, and a much later reply from Leiper to an enquiry concerning events during this period, throw some light on the way in which Rose reached these conclusions. Already on January 2nd, 1920, Leiper reported to Michelli, still Secretary to the Seamen's Hospital Society as well as to the LSTM, that he had 'had the privilege' of showing the new premises in Endsleigh Gardens to Rose. Expressing interest in plans for a new enlarged School of Tropical Medicine in central London, Rose invited Leiper to spend Saturday evening with him at the Grosvenor Hotel. During this visit Rose quizzed Leiper about the history and development of the School since its beginnings in 1899, and his own views regarding its future growth. Leiper told Michelli: 'He was very interested in the proposal to re-establish on a better footing the course of Tropical Sanitation'. Rose also enquired about the financial position of the School. Leiper continued:

> 'I gave him the fullest information that I had on the subject, it being understood that the views expressed by me were those held by me personally, and were not for official publication. It was obvious from the intimate cross questioning to which he submitted me that the Health Board desired to have for future reference as much information as could be obtained ... as I am to see Dr.Rose again later, I thought it best to be as helpful as I could without making any enquiries as to the aid that the Rockefeller might ultimately be willing to give us'.[19]

The results of a second meeting with Rose were recalled by Leiper thirty years later, in a reply to an enquiry from R.L.Sheppard, Secretary of the Bureau of Hygiene and Tropical Diseases:

> 'One evening [Rose] invited me to dinner at the Savoy Hotel and afterwards in his private sitting room he told me to relax and 'dream' what I should do if I had unlimited funds! My dream covered only £250,000. The proposal I made was to make an Imperial School of Hygiene ... My proposal was briefly to combine the London School of Tropical Medicine, the Public Health Dept. of University College and the Bacteriological Dept. of King's College in one school. [I dropped a brick as regards Kings College for the Bacteriological Dept. there was a part of the Under-graduate Medical School, whereas the LSTM and Public Health Dept. Univ. College were postgraduate units and the idea of course a postgraduate School ...] In the summer of 1920 (?) the President of the Rockefeller Foundation came to London and at a reception at University College he asked a group of the Professorial Staff, including Elliott, "what they thought of Leiper's idea"! Throughout the informal talks I had kept Dawson Williams

[editor of the *British Medical Journal*] informed ...'.[20]

Leiper's informal information was, at Rose's request, presented as a written proposal in April; Leiper also attempted, but failed, to interest the University Grants Committee (UGC) in support for clinical teaching at the School.[21] Little more happened on an official level for the rest of that year; but right from the beginning of the following year, several events took place which were to be of crucial importance for the IHB's plans for extension of its public health campaign, and for the future of the LSTM.

The Athlone Committee began its deliberations in January, 1921; at the same time, Leiper was busy shaping his plans to fit the Rockefeller outlook, and to narrow the gap between his 'dreams' for an 'Imperial School of Hygiene' on the one hand, and what he knew to be current Rockefeller policy on the other. He submitted informal suggestions to Vincent, who at the time was staying at the Hotel Cecil in London. He wrote of his hopes for ' ... integration of Public Health Studies by the creation in *close proximity* or even *contiguous with the School* and the College [UC] of an *Institute of Hygiene and Parasitology*, with chairs of Public Health Administration, Tropical Sanitation, Helminthology, and Protozoology, *in the first instance'*. [our italics]. Vincent's reply, on Hotel Cecil stationery and dated January 11th, expressed interest and explained that he and Rose would be in London again in June, concluding 'Looking forward to seeing you in June'.[22]

By June, when the Colonial Office Conference convened in London, Leiper was half-way across the world, carrying out an extensive filariasis survey in British Guiana;[23] but in the meantime he had, on his way, seen Rose on several occasions in New York, where he was held up, albeit staying comfortably at the Lotus Club, awaiting passage to Trinidad and Demerara, while one ship was cancelled and another delayed. During this time, he kept in constant contact with Michelli at the Seamen's Hospital Society. Michelli kept Leiper informed of the developments at home; Leiper reciprocated with details of his experiences in New York. He used his time there well, and in several conversations with Rose he had formed 'a very clear idea now of the ground and it is so provoking that I have to go on to British Guiana instead of returning home'.[24] Advising Michelli to work through Patrick Manson and George Newman, he outlined plans for 'a big centre of Hygiene in London which would provide for both the home Public Health and the Tropical'. This, be believed, would interest the Rockefeller Foundation to the extent that they would 'come in and provide not only a home but also adequate means of development for a well considered scheme'. Such a scheme, according to

Leiper, would involve bringing together 'for a joint development of Public Health', Bacteriology (Hewlett) and Hygiene and Sanitation (Simpson), both from King's College; Public Health Administration (Kenwood) from University College; and Parasitology (Leiper, Alcock, and 'Dr. Thomson') from LSTM. These subjects could then 'form a nucleus of an "Imperial Hygiene Institute"', providing instruction and research required for the DPH and the DTM.[25]

Leiper went on to specify the subjects to be covered in such an institution; it was a list which contained elements that would prove prophetic with regard to the concerns of the future LSHTM:

1) Public Health Administration and Law
2) Hygiene and Applied Sanitation
3) Immunology and Bacteriology
4) Dietetics and Deficiency Diseases
5) Industrial Diseases
6) Public Analyst's work, Maternity, Infant Welfare, Applied Biology (Protozoology, Helminthology, Entomology, Phytology).

To this Leiper added the comment that 'Biochemistry and Physiology are dealt with sufficiently in University College and the Medical School, and in the Wellcome Physiology and Chemistry laboratories'. Summing up the impressions gleaned from his conversations with Rose, he concluded his more than five pages of tentative plans by giving the exact dates for Vincent's and Rose's stay in London in late May and early June, adding the pregnant comment:

> 'I think you should indicate briefly to Sir Herbert [Read, who would be at the Colonial Office Conference while Leiper was still away in South America] my view that the Rockefellers are withdrawing from direct part in tropical campaigns and are tending to a policy of doing these through well founded Institutions and that they appear to regard the possibilities of one arising in London and calling for support and encouragement as full of interesting possibilities [sic]'.[26]

On the eve of final departure for South America ten days later, and having had yet another chat with Rose, Leiper wrote again to Michelli, urging action on planning through George Newman, and for the Seamen's Hospital Society to secure vacant property in Endsleigh Gardens for expansion, before the visit of 'the Rockefeller people' in June. Purchase of that particular property fell through;[27] but by the time this became clear, another possible and eminently suitable site was becoming available.

Leiper's proposals were not without their flaws. As he himself was to point out later, the Medical School at King's College was an undergraduate institution, and therefore could not have any place in a postgraduate venture. On the other hand, both Simpson and Hewlett were not just professors there; they had been associated with the LSTM from its very beginnings, lecturing on tropical hygiene and on bacteriology, respectively; Simpson had been building up an expanding course over the years.[28] However, they were both approaching retirement age. Nonetheless, individuals apart, the subjects mentioned by Leiper as constituents of the concerns of the proposed institution, show his awareness of the importance of new disciplines which were only just beginning to emerge, but which were to play fundamental roles in future schemes at the new School, most especially nutrition and industrial (occupational) health. Surprisingly, he did not mention in this connection the MRC, which with its epidemiology and medical statistics was to form a major and integral part, through Greenwood and Bradford Hill, in the work of the London School of Hygiene & Tropical Medicine, and of the growing Public Health movement in the twentieth century, nationally and internationally.

In the end, the structure of the LSHTM was to integrate elements from all three sources: Leiper's ideas, the Athlone Committee's Report, and the conclusions reached by the Colonial Office/Rockefeller Conference in the summer of 1921.

The Report of the Athlone Committee was published at the end of May, 1921. The committee, appointed by Addison in 1921 (p.00), was chaired by the Earl of Athlone (1874–1957), brother of Queen Mary, who had assumed that title in 1917, and who was later (1932–55) to be Chancellor of the University of London. The committee's remit was 'To investigate the needs of medical practitioners and other graduates for further education in medicine in London, and to submit proposals for a practicable scheme for meeting them'. Its recommendations included the establishment of a School of the University of London, attached to a centrally situated hospital and devoted exclusively to postgraduate medical education.[29] It was the latter point which concerned matters so far informally under discussion between Rose, Vincent, and Leiper. The ultimate recommendation of the Athlone Committee read:

An Institute of State Medicine should be established by the

University of London in which instruction should be given in Public Health, Forensic Medicine, industrial Medicine, and in medical ethics and economics.[30]

With regard to the funding of this ambitious scheme, the Committee felt it could and should be supported only through State aid and private endowment, as rate payers must not be expected to contribute to 'a series of institutions of a national character'. As for the proposed Institute, 'We are hopeful that assistance towards its foundation and for its endowment might be forthcoming from funds other than those of the State, ...'. The Senate of the University welcomed the proposals, 'provided the *necessary financial assistance* is forthcoming in respect of capital outlay and annual charges'.[31]

Ten days after the publication of the Athlone Report, the Colonial Office opened their Conference on Tropical Diseases, with invited representatives of the Rockefeller Foundation: George Vincent, Wickliffe Rose, and Victor Heiser.[32] Leiper was not a member of the conference; according to Acheson and Poole 'there was no place at a conference of national policy makers for Professor Leiper ...'. In any case, at the time the conference convened, Leiper was in British Guiana and the Caribbean, engaged in a major survey of filariasis, and other helminthological researches.[33] Throughout this time, he was in contact with the Seamen's Hospital Society, where Michelli kept him informed of developments at home. It is clear from Leiper's letters to Michelli that when passing through New York in March, he was repeatedly in touch with Vincent, and also with Wickliffe Rose, both before and after the June conference. Already in March, 1921, about to leave New York for southern latitudes, Leiper was well aware that to obtain Rockefeller support for Manson's School, it would have to be incorporated in a much broader scheme for an 'Institute of Hygiene' as described above. He was completely *au fait* with prevailing policies at the Rockefeller Foundation, and had adjusted his own plans and suggestions accordingly.

In meetings between June 10th and 17th, the members of the Colonial Office Conference applauded the conclusions of the Athlone Report. Wickliffe Rose warned that research work 'is expensive', and that the war had emphasised more than ever the importance of team-work. Sir William Leishman, with his vast tropical experience, spoke of the importance of using the knowledge accumulated in so many studies for immediate benefit of local inhabitants in areas where epidemics broke out; and Vincent, taking his cue from Leishman's further suggestions, observed that 'fundamentally the problem of public health in the temperate and the tropical zones was one'– a remark which would prove prophetic for the concerns of the future LSHTM.[34]

In their summing up, the Colonial Office team and the American visitors found themselves in perfect agreement in their belief in the importance of a potential 'Central Institute of Hygiene and Public Health in London', closely linked to the London School of Tropical Medicine, which should be expanded to provide additional facilities for training and research, particularly in tropical hygiene. The Rockefeller philosophy was then cautiously explained by Wickliffe Rose:

> ... that he and his colleagues were not in a position to commit the International Health Board, but that they could form an idea as to whether any proposals now put forward would fit in with the general policy of the Board. ... He felt that something in the way of a Central Institution, such as had been mentioned, would be a most useful beginning, and ... would be ... a great dynamo that would vitalize and inspire public health work ... throughout the world ... a centre of public health in London ... would be of inestimable benefit generally.[35]

Following the publication of the Athlone Report and the conclusion of the Colonial Office Conference, with its qualified support from the Rockefeller visitors, Alfred Mond, as the newly appointed successor to Addison as Minister of Health, a month later set up ' ... a Committee under my Chairmanship to draft a provisional scheme for the Institute of State Medicine recommended by the Post-Graduate Medical Committee'. The son of Ludwig Mond, co-founder of Brunner Mond & Co., Alfred Mond combined a life-time as managing director of the firm, which under his leadership became Imperial Chemical Industries (ICI) in 1926, with a political career as Liberal MP (1906–30).[36] After yet another month, of accelerating activity in and out of committee, behind the scenes and in front, Mond sent Vincent a 'provisional memorandum' on the Institute of State Medicine, adding that 'You will notice that we prefer the title "School of Hygiene" but it is of course the institution that matters not the title ... If the Rockefeller Trustees should consider that the scheme is one *prima facie* deserving their support ...'. Fisher has commented that the emphasis on 'School of Hygiene' was meant as a concession to the Rockefeller Foundation's vision of an international school rather than a 'local organisation'; and at the same time, Mond made it clear that it would be wholly impossible for the British Government or the University of London to finance such an institution unaided.[37]

In reply, Vincent wrote Mond a friendly, personal letter, speaking of his gratification to know 'that substantial progress has been made', and that he must await a meeting of his Trustees before any assurances could be given.[38] By the following February, the Rockefeller Trustees had indeed offered the financial support needed, and Vincent and Rose again travelled to London to work out details of a suitable agreement. On March 1st, 1922, George Newman wrote a memorandum to his Minister. It was now headed:

The Rockefeller School of Hygiene

(The Rockefeller Foundation later made it clear that they did not expect, or want, inclusion of their name in any way, official or otherwise). Newman wrote:

> I explained [to Sir James Michelli] briefly the history of the negotiations which had resulted in the Rockefeller offer, and that among the *conditions* which affected it were (a) that the maintenance of the Institution should be found in this country, and (b) that the School should serve as a *Central Institution* with which should be co-ordinated existing Institutions which were doing hygiene work effectively. Among these Institutions I cited the Medical Research Council, the Lister Institute and the Tropical School of Medicine [*sic*].[39]

Newman did not mention the Royal Institute of Public Health, an establishment largely concerned with the training of DPH students which never succeeded in becoming a recognised part of the University of London, although authorised to award the DPH. Its number of students were low, but the Institute resisted any suggestions of cooperation with the developing School.[40]

In addition to the delicate negotiations between the various committees representing the British Government, its Ministry of Health, the University of London, and the Rockefeller Foundation officials, there was also the question of site of the proposed new School. It was by now understood that any arrangements must include provision for the London School of Tropical Medicine, and that the planned complex must be situated within the area also meant for the new buildings proposed for the University of London i.e., Bloomsbury. In the spring of 1921, Leiper and Michelli had fought a losing battle to acquire vacant property in Endsleigh Gardens, near the School buildings, for expansion. Now, a year later, all eyes were on a site on the corner of Gower Street and Keppel Street, owned since 1913 by a committee formed to build a 'Shakespeare Memorial Theatre'.[41] In existence since 1904, and merged in 1908 with the 'National Theatre Committee', its aim was to create a National Theatre, with a resident company, with an endowment sufficiently large to ensure complete integrity in its artistic policy: keeping in its repertory the plays of Shakespeare and other English classics, as well as more recent works, English and foreign. Fund-raising for the rather grandiose scheme was interrupted by the war in 1914; during the war years the site was used for the entertainment of troops in makeshift 'Shakespeare huts' erected by the YMCA. Following the end of the war, the huts were used for the accommodation of Indian students. Throughout 1919, 1920, 1921, and 1922, attempts were made to raise enough funds to make it possible to realise the original plans for the theatre. It became increasingly clear that this was a vain hope. By March, 1923, less than a fifth of the £500,000 needed had been collected, and after some legal wrangles the Executive Committee had little option but to accept the offer from the International Health Board, in the person of Wickliffe Rose during his visit to London in April, 1922, of £52,000 for the site.[42]

The final offer from the Rockefeller Foundation for the site concluded anxious weeks of uncertainty over the willingness and ability of the post-war British Government to meet its required contribution of an annual £25,000 of maintenance expenses.[43] Remaining difficulties regarding the purchase of the Bloomsbury site and other arrangements were ironed out before the end of 1923 in discussions and correspondence between the University, the Ministry of Health, and the Rockefeller Foundation.[44] By January, 1924, the 'Draft of Suggested Charter for School of Hygiene' was complete. It was given final approval by H.M.King George V in Council on April 1st, 1924. The position of the new School as the country's Central School of Public Health and Hygiene was sealed by the Royal Charter's point 1, *viz.* that

> all the persons ... in accordance with this Our Charter ... members of the Board of Management ... shall be one body corporate and politic under the name of the London School of Hygiene and Tropical Medicine for the purpose of promoting the study of and education in *public health, hygiene, State medicine,* and *tropical medicine* in Great Britain, the British Dominions, Colonies and Possessions, and in other countries, having a perpetual succession and a Common Seal ....

Paragraphs 11 and 12 of the document refer to the accountability of the Board of Management to 'Our Treasury' with regard to 'any moneys provided by Parliament'.[45]

With the Charter in place, much remained to be determined concerning the structure, both internal and external, of the new institution. Already six months before the signing of the Charter, Andrew Balfour had been appointed Director of the developing School by the Transitional Executive Committee on October 26th 1923. The close interest shown by the Rockefeller Foundation in the events and documented by a number of telegrams and letters preserved in the Rockefeller Archives has been mentioned at the beginning of this chapter. Immediately after his appointment Balfour left for Bermuda, to undertake a 'sanitary survey' at the request of the Governor, with the sanction of the Colonial Office. Once back in London he faced a daunting task, which he attacked with zest and vigour, but which in the end would break his health. The formal contract between the University of London, the Rockefeller Foundation and the Ministry of Health had been signed on June 25th, 1923; on March 31st, 1925, Andrew Balfour could watch the School's Seal being placed on the document of the Deed of Covenant by which the Foundation transferred the Bloomsbury site to the School, and the following year, the Foundation Stone was laid by Neville Chamberlain (1869–1940). By a neat twist of history this second son of Joseph Chamberlain, who at the Colonial Office had done so much to further the founding of the original School of Tropical Medicine, was by now Minister of Health. The appointment of the Director was one thing; but the choice of members of the governing body was the responsibility of the ministry of Health, and was not unanimously welcomed. An editorial in the journal *Public Health* aired the pique and bitterness of the Society of Medical Officers: 'As the representative body of the Public Health Service the Society of Medical Officers had expected that it would be their privilege to have a *real share* in the management of a School in which they would have a more direct interest than any other section of the community. ... their claims to representation on the Board of Management of the School were ignored by the Ministry of Health, and they were offered only a single seat on the Court of Governors, *a decorative body* of thirty-four persons who will probably meet once a year to applaud the decisions of the Board of Management. ....On these grounds the Society asked to be excused from making a nomination to the Court of Governors. ...'.[46]

Physically, the School was built over a period of three years between July, 1926, and July, 1929. The office of P.Morley Horder and Verner O.Rees, in St.James's, won a 'limited competition' among architectural firms selected for their experience in laboratory design.[47] The plans were the work of the junior partner, Verner Rees, who consulted Balfour, and newly appointed staff members, in order to make those plans fit the requirements of the teaching and research scheduled to take place there once the building was finished. Bradford Hill later recalled that the architect took particular pride in the main library, which ' ... would be the showpiece of the School and suitable for functions, receptions, and the like [the main reading room is still occasionally used for such purposes]. This would entail slightly less space for the books to which Major Greenwood said 'perhaps we could keep all the books elsewhere?' – which must have endeared him to the architect. The Rockefeller Foundation officials, who had so generously contributed to realisation of the project, never made their influence felt during this period. They watched the progress of the building works whenever they were in London, but only as disinterested observers; at no time did they make any suggestions, or in any way try to interfere. Once they had secured the Bloomsbury site, and provided additional means for buildings and equipment with their grant of $2,000,000, and also extracted the promise of future maintenance support from the British Government, they were happy to take a back seat.[48]

PROBLEMS OF SCHOOL AND HOSPITAL

Before plans could be finally put into practice, there remained the question of incorporation of the activities of the School of Tropical Medicine in the overall scheme of development for the new School of Hygiene. Back in January, 1921, Leiper had talked of his 'vision' of an institution to match 'the School at Baltimore on the other side of the world'.[49] Now, with the plans under way, there were problems with the interrelationship of Manson's School and the Hospital for Tropical Diseases, with its separate funds and organisation, administered by the Corporation of the Seamen's Hospital Society. Arthur Robinson, Chairman of the 'Site and Planning Committee', had a number of meetings with Michelli; but the Seamen's Hospital Society was not yet ready to consider outright amalgamation, which would involve geographical separation of the school from the hospital, since the Endsleigh Gardens site was no longer available. Michelli, who personally favoured full cooperation, feared opposition from the hospital's medical staff, and from Read and Manson. Nothing daunted, the Planning Committee provisionally built inclusion of the Tropical School into their contingency plans and financial estimates.[50] On

April 1st, 1922, Manson wrote a friendly, personal letter to Wickliffe Rose, setting out his views of the *pros* and *cons* for amalgamation; the two men had discussed the matter the previous week. Manson appeared to be at last satisfied that the Rockefeller scheme would 'help and not suppress the School or compete with it'. It has been seen as Manson's final blessing for the new School. He died the following week.[51]

Absorption of Manson's School into the new London School of Hygiene and Tropical Medicine officially took place on August 1st 1924.[52] The date marked the end of the long stewardship of the LSTM by the Seamen's Hospital Society, and the physical separation of the Hospital for Tropical Diseases from the School it had given houseroom, and unstinted support, for a quarter of a century. Even then, the change-over was not without its problems. The following year, the Board of the Society, which had initially insisted that the LSHTM Charter must require the School to use material in the hospital for its clinical teaching, was beginning to make difficulties. In the words of Arthur Robinson, 'they are not in fact behaving very well'. They complained that the hospital was 'out of their way', difficult to administer, and too costly for their present funds. In fact, they wanted to pull out of existing arrangements with the School if not before, at least by the time the new buildings were opened.[53]

This prompted the School, supported by the Ministry of Health, to begin looking into possibilities for building a modern hospital, an 'Imperial Hospital for Tropical Diseases' that would meet their clinical needs in a way which the existing one could not. At the Ministry of Health, Neville Chamberlain appointed a committee, chaired by Alfred Mond, to 'consider and report how the necessary clinical and pathological facilities for the study of tropical diseases can best be secured to the London School of Hygiene & Tropical Medicine'.[54] An adequate 'Imperial Hospital' would be expensive; funds were to be sought from the Rockefeller Foundation and the British Red Cross. Negotiations were begun with the Bedford Estate concerning purchase of an additional site in Malet Street. Throughout 1926–7 the negotiations went on, to find the money, to secure a site, and also to gauge the climate of opinion among the main London hospitals who had themselves an interest in tropical diseases. Their responses were on the whole discouraging, some even reflecting arguments used against Manson's ideas for his original School in 1898: a central hospital might deprive other medical schools of interesting cases and valuable teaching material. Asked for their opinions in January, 1927,

St.Thomas's did 'not think it practicable';

Guy's and UCH were 'unable to give a straight yes or no to undertaking to transfer tropical disease cases to a Central Hospital for Tropical Diseases';
Middlesex's answer 'must be in the negative';
only Bart's and the London could 'agree in principle'.[55]

At the beginning of October, 1927, *The Times* carried a critical leader, comparing plans for a new hospital in London unfavourably with the existing Seamen's Hospital Society one, which would be in danger of being 'overshadowed by another institution lacking either its traditions, its voluntary basis, or its strictly national character'. This outburst brought an immediate response from the highest level, in the form of a letter to the Editor from Neville Chamberlain, accompanied by a personal note to Geoffrey Dawson, warning him to exercise 'considerable caution' with respect to information from the Seamen's Hospital Society if indeed that was the 'inspiration for the leader in question'.[56] Shortly afterwards, the ambitious project was shelved indefinitely. The Seamen's Hospital Society had decided after all not to close down Endsleigh Gardens, and plans for purchasing an adjacent hospital site in Bloomsbury were abandoned.[57]

The first Annual Report to the Court of Governors of the London School of Hygiene & Tropical Medicine was published in October, 1925, signed by Alfred Mond as Chairman of the Board, and by R.W.Harris as Secretary of the new School.[58] It was a workmanlike report, concerned with the practical details of creating the framework for an institution on a scale and of a character not before seen in Britain (although to describe it, as one recent historian has chosen to do, as 'ostentatious' seems a curious misuse of the English language).[59] The purposes of various committees appointed to oversee developments are self-explanatory: there was a Finance Committee, an Education Committee, and a Building Committee, all accountable to the Board of Management. The architects invited to submit designs for the new buildings in the autumn of 1924 were eventually given a deadline of the end of April, 1925; they were also reminded that the proximity of the site to the British Museum should be kept in mind when designing the façade of the building, a fact which may also have influenced the authorities when they adopted the image of an ancient Sicilian coin, believed to have been struck in celebration of deliverance from pestilence, as the Seal of the School. This first report is not surprisingly much occupied with details of arrangements for the building, the choice of architects, engineering services, surveyors, etc., and financial problems – the sterling value of the Rockefeller grant had to be adjusted, as sterling had been rising steadily against the dollar since the grant was originally made in February, 1922.[60]

While the Building Committee was dealing with the myriad practical problems, the Education Committee and the Director, Andrew Balfour, were occupied with the organisation of teaching and research in the developing institution. When appointed Director of the IHB in 1913, Wickliffe Rose had begun with a fact-finding tour in Britain and British colonies and possessions. Now Balfour, who officially took up his duties on January 1st, 1924, reversed the process, beginning with a tour of the North American continent. From January 4th to 7th he was in New York as guest of the Rockefeller Foundation.[61] Vincent and Russell, who had taken over as Director of the IHB in 1923, took great pains to show him everything they thought would be of use to the LSHTM, asking his advice on the contents of malaria films for 'teaching and propaganda purposes', copies of which were later presented to the School. A high point of the visit was a tour of the Rockefeller Institute for Medical Research with Simon Flexner and his staff. It continued at a rapid pace; before Balfour left on his return journey to Southampton from New York on February 2nd, he had inspected the quarantine service on Ellis Island, and visited vaccine institutes, research laboratories, and State Health Boards in Boston, Toronto, Montreal, and Washington. Perhaps most important of all was his last port of call, to Baltimore and the Johns Hopkins School of Hygiene and Public Health, the institution Leiper had hoped for London to match as long ago as January, 1921. Balfour returned home with much valuable information on the twin subjects of the School coming into existence under his direction: tropical medicine and public health.

Until 1927, only what was now styled the 'Tropical Division' was a working part of the LSHTM. In this first report of his, Balfour described the activities and negotiations which during 1924–5 helped to ease the LSTM into its new identity as the Tropical Division of the LSHTM. He noted with some satisfaction that student attendance was at an all-time record high, that 68 out of 115 students had obtained the DTM&H, and four out of six examined had gained the MD(London) in Tropical Medicine. The research work in the four departments making up the Tropical Division (Entomology, Protozoology, Helminthology, and Pathology and Bacteriology) under Leiper was published in a total of 32 papers; the Director himself listed 11 publications; and the clinical papers amounted to a total of eleven, several 'in the press'.[62]

The 1924–5 Report also contains a short paragraph stating that it 'is not intended to deal here with the work of the Institute of Agricultural Pathology, which forms part of the Helminthological Department, for it is concerned with home conditions. ...'. This might seem a rather ungracious way of introducing what became the School's first field station on home ground; amends were made in the following year's Report:

> As explained in last year's report, the Institute of Agricultural Parasitology, with headquarters at Winches Farm, on the outskirts of St.Albans, though it is under Professor Leiper's guidance, is only concerned indirectly with the work of the Tropical Division of the School. At the same time, experience is showing that this important Institute deals with matters which have a distinct bearing on tropical pathology, especially tropical comparative pathology. Hence there need be no apology for the addition of a note stating that excellent progress has been made in equipping the abovementioned farm as a field station, where work is already carried out on problems affecting the health of domesticated animals and of economic plants. Further reference will be made to this work under the heading "Research", but it may be said that the School had benefited by the generous gift of the Ministry of Agriculture, and that the future of the Institute seems assured.[63]

The Institute of Agricultural Pathology was another example of Robert T.Leiper's talent for innovation and organisation, and his eye for research areas in need of development. In 1921, at the height of his activities to secure development for Manson's School, at the same time as carrying out helminthological surveys in far-flung corners of the world, he had also found the time to begin to turn his attention to the effects of parasites in farm animals. An early interest in zoology had developed into a talent for experimental physiology and discovery of animal parasites while still an undergraduate medical student at Glasgow.[64] By 1924, Ministry of Agriculture grants made it possible for Leiper to acquire a field station on the site of Winches Farm at St.Albans. It eventually became an integral part of the School, and its specialist research and advanced teaching will be discussed in a subsequent chapter.

By the time the 3rd Annual Report to the Second Court of Governors (largely identical with the preceding First Court) appeared at the end of September, 1927, the future structure of the School was becoming clear. Administratively, teaching and research would be grouped in six 'Divisions'. The 'Tropical Division' now spawned two new Divisions: 'Tropical Medicine and Hygiene' under Balfour, and 'Medical Zoology' under Leiper, which comprised departments of Entomology (P.A.Buxton), Protozoology (J.G.Thomson), and, of course,

Leiper's Helminthology. This was little more than reorganisation of the LSTM's parasitology and tropical hygiene. A radical new departure came with two Divisions added in October, 1927. A Division of Bacteriology and Immunology presided over by W.W.C.Topley in a University of London Chair (Faculties of Science and Medicine) became reality on October 1st 1927. It offered a course leading to a Diploma in Bacteriology, open to graduates in medicine, science or pharmacy, and others deemed to be equally qualified. Housed in temporary accommodation, the Division was nevertheless able to report a successful conclusion to its first year's work when all five students taking the examination gained the Diploma in Bacteriology. Also in October, 1927, advanced courses began in Epidemiology and Vital Statistics, the third Division to be recognised in the University Faculties of Science and Medicine. These courses were initially given at the National Institute of Medical Research (NIMR) in Hampstead, courtesy of the MRC. It was an arrangement which allowed Major Greenwood, appointed to the University Chair of Epidemiology and Vital Statistics from October 1st, 1927, to continue, with his staff, the ongoing work for the MRC and Ministry of Health.[65] Thus by the end of the academic year in July, 1927, three of the planned six Divisions were working, although in temporary accommodation. As for the fourth Division, of Public Health, the long search was on for a Professor to occupy the proposed University Chair to be established 'in the great group of subjects comprising the Principles and Practice of Preventive Medicine ... and General Sanitation and Public Health Administration. The proper organisation of this important Division will take considerable time and involve consultation with Local Authorities and other bodies, e.g. in regard to the outdoor courses of study for prospective Medical Officers of Health'.[66] The first step would be the appointment of a Professor-designate, to begin helping with the organisation of the Division of Public Health. The search for a professor ended with the appointment of William Wilson Jameson (1885–1962), to take up his appointment on January 1st, 1929. In the event, the major part of the organisation and arrangements necessary to put the new Division in working order for the beginning of the academic year of 1929–30, in the new building, fell to Jameson; and with Balfour's health fading, he was soon to have to take over the duties of Dean of the LSHTM as well.[67]

The choice of Balfour as Director to oversee the formative years of the LSHTM had been a wise one. He had proved his organising and administrative abilities, first as Director of the Wellcome Tropical Research Laboratories at Khartoum from 1904 to 1913; and subsequently in London as Director of the Wellcome Bureau of Scientific Research from 1913 to 1923. An athletic Scot and outstanding rugby player, from his early youth he drove himself hard in all he undertook; and like Ronald Ross, he also tried his hand a novel writing. Already at Khartoum he had at one point been forced to take a six months' leave of absence when suffering from the kind of nervous exhaustion which would later be exacerbated by his dealings with what Sidney Chave called the 'prima donnas' on the staff of the LSHTM (others have suggested that 'warring generals' might be more appropriate). At the same time he himself was not entirely free from a touch of 'prima donna' attitudes – in Khartoum he had ruled the institution with an iron first, and had conducted an acrimonious dispute with J.B.Christopherson, then Director of medical services for the Sudan Government, over the naming of a parasite. In 1914 he joined up, serving in France and with the RAMC (he had served as a surgeon in Pretoria during the South African War). As a member, and eventually President of, the Medical Advisory Committee to the Mediterranean Expeditionary Force, he perfected his experience of disease control in tropical and sub-tropical conditions on a wider front. In his student years, always eager to improve his knowledge beyond his medical degrees, he had taken the DPH at Cambridge, and later a B.Sc. in Public Health. Long before there had been any plans for a LSHTM, he had accumulated overwhelming credentials for the post of its Director.[68]

Throughout the years of building and organising and coordinating old and new departments, Balfour never spared himself and his physical and nervous energies. Nor did he neglect his writings and other interests; and in the end he had stretched himself beyond the limit. He wrote his last Report, for the year ended July 31st, 1929, in August, 1929. The School had been opened on July 18th by the Prince of Wales, although the new building was not yet entirely complete.[69] This 1928–9 Report notes the acceptance of the recommendations for the public health curriculum by the School Council, and announces the beginning of a 'scheme of study in public health, framed on different lines from any course hitherto in vogue, to come into operation in October'.[70] Very shortly afterwards, Balfour's health broke down irretrievably. Wilson Jameson signed that year's Report as 'Dean (acting in Sir Andrew Balfour's absence)'; and on January 30th, 1931, Andrew Balfour paid the ultimate price for continued overwork, when his frozen body, a sash-cord around the neck, was found in the grounds of the Cassell Hospital in Penshurst, Kent, where he was being treated for clinical depression. As Jameson took over as the first 'Dean' of the new School, and the first in a long line of Deans who did not necessarily have any tropical experience, the *Daily Express* attempted to link Balfour's suicide to the unhappy incident of the death of a technician, who had become infected with yellow fever in the laboratories of the Hospital for Tropical Diseases in Endsleigh Gardens.[71]

NOTES

[1] Third (1926-7) and Fourth (1927-8) *Annual Report to the Court of Governors,* LSHTM.
For the School's position in the general history of health education see: Elizabeth Fee and Roy M.Acheson (eds), *A History of Education in Public Health,* OUP 1991; here the School is consistently described as 'the national school of public health', *ibid., passim.*

[2] Heiser to Russell, 19 Oct.1923; Robinson to Russell, 26 Oct.1923; Russell to Balfour, 26 Oct.1923; Vincent to Balfour, 2 Nov.1923; RFA, LSHTM, 401 Balfour; copies, LSHTM.

[3] Donald Fisher, 'The impact of American foundations on the development of British university education, 1900-39', Ph.D. dissertation, University of California, Berkeley, 1977; *idem,* 'Rockefeller philanthropy and the British Empire: the creation of the London School of Hygiene & Tropical Medicine', *Hist.Educ.,* 1978, *7:*129-43;
idem, 'The Rockefeller Foundation and the development of scientific medicine in Great Britain', *Minerva,* 1978, *16:*20-41; Roy Acheson and Penelope Poole, 'The London School of Hygiene & Tropical Medicine: a child of many parents', *Med.Hist.,* 1991, *35:*385-408.

[4] Leiper correspondence with Michelli, Dawson Williams, Vincent, Heiser, and Rose, LSHTM archives, MSS FA: D1(25-8) and MSS FA: D3(13), etc.

[5] John Ettling, *The germ of laziness. Rockefeller philanthropy and public health in the New South*, Cambridge, Mass., Harvard University Press, 1981, pp.58-72, and 178-86.

[6] Ettling, op.cit., pp.9-21, and 97-8;
Raymond Fosdick, *The story of the Rockefeller Foundation,* London, Odhams, 1952.

[7] cf. Chapter 2 above, pp.14-17.

[8] Quoted by Fisher, op.cit. note 3, from F.Gates, 'Philanthropy and Civilization', 1923, in the Gates Collection in the Rockefeller Archives.

[9] Mond (Minister of Health April, 1921-October, 1922) and Newman were to be powerful influences in developments concerning the future of medical education in general, and the School in particular; D.Fisher, op.cit., note 3.

[10] Fisher, *Minerva* op.cit. note 3, pp.21-2;
G.C.Cook, 'William Osler's fascination with diseases of warm climates', *J.Med.Biogr.,* 1995, *3:*20-9.
M.E.Gibson, 'The Ross/Osler correspondence', *ibid.,* 1993, *i:*117-24.

[11] Fisher, note 10 above, pp.28-32.

[12] SHSMB *15*, pp.437 (12 July, 1918).
[13] SHSMB *16*, pp.33-4 and 46-7 (9 January, 1919).
[14] SHSMB *16*, pp.90-2 (26 June, 1919); and p.161 (12 February, 1920).
[15] 'Tropical medicine in London', *Br.med.J.* 1920, *ii:*789, (20 November, 1920).
[16] Vincent to Leiper, 29 November, 1919, LSHTM, FA: D1 (25).
[17] Fisher, *Hist.Educ.*, op.cit. note 3, p.132.
[18] *ibid.*, p.133.
[19] Leiper to Michelli, 2 January 1920, LSHTM FA: D1 (26).
[20] Leiper to Sheppard, 15 November 1950, LSHTM, no ref.no.
[21] Fisher, *Hist.Educ.* op.cit. note 3;
'Memorandum of a conversation with Dr.Dawson Williams [ed., *BMJ*], Saturday 8 February, 1920, LSHTM FA: D1 (27). The same LSHTM file also contains copy of memorandum to the UGC on new needs of the LSTM, 1920.
[22] Leiper to Vincent, 9 January 1921, and Vincent's reply, 11 January, 1921, LSHTM FA: D1 (25); Acheson and Poole write of the latter '[Vincent's] reply, which was probably in manuscript, has not been preserved' – it is, in fact, in the LSHTM archives.
[23] *Helminthological researches in the Caribbean area. Under the direction of R.T.Leiper,* London School of Tropical Medicine Research Memoir 7, 1924.
[24] Leiper to Michelli, marked <u>Personal</u>, from the Lotus Club, New York 14 March, 1921, p.1, LSHTM FA: D3 (13).
[25] *ibid.*, p.2.
[26] *ibid.*, pp.5-6.
[27] Wickliffe Rose to Michelli, 10 June and 7 July, 1921; Leiper to Michelli ('<u>Purely Personal</u>'), from Vancouver, 16 August and 17 August, 1921, LSHTM FA: D3 (13).
[28] Cf. Chapter 1, p.27 and note 72; for syllabuses compare *prospectus* for 1907 and for 1914.
[29] *Report of the Post-Graduate Medical Committee, May, 1921,* London, HMSO, 1921;
LSHTM MSS FA:D1 (15);
ULSM 20 July 1921, 4662.
[30] *ibid.*, Athlone Report p.26.
[31] *ibid.*, Athlone Report p.24.
[32] *Confidential Summary of Proceedings at a Conference between the Colonial Office and Representatives of the Rockefeller Foundation,* Colonial Office, July, 1921. The Chairman was the Parliamentary Under Secretary of State for the colonies, E.F.L.Wood, and the British members

included Herbert Read and four Fellows of the Royal Society: Rose Bradford, Walter Fletcher, Leishman, and Arthur Shipley.
[33] The survey (note 23 above), first requested by the Governor of British Guiana in 1914 because of the crippling effects of filarial disease in the native population, was conducted by Leiper and John Anderson, Wandsworth Scholar at the LSHTM. Nightly domiciliary visits, necessary for statistical purposes, were carried out by Drs. Chung Un Lee and Mohammed Khalil el Kalik, whose assistance was necessary to make such visits acceptable to the largely Chinese and Mohammedan population.
[34] Colonial Office Conference Summary, note 32 above, 1st meeting, 10th June.
[35] *ibid.*, 3rd meeting, 15th June.
[36] PRO, MH 58/248, July, 1921.
On Alfred Mond and ICI:
W.F.L.Dick, *A hundred years of Alkali in Cheshire,* Birmingham, Imperial Chemical Industries LTD Mond Division, 1973, pp.40-6; and Erik Bergengren, *Alfred Nobel: the man and his work,* London etc., Thomas Nelson and Sons Ltd, 1962.
Alfred Moritz Mond became 1st Lord Melchett in 1928, and a Fellow of the Royal Society in the year of his death, 1930.
[37] PRO, MH58/248, August, 1921;
Fisher, *Hist.Educ.*, 1978, op.cit. note 3, pp.136-7.
[38] Vincent to Mond, 12 November, 1921, PRO, MH58/248.
[39] Memorandum from Sir George Newman, 1 March 1922, PRO. MH58/251 (1).
[40] C.D.L.Lycett, *The Royal Institute of Public Health and Hygiene,* London, The Institute, c1986;
'LSHTM Liaison with Royal Institute of Public Health', PRO, MH58/256.
[41] C.M.Clark and J.M.Mackintosh, *The School and the Site,* LSHTM Memoir 9, London, H.K.Lewis & Co.Ltd., 1954, pp.53-7; Document *re* legal aspects of sale, and role of Charity Commissioners, of the site to the Rockefeller Foundation by the Shakespeare Memorial Trust, filed in the High Court Chancery Division 28th March 1923, 1923 L.No.890, LSHTM archives.
[42] *ibid.*, p.10 of High Court Document.
[43] Fisher, *Hist.Educ.*, 1978, op.cit. note 3, p.138.
[44] ULSM Oct.1922–Sept.1923, ST2/2/39, 119–24; and ULSM Oct.1923–Sept.1924, ST2/2/40.
[45] Published marked <u>Strictly Confidential</u> as Appendix A.C.2 to ULSM Oct.1923–Sept.1924, ST2/2/40, 2766.

⁴⁶ *The School and the Site,* op.cit. note 41, p.57;
Indenture *re* the covenants between the LSHTM and the R.F., witnessed by the Seal of the LSHTM, London, 31 March 1925. File LSHTM 401, RFA, copy LSHTM Archives;
Public Health, 1924–5, *38:*233.
⁴⁷ LSHTM First *Annual Report to the Court of Governors,* 1924–5, pp.5–6; LSHTM archives, D13, D70, D75.
⁴⁸ *The School and the Site,* op.cit. note 41, pp.59–61;
ABH January 1988, p.1.
⁴⁹ Leiper to Vincent, 9 January 1921, p.6, LSHTM FA: D1 (26).
⁵⁰ Newman Memorandum, 1 March 1922, PRO, MH58/251; Fisher, *Hist.Educ.* 1978, op.cit. note 3, p.139.
⁵¹ Manson to Wickliffe Rose, 1st April 1922, LSHTM FA: D1 (26).
⁵² Michelli to Leiper, 24 July, LSHTM FA: D1 (25); *The School and the Site,* op.cit. note.41, p.55.
⁵³ Arthur Robinson to Minister of Health, 2 June 1926, PRO. MH58/243 (1).
For the impact of these decisions and the outcome of the negotiations, as seen from the viewpoint of the clinicians involved in the work of the Hospital for Tropical Diseases, see G.C.Cook, *From the Greenwich Hulks to Old St.Pancras,* London, Athlone Press, 1992.
⁵⁴ Report of Committee, 19 November 1926, PRO MH58/243 (2).
⁵⁵ Report, January 1927, PRO, MH58/243 (3).
⁵⁶ *The Times,* 3 October 1927; Chamberlain to Dawson, PRO, MH58/244.
⁵⁷ *The School and the Site*, op.cit. note 41, Appendix IV, pp.104–5.
⁵⁸ First *Annual Report*, October, 1925.
⁵⁹ M.Worboys, 'Manson, Ross and colonial medical policy: tropical medicine in London and Liverpool, 1899–1914', *in:* R.MacLeod and Milton Lewis (eds), *Disease, Medicine and Empire,* London and New York, Routledge, 1988, p.32.
⁶⁰ 'Seal and Shield of the School' LSHTM FA: D3 (18); *Annual Report,* note 58 above, pp.5–8.
⁶¹ *ibid.,* 'Report of the work of the Tropical Division for the year ended July 31st, 1925'.
⁶² *ibid.,* 'Appendix', pp.14–16.
⁶³ LSHTM *Annual Report,* November 1926, 'Report of the work of the Tropical Division', pp.8–9.
⁶⁴ P.C.C.Garnham, 'Robert Thomson Leiper 1881–1969', *Biogr.Mem.Fellows R.Soc.,* 1970, *16:*385–404, p.386;
R.T.Leiper, 'On an acoelous turbellarian inhabiting the Common heart

urchin', *Nature,* 1902, *66:*641.

[65] LSHTM *Annual Report,* September, 1927, pp.11-12.

[66] *ibid.,* p.12.

[67] By July, 1930, Jameson was 'acting Dean' in Balfour's absence; he became Dean following Balfour's death on 30th January, 1931. LSHTM *Annual Reports* for 1929-30 and 1930-1.

[68] 'Sir Andrew Balfour', *J.Trop.Med.Hyg.,* 1931, *24:*63-4; *Br.med.J.,* 1931, *i:*245-6; *Lancet,* 1931, *i:*325-7;

E.M.Tansey and R.C.E.Milligan, 'The early history of the Wellcome Research Laboratories, 1894-1914', *in: Pill Peddlers: Essays on the history of the pharmaceutical industry,* J.Liebenau, symposium organiser and chairman; G.J.Higby and E.C.Stroud (eds), Madison WIS, *Amer.Institute Hist.Pharmacy,* 1990, pp.91-106;

Sidney Chave, 'The School through fifty years', LSHTM MSS Collection, acc.no.83461, 1976; cf.Chap.10 note 5;

'John Brian Christopherson', *Lancet,* 1955, *ii:*255-6; and *Br.med.J.,* 1955, *ii:*327-8;

W.E.Ormerod, personal communication 1995.

[69] *The School and the Site,* op.cit. note 41, pp.64-5.

[70] *ibid.,* pp.62-3.

[71] Whereas all professional journals treated the cause of Balfour's death with restraint *The Times*, perhaps surprisingly for the time, bluntly reported his fall from a window in the nursing home where he was being treated:

G.C.Cook, 'Fatal yellow fever contracted at the Hospital for Tropical Diseases, London, UK, in 1930', *Trans.R.Soc.Trop.Med.Hyg* 1994, *88:* 712-13, footnote p.713.

4
EPIDEMIOLOGY AND MEDICAL STATISTICS

The simultaneous appointments in October, 1927, of W.W.C. Topley (1886-1944) and Major Greenwood (1880-1949) as professors of, respectively, Bacteriology and Immunology, and Epidemiology and Vital Statistics, marked the beginnings of new appointments and the establishment of new departments, or 'Divisions', in the developing School.[1] It also introduced a new era in epidemiological concepts on two fronts: collaboration between the two new professors and their respective staff members consolidated the subject of experimental epidemiology, initiated by Topley and now given additional substance through Greenwood's mathematical expertise in statistical treatment. At the same time, Greenwood's humanising influence on the cold logic of emerging medical statistics, gradually making the subject acceptable to a reluctant medical profession, also gave it an added dimension and a new direction towards what could be called the third era of epidemiology. To justify this interpretation, it is necessary to consider briefly the progress of the science of epidemiology prior to the 1920s.[2]

The classical epidemiology of the Hippocratic *corpus*, and of Galen and Fracastoro, was developed in the seventeenth and eighteenth centuries with the introduction of Graunt's own numerical analyses of Bills of Mortality, with Sydenham's elaboration on Hippocratic foundations of ideas of 'epidemic constitutions', with Rammazini's treatise on *Diseases of Workers,* and with his and Lancisi's enforced concern with the devastating cattle plagues of the eighteenth century. It was in the nineteenth century that higher mathematics began to contribute to analysis of medical observation, with the work of French mathematicians and physicians. At the same time, in France and in Germany, increasing preoccupation with public health as influenced by social conditions, reflected the political concerns of an age of political upheaval, and of men such as P.C.A. Louis (1787-1872), L.R. Villermé (1782-1863), and Rudolf Virchow (1821-1902). In a Britain enjoying far more political stability than her continental neighbours, the development of nineteenth-century epidemiology was closely connected with the establishment of the office of Registrar – General of Births, Deaths, and Marriages, and the methodology of statistical analysis developed by William Farr (1807-83), Compiler of Abstracts for that Office. By mid-century, London had acquired two societies which were to play influential roles in shaping changing patterns of development in epidemiological studies: 'The Asiatic Cholera Society', which had John Snow (1813–58) among its founder members, and which would soon change its name to the more general sounding 'Epidemiological Society'; and the 'Statistical Society', later the 'Royal Statistical Society', which counted both William Farr and Edwin Chadwick (1800–90) among its members. As the century progressed, members of both societies began to extend their concerns from epidemiological problems in Britain, with indigenous and imported diseases, to similar problems in other parts of the Empire.[3]

Finally, towards the end of the century, the science of epidemiology was radically to change direction under two major influences. The germ theory developed, in the capable hands of Louis Pasteur (1822–95), Robert Koch (1843–1910), and their disciples, into a broadly based, scientific bacteriology, and furthermore did so in parallel with matching developments in biometrics, the branch of statistics concerned with biological variation and inheritance, pioneered in Britain by Francis Galton (1822–1911) and Karl Pearson (1857–1936).

As Paul Fine has pointed out, the epidemiology inspired by the results of the founders of bacteriology in the later nineteenth century, was firmly rooted in a practical approach to control of specific diseases caused by specific agents. The 'pure theorists' could begin to function only when interest shifted from the hectic pursuit of individual disease agents of early bacteriology to a more global approach, allowing analysis of information gathered on a broad basis, and concerning disease patterns in relation to 'time, space and populations'.[4] He singled out three British 'theorists', who bridged the gap between the era of 'bacteriological' epidemiology and that of the more comprehensive, later twentieth century, epidemiology concerned with chronic as well as acute infectious diseases, and environmental causes.

In chronological order of their influential papers, William Heaton Hamer (1862–1936) was the first. Hamer was a London physician who, having gained his M.D. at St.Bartholomew's Hospital Medical School in 1890, joined the medical service of the London County Council two years later. He eventually became its Medical Officer of Health and School Medical Officer. In 1906, in the Milroy Lectures, he produced a mathematical formula to explain the regularity of recurrence of measles epidemics. Greenwood called these Milroy Lectures ' ... in a sense, [Hamer's] most original contribution to epidemiological science ... a mathematical demonstration of the fact that the main features of the periodicity of measles in London could be referred to the ebbing and flowing of the susceptible population'.[5] Fine suggested that the 'discrete time model' proposed by Hamer clearly expressed 'one of the most important themes in all mathematical epidemiology, the so-called "mass action principle"'. Ronald Ross, who also counted theories of epidemics among his many varied interests, two years later published his version of an algebraic expression for endemic malaria, and proceeded to explore other aspects of the mass action principle, eventually producing a 'theory of happenings' for epidemiological phenomena.[6] Ross's contributions to mathematical epidemiology rivalled in importance his earlier, better known and Manson-inspired, experimental studies on the transmission of the malaria parasite.

The third of the early theorists, and the main object of Fine's study on the impact of early mathematical theory on developing epidemiology, was John Brownlee (1868–1927); and with Brownlee we arrive at a formative influence on Major Greenwood during his years at the MRC which, in the year of Brownlee's death, merged into the long period of his dual responsibilities to the LSHTM and the MRC. Scots born and educated at Glasgow, Brownlee spent two years in Guernsey as Medical Officer of Health before returning to Glasgow and clinical and administrative posts at the Belvedere and Richill Fever Hospitals. During these years he built up a reputation for excellence in statistical epidemiology which led, in 1914, to his appointment as the first Director of the Statistical Department of the newly established Medical Research Committee, which five years later became the Medical Research Council (MRC). Brownlee's statistical epidemiological work was based on attempts to translate Farr's much earlier descriptive technique for mortality curves into a valid theoretical principle for the transmission of infection in epidemics. His ultimate goal, never quite attained, was to interpret the phenomena of life – and of epidemics in particular – in terms of biochemical reactions, described in mathematical language. A year after Brownlee's death, Greenwood published a paper on '"Laws"of mortality from the biological point of view' as an affectionate memorial tribute to Brownlee's work in this area. In this part of his life-work, Greenwood wrote, Brownlee 'approached the problem with an erudition, both biological and mathematical, to which I have no pretensions and, had his power of exposition been equal to his natural sagacity and learning, there would have been small need of any other writer'.[7]

That was Greenwood's mature assessment of Brownlee's work, at the end of their joint endeavours at the MRC. As a young man, Greenwood had been influenced by quite other forces. It was as a pupil of Karl Pearson and of the physiologist Leonard Hill (1866–1952) that he first began to make his very considerable contributions in epidemiology and medical statistics. Pearson was a man driven by an obsession with logic and pure mathematics, with less time for general biological and human aspects. Greenwood on the other hand was to become the humanising influence, who would apply the coldly efficient biometrics he had been taught in a wider clinical and social context, to make the use of statistics in medical science acceptable to the medical profession. Brought up in a family of general practitioners and expected to take over, in due course, the family practice in London's east End, the young Greenwood was rescued from a future which did not appeal to someone of his scholarly bent by this two mentors. The strict discipline of Pearson's 'idolatry of measurement as an end in itself',[8] and the imaginative experimental science carried out in Hill's physiology department at the London Hospital, combined to make him an ideal choice when Charles Martin (probably influenced by Hill) appointed him as the Lister Institute's first professional statistician in 1910.[9]

The 1914-18 war affected the careers, in one way or another, of a whole generation, in all walks of life. Greenwood, in his early thirties, having served in the RAMC from 1915-16, was drafted into the research team of the Health of Munition Workers Committee (HWMC) through Leonard Hill, who was a committee member. The HMWC was a government committee, established to advise on questions of industrial fatigue, hours of work, suitable diets, etc., anything which would boost the efficiency of wartime workers in the munitions industry. From 1918 onwards, the committee's work became the domain of the Industrial Fatigue Research Board (IFRB); work which initiated the modern approach to the epidemiology of occupational health, and which in time was to spawn a separate department, and even a TUC Institute, concerned with such problems at the LSHTM. By the time the HMWC was replaced by the IFRB, Greenwood was working for the Health and Welfare Section of the Ministry of Munitions. When a Ministry of Health was created in 1921, Greenwood became its first senior Statistical Officer. With him, medical, epidemiological statistics arrived at government level in Britain.

Greenwood had left the Lister Institute in 1919, to become officially 'attached' to the MRC's Department of Applied Physiology, whose Director was his old friend and mentor, Leonard Hill, rather than to Brownlee's Statistical Department.[10] It was as representative of the Section of Medical Statistics of the Ministry of Health and of the Committee on Industrial Health Statistics of the MRC that Greenwood entered into collaboration with W.W.C.Topley, then pursuing his pioneering studies in experimental epidemiology, with MRC grants, at the University of Manchester.[11] The MRC Report for 1922-3 stated:

> The important studies in experimental epidemiology to which the Council have for some years given support have been continued by Professor W.W.C.Topley in the Department of Bacteriology and Preventive Medicine in the University of Manchester. The importance of the *statistical aspect* of these investigations is increasing as the experimental data accumulate, and Dr.Major Greenwood and Miss E.M.Newbold are cooperating with Professor Topley from this point of view. ....[12]

In 1925, the MRC's *Annual Report* clarified Greenwood's position *vis à vis* Brownlee:

> Dr.Brownlee of course directly represents the Council's Statistical Department. Dr.Greenwood who, by arrangement with the Ministry of Health, has carried out much of his statistical work as Medical Officer to the Ministry within the National Institute since 1920, represents the Ministry upon the Committee and is Chairman of it. ....[13]

Two years later, Brownlee died;[14] and Greenwood and Topley became colleagues at the LSHTM as professors of, respectively, Epidemiology and Vital Statistics, and Bacteriology and Immunology. In these positions, they were to continue their collaborations in the subject which so eminently combined the research interests of their two 'Divisions', and their continued loyalties to the MRC: experimental epidemiology. In a special report published in 1936 they acknowledged that 'The cost of these necessarily prolonged investigations has been provided during a period of eighteen years by the Medical Research Council ... '. Five years earlier, Greenwood had explained his approach to this version of epidemiology in the Herter Lectures, on which he subsequently based his textbook *Epidemics and crowd-diseases*. Dedicated to the 'Tea Club' of the Division of Epidemiology and Vital Statistics, the text also contains the key to growing acceptance in work on experimental epidemiology of random use of 'herd disease' and 'crowd disease' in man and in animals.[15]

Greenwood's work at the MRC and the Ministry of Health would prove to have been perfect preparation for the post as head of the Division of Epidemiology and Vital Statistics when he was appointed in 1927. The Division was an essential cog in the wheel of the developing School; but with another two years of building works still to be completed, there was as yet no permanent home for the Division on the Bloomsbury Site. The MRC came to the rescue with extended hospitality; and while Bacteriology struggled in the unlikely surroundings of the Institute of Historical Research in Gordon Square, the Division of Epidemiology and Vital Statistics of the LSHTM began work in temporary accommodation at the MRC's National Institute for Medical Research in Hampstead. Here Greenwood and his staff, most of whom followed him to the School as full or part-time Assistants, could continue work in familiar surroundings; and of course Topley's experimental work moved with him from Manchester to London. By this time, singly and collectively, Topley in Bacteriology and Greenwood in Epidemiology and Statistics, had more than established their claims to be regarded as outstanding representatives of their respective fields, and eminently suited to lead their new departments at the School.[16]

The indivisibility of work in statistical epidemiology at the new School and for the MRC was made plain in Greenwood's first report in his new position, for the academic year 1927–8. He wrote:

> Having regard to the very close association between the Staff of the Division and that of the Medical Research Council's Statistical service, it is neither possible nor desirable to attempt to distinguish between work which is wholly school work and investigations originally set on foot either by the Ministry of Health or the Medical Research Council. The whole of the workers have shared in all the activities of the Division.[17]

Teaching of course was another matter. In that first year, three courses were given, each of three months' duration, as had been usual in other subjects in the old tropical school. The total number of students was seven, all medical graduates. With seven distributed between three courses, they must have enjoyed a high degree of individual attention during their twenty-five lectures and ninety-eight hours of practical work. Seminars with discussions were an integral part of the courses, and the year's work was regarded as a success, although Greenwood felt that adjustments might have to be made in 'framing the regular curriculum'.[18] The only full-time appointment made, in addition to Greenwood himself, in that first year was of Miss H.M.Woods, who had been his assistant at the MRC; to her fell the burden of running the practical classes. Although the number of students was small, setting up such classes for the first time must have required considerable courage and ability on the part of Miss Woods, hitherto engaged exclusively on statistical analyses.

Research was not neglected in the new Division, as witnessed by the number of papers published during the year, which covered a wide range of subjects. An extensive report was being prepared on data collection over a period of nearly twenty-five years and relating to cases of Scarlet Fever and of Diphtheria admitted to the Eastern Fever Hospital. Another protracted investigation in hand was a statistical analysis of anthropometric data concerning 12,000 elementary school children from various parts of England and Wales, a major undertaking planned under the direction of a 'strong committee' presided over by George Newman.[19] In addition to the continuing collaboration on experimental epidemiology, the Division had also been concerned with Greenwood's erstwhile interest in infant and puerperal mortality; and among other responsibilities remained weekly reporting of notifiable diseases to the Ministry of Health. New names appeared as 'teaching assistants' at the beginning of the Division's life: Miss E.M.Newbold, Dr.P.McKinlay, and Dr A.B.Hill. They were to play their parts in the work of the School, none more so than Bradford Hill, the son of Greenwood's mentor, Leonard Hill. It was a family connection which would be continued through several generations.[20]

The young Austin Bradford Hill (1897–1991) had every intention of following his father into the profession of medicine when in 1915 he was approaching the end of his years at school. He has disarmingly described himself at the time as '...head of the school, captain of football (soccer), in the cricket XI, champion cross country runner – and a prig'.[21] With youthfully romantic ideas of flying for his country, and no desire to be handed white feathers in the streets of London, he enlisted in the Royal Navy Air Service, deferring plans for entering medical school. It would turn out to be a fateful decision. On duty in the Aegean, in 1917, tuberculosis caught up with him. Severely affected, he was invalided home, and not expected to survive, as evidenced by the 100 per cent disability pension he was awarded, and which he proudly collected until the end of his very long life. For two years he was confined to bed. Then, slowly recovering in spite of all the odds, but still unfit for medical studies, he used his convalescence to obtain an external degree in economics at the University of London. Although he later claimed to have forgotten most of this,[22] Major Greenwood considered it a good enough qualification for work in statistics, and arranged with Walter Fletcher for an MRC grant for an inquiry into 'internal migration' from rural villages in Essex into the towns.[23] From such humble beginnings grew the career of one of the most influential forces to shape medical statistics of chronic non-infectious diseases, and of therapies, and the corollary of clinical trials, in the twentieth century.

The Essex results were analysed at the NIMR in Hampstead in

1923, and Hill's successful report led to an appointment with the IFRB, and a series of investigations regarding occupational diseases in such varied activities as cotton spinning and weaving, printing, and driving of London buses.[24] This early experience was to bear fruit much later when, as Dean of the LSHTM towards the end of his career in the School, Hill played a crucial role in setting up a Rockefeller Unit of Occupational Health at the School. Between 1922 and 1932, he remained an employee of the MRC while working with Greenwood at the LSHTM, until he was appointed reader in the School,[25] cementing the lasting MRC/LSHTM connection. In the School Report for 1928–9, Greenwood wrote:

> During the past academic year the staff of the Division of Epidemiology and Vital Statistics have continued to enjoy the hospitality of the National Institute of Medical Research. From August, 1929, the divisional staff will be the hosts and not the guests of the Medical Research Council's investigators, but there is no doubt that the spirit of co-operation – a co-operation so close that no real distinction can be made between the work of members of the two staffs – will not be weakened by the change of domicile.[26]

In this Report, Greenwood took the opportunity to remark on the end of the 'period of transition', and on the lessons learned by staff during their novel teaching duties. The relatively small numbers of students in the first two years – seven in 1927, and a total of twelve in the second – had allowed staff to find their feet and prepare themselves for handling larger classes in the future. The list of papers published by members and associates of the Division also testified to a successful year. There was just one note of warning in Greenwood's report, one that would be echoed from other departments over the years. Greenwood concluded his report in 1929:

> Having regard to the fact that the School has an international character, there is one result of our experience which is perhaps worth mention. We have found that foreign students often come to us with a knowledge of English quite insufficient to permit them to follow lectures properly. When the students are so few that much individual attention can be given, the difficulty created is not insuperable. But with larger classes it must result in waste of time and money. Insufficient attention seems to be given to this point in the selection of candidates for travelling studentships. On the

other hand, very few English speaking students seem to be able to consult German or French sources of information.

In addition to the 'visiting lecturers' from the staff of the MRC, Greenwood's department acquired a second full-time Assistant Lecturer to join Miss Woods in the academic year 1928-9. He was Mr.P.G.Edge, who seems to have had no statistical qualifications, and it is not clear what his background was. If one can rely on Bradford Hill's late recollections, occasionally bordering on the frivolous, he was 'probably another of Greenwoods relations'.[27] In any case, Edge (in subsequent reports, he is styled 'Major Edge', a military title and not a given name as was the case with Major Greenwood) soon picked up the tools of his trade, and in addition to teaching duties frequently undertook work abroad, performing statistical surveys and advising on census taking.[28] He retired in 1945, and died in 1976. The dual staff arrangement continued successfully until Greenwood's retirement at the end of World War II. On that occasion he wrote of the School's 'heavy debt of gratitude to the Medical Research Council. Without the Council's unfailing support, we could have done but little.'[29]

With this final cordial acknowledgement to his staff, to the School, and to the MRC, Greenwood put the seal on what had not always been easy relations. There had been controversies, and Greenwood was not the man to mince words in difficult situations. Ever since he had first accepted C.J.Martin's offer of the appointment as 'Statistician or Medical Statistician' at the Lister Institute, in October, 1909, at a salary of £400 per annum,[30] he had written spirited letters on matters deserving consideration. In 1914, Greenwood joined with enthusiasm in the not entirely amiable discussions when the Governing Body of the Lister Institute approached the newly established Medical Research Committee[31] offering, 'under certain conditions', to hand over the Institute with a view to giving it to the Nation as a 'Central Institute under the control of the Committee'.[32] The arrangement would have involved disposal of the Committee's Mt.Vernon Hospital buildings and site, already acquired and in the first stages of development into a National Institute for Medical Research. Negotiations concerning amalgamation took place throughout the early summer of 1914, and included consideration of an offer, made on May 18th, by Lord Iveagh, already the principal benefactor of the Lister Institute, to build a 50-bed Research Hospital adjoining the Institute. But this was 1914, and by August Europe was at war. In November amalgamation talks were suspended, never to be resumed. Surviving correspondence between Charles Martin and J.Luard Pattison

(Director, and Hon. Treasurer, respectively, of the Lister Institute), and referring to the conflicting views of Bradford Rose, Roscoe, Osler, and Leishman, suggests that the chances of success were never very high.[33] Major Greenwood also had his say in the matter. Writing to Martin he put forward several pages of criticism of the proposals, and incidentally of the Institute which had launched him in his career by initiating a department of medical statistics. His rather rambling comments culminated in a conclusion which certainly did not anticipate the dual role which, in the following decade, the LSHTM, a School of the University of London, and the MRC's National Institute for Medical Research, would play in furthering developments in medical statistics under his own leadership. He wrote:

> These are the broad considerations which incline me to think that if the Lister Institute is to be merged it should be merged in the *university* and *not in the National Institute*. Such a step would enlarge our possibilities for good without destroying our peculiar virtues; the risk of hardening into a sort of *scientific Harrods Stores* with a large output of second rate work, a big animal with a small soul, would be minimised.[34]

The ten-year period from the opening of the new buildings in Keppel Street in 1929, to the outbreak of war in 1939, was one of steady development of teaching and research in epidemiology as in all other departments of the School. Student numbers continued to rise. Basic epidemiology was taught as part of other courses: the D.P.H. class; the Tropical Hygiene class; the Industrial Psychology class (Millais Culpin from the I.H.R.B. joined the School as lecturer in 1929); students from University College. Advanced courses were taught for students specialising in epidemiology.[35]

From the academic year 1935–6, there was a change in the system of teaching. Until then, emphasis had been on a heavy schedule of lectures, in the absence of modern textbooks. Now several such texts were available, and the courses were reorganised to increase the time spent in seminars, with opportunities for informal discussion, while reducing the number of formal lectures. Postgraduate students could now benefit from reading textbooks for themselves, and the courses were adjusted accordingly.[36]

On the research front, statistical analyses of data from home and abroad were prominent. P.G. Edge continued and extended his work on medical-statistical reports coming in from tropical areas, useful reference points for teaching in the tropical hygiene classes. Others were at work on statistical aspects of such varied subjects as experimental carcinogenesis, school epidemics, measles prophylaxis, and diabetes mortality data. Bradford Hill, appointed Reader in the School in 1933, worked in the mid-1930s on mortality rates from tuberculosis in young adults; English rates compared unfavourably with those on the European continent, where BCG-vaccines were widely used. As a survivor of the disease, Bradford Hill must have felt a particular interest in this subject.

As the decade was drawing to its close, the threat of war loomed large in Europe. When the threat became reality on the eve of the autumn term in 1939, all regular teaching was suspended. Instead, short intensive courses in tropical medicine and hygiene were given for those about to depart for service in tropical areas. Throughout World War II more than 2,000 men and women attended such short courses. Two courses of a fortnight each were specially arranged for sixty RAMC officers about to leave for Africa and the Near East.

One student who was later to leave his mark on epidemiology has left a record of attendance at a course on 'diseases in other parts of the world' after volunteering for service overseas in the early days of World War II. A.L.Cochrane's (1909–88) course was completed the night the first bombs fell on London; he then saw action as medical officer in Egypt and Crete, and subsequently spent four years in German POW camps. After a short period of rehabilitation at the end of the war, he returned to the LSHTM, the recipient of one of the first Rockefeller sponsored fellowships in preventive medicine. It began with the DPH course at the School during the academic year 1946–7, where he was taught medical statistics by Bradford Hill and the newly arrived Donald Reid, followed by a year's training in the United States. For Cochrane it was a valuable introduction for his later life's work with the MRC's Pneumoconiosis Research Unit in Wales. The School Report for 1939–40 began and ended on a sombre note. In his last Report as Dean before leaving for duty as Chief Medical Officer of the Ministry of Health, Wilson Jameson concluded with the understatement: 'The year has been a trying one for everyone.'[37]

The next five years were of course no less trying. Quite apart from personal effects on staff and students, there was extensive bomb damage in the Malet Street wing when the School received a direct hit in May, 1941. None of four people in the building at the time, including Brigadier George Singleton Parkinson, who had succeeded Wilson Jameson as 'Dean of the School for the duration of the war', was hurt; but the Museum and its collections of teaching aids were extensively damaged, as were furniture and contents in the departments housed in the wing affected.[38]

The Epidemiology Division was affected in a different way, when Major Greenwood became involved in internal intrigues concerning the succession to the Deanship. In August, 1943, Brigadier Parkinson (1880–1953) was appointed Director of the Public Health Sub-Commission of the Allied Military Government in North Africa and Italy, and so was obliged to relinquish his position as 'Dean of the School for the duration of the war'. At the end of the month, Major Greenwood wrote a letter to Sir Edward Mellanby (1884–1955), then Secretary to the MRC and a member of the School's Board of Management (1933–52). It was marked '**Confidential**', as are many of Greenwood's surviving letters, for obvious reasons; in it he presented the situation as perceived by him from inside the School, and emphasised the need for an acting dean to take it through until the end, not yet in sight, of the war.[39]

The choice appears to have been between the School's two senior professors: R.T.Leiper, who had worked in Manson's School since 1905, since 1920 as 'University Professor'; and Greenwood, his equally distinguished contemporary, who had been with the School of Hygiene and Tropical Medicine since 1927. They were both strong characters – named by Sidney Chave thirty years later among the 'prima donnas', whose antics had contributed to Balfour's terminal decline;[40] and both held strong personal views on their attitudes to the vacant position. We do not have a corresponding letter from Leiper, but Greenwood's is quite sufficiently revealing. For himself, he was reluctant to add further administrative duties to an already taxing load of statistical wartime work, and would be prepared to do so only until a professor of public health and future dean could be appointed, as soon as possible. Leiper on the other hand – although Greenwood calls his 'communication ... as cryptic as his communications usually are' – insisted on becoming 'not acting dean but unqualified dean', and so would in the event hold office until 1946, when he would retire under the age limit at 65. The situation afforded Greenwood an opportunity for saying a few harsh words about the Committee of Management and the Chairman of the Court of Governors, and the inefficient way the matter was being handled. His final salvo was reserved for Leiper:

> I don't think I am doing Leiper an injustice in saying that (1) he has a lust for power, (2) he never forgets or forgives what he conceives to be a personal injury. He has some obscure quarrel with Topley, he probably despises most of his colleagues and he

neither has nor professes to have any interest whatever in the public health as distinct from the tropical side of the School's work. In spite of all this, I don't believe a man of 62 [Leiper was one year younger than Greenwood] can do much irreparable harm, ...'[41]

Although there is some evidence that relations at the MRC between Mellanby and Greenwood were not always trouble-free,[42] – Greenwood began the above letter: 'You and I, being different human beings, do not agree on everything ...' – and although Leiper in the end may have softened his conditions,[43] the Management Committee appointed Greenwood 'acting dean' at the end of September, 1943.

The longed-for appointment of a Professor of Public Health who would also be Dean was not long in coming. J.M.Mackintosh (1891–1966) took office as professor of Public Health on October 1st, 1944, and as Dean on January 1st, 1945. After little more than a year, Greenwood was freed of the responsibilities of an 'acting dean', with two terms left until his official retirement from the Chair on September 30th, 1945. The succession had been secured with the appointment of Bradford Hill to be effective from October 1st, 1945; but whereas Greenwood retired to become Professor Emeritus of Epidemiology and Vital Statistics, Bradford Hill stepped into a new University Chair of Medical Statistics.[44] What had been the 'Division' of Epidemiology and Vital Statistics since 1927, had become the 'Department' of Epidemiology and Vital Statistics ten years later, following the Board of Management's decision to reorganise the erstwhile 'Divisions' into 'Departments'.[45] In 1945, it emerged as the Department of Medical Statistics, under Professor Bradford Hill. It was a change in name rather than direction or scope, and any semantic confusion was resolved when D.D.Reid (1914–77), a former Squadron-Leader brought into the department as a lecturer by Bradford Hill, was promoted to Reader in Epidemiology and Vital Statistics in 1948; from the following year onwards, the Department was titled 'Medical Statistics and Epidemiology'.[46]

Terminology apart, the change-over in directorship of the department was painless and well-nigh seamless. In his last Report, Greenwood had emphasised the success over nearly twenty years of the close and harmoniously executed cooperation between the department and the MRC's Statistical Committee under his chairmanship. The following year, the Department's Report stated:

It is a matter for much satisfaction that following [Greenwood's] retirement from the Chair of Epidemiology and Vital Statistics this arrangement is being continued, Professor Bradford Hill taking over the direction of the Medical Research Council's unit as well as of the Department of Medical Statistics; the change of title briefly indicates the widening range of work and interests.[47]

This close working relationship, first established in the 1920s, between the Medical Research Council, the Ministry of Health, and the London School of Hygiene & Tropical Medicine, and initially centred on the person of Major Greenwood, meant that the science of epidemiology and medical statistics came to form a framework for new and better informed policy-making in public health. To this end, the working relationship was of course extended in the 1930s in a *rapprochement* with the new Department of Public Health, where Wilson Jameson (1885–1962), the administrator *par excellence,* developed the DPH course until, after the outbreak of war, he was invited in 1940 to become Chief Medical Officer to the Ministry of Health. Here, in addition to wartime responsibilities, his organising skills were to face their sternest test in the role he played in the development of the National Health Service (NHS) between the publication of the White Paper in 1944 and the introduction of the NHS in 1948.[48] It is necessary only to look at the papers published by members of the groups, however affiliated, under Greenwood and Bradford Hill to realise the influence of epidemiological statistics on public health policies between the wars, and after, even well before the pioneering work on smoking and lung cancer had been thought of, much less had begun to influence the lifestyles of nations in the Western world. From early work on industrial fatigue and incidence of tuberculosis in workers, and mortality in infants and young children, to the extended studies in experimental epidemiology and herd immunity with Topley and his team, the statistical analyses carried out by department staff were all complementary to problems in public health.[49]

Instead of listing at length titles of papers published by members of the department and of the MRC Statistical Unit, their wide-ranging concerns can be indicated by the variety of the MRC's Principal Committees and 'Particular Investigations' with which Bradford Hill was involved. They included committees on Industrial Pulmonary Diseases, Occupational Health, Air Hygiene, Social and Environmental Health, Cortisone Treatment of Chronic Rheumatic Diseases, Tuberculosis Chemotherapy Trials and Tuberculosis Vaccines Clinical Trials, Antibiotics Clinical Trials and Clinical Trials of Influenza Vaccine, Tuberculin Sensitivity Surveys, and Whooping Cough Immunisation.[50]

Shortly after taking over as head of the Department of Medical Statistics Bradford Hill, the indefatigable research statistician, was faced with an administrative problem of no mean proportion, and one which aroused all his considerable combativeness. In his own words, 'The foundation of the NHS led to complications of its coordination with the London hospitals' medical schools which were schools within the University.'[51] The LSHTM in particular was affected by the consequent division of departments into 'clinical' and 'pre-clinical'; those whose concerns were perceived as being 'outside medicine' were designated 'non-clinical'. As far as staff members were concerned, the distinctions were related to their pay scales, with medically qualified staff enjoying a higher scale than that applying to colleagues, in identical positions, who had graduated in other disciplines.[52]

Within the LSHTM, this labelling was administered in a way which, even in retrospect, appears to have been somewhat arbitrary, and which was certainly unacceptable to Bradford Hill. Clinical Tropical Medicine was of course unquestionably 'clinical'. The only other department so labelled was that of Public Health whose Professor, James M.Mackintosh (1891–1966) at the time, was also Dean, and so responsible for the decisions made together with the Principal of the University, Douglas W.Logan (1910–87). All other LSHTM departments were 'pre-clinical' - except Medical Statistics, which was regarded by Logan as being the equivalent of the departments of statistics at UCL and the LSE, and hence 'non-clinical'.[53] It was a decision which was intolerable to Bradford Hill; one which would destroy plans for development of the department and the associated MRC Statistical Research Unit. He needed to attract new staff from among physicians and mathematicians alike to take part in the work he planned. In a memorandum to the Dean – J.M.Mackintosh had been succeeded in 1950 by Andrew Topping (1890–1955, full-time Dean 1950-5) – he set out his case and threatened resignation and migration to the MRC if his department was not made 'pre-clinical'. Negotiations with the University had immediate results, and the department became 'pre-clinical', enabling Bradford Hill to assemble and maintain on his staff a felicitous mixture of medically and mathematically trained statisticians, including among others D.D.Reid, MD, Ph.D.; J.Knowelden, MD, DPH; J.O.Irwin, MA, D.Sc., Sc.D.; P.Armitage, Ph.D.; W.R.S.Doll, MD, MRCP; and I.Sutherland, D.Phil.[54]

It was a mixture of minds and talents which had already begun to prove its worth under Greenwood; under the inspired leadership of Bradford Hill, its widening range of concerns in the post-war world strengthened the department's stature and influence in step with its growing contacts abroad. The progress and widening scope were reflected not only in the variety of research projects undertaken by the special cooperative working relationship between the department and the MRC's Statistical Research Unit, but also in the way in which the department adjusted its teaching to changing requirements for new CPH and DPH courses introduced after the war.[55] In the year the department changed its name to 'Medical Statistics and Epidemiology', Bradford Hill emphasised in his annual report that the change in title was a corollary of a growing need to teach medical statistics as an integral part of the rapidly expanding field of epidemiology.[56] Donald Darnley Reid (1914-77), newly appointed University Reader in Epidemiology and Vital Statistics, was responsible for development of new courses along such lines. His course given within the DPH curriculum was designed to be in parallel with the course in medical statistics, thus illustrating the application of those methods, and indeed of scientific ideas generally, to epidemiological investigations.

These adjustments in the teaching within the department were of course only a reflection of developments which had been taking place in its research over the years. Some early studies by Bradford Hill would eventually be seen to belong in a separate category, that of occupational health. In time, occupational health would enjoy, for a period of little more than thirty years, first a Unit, then a Department, of its own, and finally from 1968, a TUC Centenary Institute,[57] all under the direction of Richard Schilling (b.1911-97) until his retirement in 1976. The creation of this department took place, fittingly, in 1956, during the two years when Bradford Hill was 'acting dean' (as Greenwood had been at the end of the war), and then Dean – the School's first Dean with no medical qualification – following the illness and untimely death of Topping.[58] The main developments in statistical, epidemiological research following World War II at the LSHTM took place during Bradford Hill's tenure as head of department, and were to a very great extent inspired by him. But in a wider context, they were also part and parcel of developments and shifts in epidemiological concepts which had been evolving since the early decades of the century, when epidemiologists throughout the Western world painfully realised that the promises of disease control at first thought to be inherent in the new bacteriology were, with a few exceptions, little more than idle hopes. J.E.Gordon has described the changing attitudes during this period as a general need to recognise that

> there is no single cause of mass disease, that causation involves

more than the agent directly giving rise to the process, that cause lies also in the characteristics of the population attacked and in the features of the environment in which both host population and agent find themselves.[59]

Through such reasoning, epidemiologists gradually came to perceive their subject as a kind of medical ecology, and herd (or community) disease as the result of ecological processes. As the century progressed, so did such informed changes in epidemiological outlook, with dramatic and wide-ranging results.

Nor were these isolated developments in Britain; they were part of a pattern, and their main exponents in the United States were associated with precisely those institutions with which the LSHTM was linked through its foundation: Simon Flexner (1863–1946) worked at the Rockefeller Institute for Medical Research, and Wade Hampton Frost (1880–1938) at the Johns Hopkins School of Hygiene and Public Health. Flexner and Frost were both among those who during their distinguished careers moved from single-minded pursuit of infectious agents to a broader view of causes and effects.[60] Bradford Hill, belonging to a younger generation with no preconceptions of the infallibility of bacteriology, was in search of the wider issues from the beginning of his career.

From their vantage points on either side of the Atlantic, Greenwood and Bradford Hill at the LSHTM, and Flexner and Frost in the United States, presided over developing epidemiology during a crucial period. Bradford Hill, by far the youngest of the four, and enjoying exceptional longevity, lived to see the developments coming close to full circle: from the Western world to the tropics, and back to a situation where mass tourism has made most problems universal; and from microbiological epidemiology to chronic disease epidemiology, and on to an era when infectious agents are being incriminated in many chronic diseases. When Greenwood, following World War II, warned of the continuing danger of mass epidemics to society, he was thinking in terms of genetic variability and mutating microorganisms causing new diseases. Present developments have proved him right; what the future holds is now anybody's guess.

The achievements of the Department of Medical Statistics and Epidemiology in the time of Bradford Hill and his dedicated staff were many and varied. They included statistical analyses of BCG vaccination as a controlling factor in tuberculosis, and of the effectiveness of inoculation procedures in the severe polio epidemics in the late 1940s and early 1950s. But the crowning achievements of Bradford Hill's career were the pioneering studies, with Richard Doll, of cause and effect in smoking and lung cancer, and the no less pioneering developments of clinical trials, and of randomisation in controlled clinical trials.[61] The work on smoking and lung cancer is perhaps the better known, having had so profound an effect on not just medical opinion and public health policies, but by extension on voluntary changes in lifestyles by large sections of populations throughout the Western world. On the other hand, it is arguable that at least as many individuals have been, sometimes unwittingly, influenced by clinical trials of new products of the chemical and pharmaceutical industries.

The work on smoking and cancer of the lung went on over a long period, and was meticulously designed and carried out. As early as 1932, questions had been asked in Parliament on this subject. In late November, 1932, when Bills were introduced with such varied contents as Slaughter of Animals, Nightwork in Bakehouses, and Vivisection of Dogs, the Minister of Health, Sir Hilton Young, was replying to questions being asked about incidence of cancer, and an increase in mortality statistics recording numbers of deaths attributed to cancer of the lung. Various tentative explanations were put forward; only towards the end of the discussion did one participant ask 'whether the increase in smoking was not one of the greatest contributory causes, and whether that also would be investigated'. The Minister, ever the cautious politician, replied that he 'would not like to give a definite answer to that question'.[62] It was only after World War II, and indications of a disproportionate rise in lung cancer mortality in women, that Bradford Hill turned his attention to statistical analysis of a possible relationship between smoking and carcinoma of the lung. The work, undertaken in collaboration with Richard Doll, was prompted by an MRC conference in 1947, convened to consider possible reasons for an alarming, overall, recent increase in deaths from lung cancer. Cigarette smoking was only one of a number of possible causes, but it was the one chosen for initial analysis by Hill and Doll, with the result which has become a classic of epidemiological investigation in the 'third age' of epidemiology.[63]

Bradford Hill has himself described the meticulous preparations and execution necessary for this classic of statistical, epidemiological study, the roles played by himself and Richard Doll in the design and implementation of the investigation, the reasons for choosing physicians as a group of subjects most likely to answer questionnaires with interest and reliability.[64] The impact of the study, the first of its kind (its American counterpart followed soon after), was unprecedented in its effects on public health policies and private habits in the second half of the twentieth century. It signalled a change, in this as in other areas of epidemiology, to a more socially conscious orientation, closely linked to the public health movement. In Britain it was reflected in the close interest taken in developments by the Royal College of Physicians, which on the advice of Sir Francis Avery Jones set up a Committee to report on smoking and atmospheric pollution, and by the MRC, which began to revise aspects of scientific policy in line with developments in clinical research. There was also response from the Socialist Medical Association, of which Greenwood had been a founding member in 1930.[65]

If the epic work on smoking and carcinoma of the lung is by now lodged in the public's consciousness as the ultimate exponent of the uses of epidemiology, to the medical community Bradford Hill's greatest contribution is his work on, and proselytising of, randomised controlled clinical trials. The type of trial still in use was introduced in 1946, initially to test the efficacy of newly developed streptomycin, which had been discovered by S.A.Waksman (1888–1973) during the war,[66] in the treatment of pulmonary tuberculosis. The trial was planned by an MRC Committee and designed by Bradford Hill as a member of the Committee.[67] Many years later he described the driving forces behind this first prototype of a controlled trial in the following words:

> ... in the late 1940s streptomycin had been developed in the U.S.A. and there was growing evidence there of its beneficial effects in Tb. Three things made a controlled trial in the U.K. possible. There was (1) myself, the Hon.Director of the S.R.U., longing for an opportunity to put into practice the kind of trial I had discussed in my *Lancet* articles (randomisation was the only missing element in those and you have to teach the clinicians to walk before they can run and I had already used it in the MRC's trial of a whooping cough vaccine, i.e. the preventive field, now for the clinical; (2) there was an M.R.C. Unit of Tuberculosis longing to perform a proper trial in that illness; and (3) *we had no streptomycin* and we had no dollars and the amount we were offered by the Treasury was enough only for, so-to-speak, a handful of patients. In that situation I said it would be unethical *not* to make a randomised C.T.– the first of its kind.[68]

Other Clinical Trials followed, and so did the inevitable discussions on the ethics involved in such trials which continue to this day. Two of Sir Austin's erstwhile close colleagues and collaborators have been and still are in the forefront of such discussions. Fittingly, one is a medical epidemiologist, the background of the other was in pure mathematics. Sir Richard Doll has had this to say on 'informed consent' and on the criteria for discontinuing an ongoing trial:

> So long as physicians limit trials to situations in which they genuinely do not know what is the best way to treat patients, weighing potential risks against benefits, it is, I believe, frequently undesirable to be explicit about the nature of the trial, just as the doctor who is not carrying out a trial is normally not explicit about all the uncertainties associated with the treatment he prescribes.
> ... Sequential analysis, which was introduced into clinical trials by Armitage, often provides a valuable safeguard against the possibility of doing unsuspected harm. ...[69]

Peter Armitage, who succeeded Bradford Hill as Professor of Medical Statistics at the LSHTM before moving on to Oxford as Professor of Biomathematics and then Applied Statistics, wrote at the same time: 'Randomisation is entirely compatible with medical ethics in circumstances when the treatment of choice is not clearly identified.' And again:

> Perceptions of precisely what randomised comparisons would be ethical are likely to vary from one country to another, and will certainly change with the passage of time as more information becomes available.[70]

Dangers inherent in drawing definite conclusions affecting clinical decisions, on the basis of small or even medium sized differences found in randomised trials involving limited numbers of patients, have been emphasised by results over the years; a dilemma addressed by Richard Peto, FRS, in the fourth Bradford Hill Memorial Lecture at the School in April, 1995. Peto is now Professor of Medical Statistics and working closely with Sir Richard Doll at Oxford, where they have followed up the studies on smoking and lung cancer by Doll and Hill from the 1950s, and added similar studies on effects of alcohol consumption in various diseases. In his Bradford Hill Lecture Peto discussed the ultimate validity of the results of randomised clinical trials, and the caution which should be exercised in the use of those results in the design of future policies.

The close relationship between formulation of public health policies and the perception of medical ethics, in this rapidly developing medical specialty, has inherent problems open to public and medical debate. Ethical considerations have naturally influenced clinical decisions for centuries. In earlier times philosophy necessarily played a major role in decision making; in today's intellectual climate, where rapidly accumulating scientific facts serve as guidelines for such decisions, an all important margin of error accentuates the dilemma of taking decisions, which by their very nature can never be anything other than controversial in their ethical content.

When Sir Austin Bradford Hill retired (he was knighted in the same year, 1961), his department underwent another change: his responsibilities were divided. Donald Reid, who had been promoted to Professor of Epidemiology two years before, became Director of the Department of Medical Statistics and Epidemiology, while Peter Armitage succeeded to the Chair of Medical Statistics.[71] At the same time, Richard Doll became Director of the MRC's Statistical Research Unit. With increasing responsibilities in an expanding field, Bradford Hill's multiple research interests and dual positions linking the LSHTM and the MRC's Statistical Unit, had been carved up into three separate positions. It was an indication of approaching expansion and diversification in the subject of epidemiology, within and without the School, which would take place over the next twenty years.

Within the School, it meant a narrowing of gaps, slow at first and accelerating only during the late 1970s and throughout the 1980s; gaps between communicable disease research and chronic disease (this term came to be used for diseases thought to be non-infectious in origin) research on the one hand, and between tropical epidemiology and epidemiology of temperate climes on the other. The first addition to the staff of the department under Reid's directorship was G.A.Rose (1926–93) who, in his own words had come 'to the department rather than the School' since, a Senior Registrar and clinician, he maintained a dual existence with St.Mary's Hospital until 1977. His heart remained always in clinical medicine, and he was acutely aware of 'the danger of being separated from mainstream medicine and clinical skills within an institution such as the LSHTM'.[72] Rose became a Reader – 'part-time'-in 1964, and in 1970 'Visiting Professor of Epidemiology and Preventive Medicine'. His particular contribution was in the development of standardised methods for research into cardiovascular disease; the 'Rose Method' was adopted by the WHO in a standard monograph.

Rose's interests tied in closely with the work of Reid during his most productive years in the 1960s and 1970s, when the department, and MRC working parties, made intensive studies of epidemiological and therapeutic aspects of cardiovascular disease, complementing similar work in the Public Health department.[73]

Chance had influenced Donald Reid's choice of a future career during World War II. Where a previous generation had been marked by experiences in the Great War, Reid's future was shaped when in September 1939, two years out of Medical School at Aberdeen, he was drafted to Bomber Command. His admiration for the courage and resilience displayed by the aircrews, and of their ability to mask the stress of their dangerous missions with their own brand of jocularity and sardonic humour in the face of appalling casualty and mortality rates, determined his choice of post-war career. The medical records he kept during the war demonstrated only too clearly the relationship between psychological effects of operational stress on aircrews, when compared with records of flights and casualties.

Encouraged by Bradford Hill to sharpen his knowledge of statistics, Reid built a career in epidemiology based on this early experience of 'psychiatric epidemiology': his wartime impressions between 1939 and 1945 did for research in psychiatric epidemiology what knowledge gained during the Great War had done for Millais Culpin and Applied Psychology at the School in the 1930s.[74]

Within the Department of Medical Statistics and Epidemiology, after 1961 as Bradford Hill's successor, Reid was occupied with epidemiological analyses of other chronic, non-communicable diseases traditionally of concern to the department: of effects of air pollution on outdoor and factory workers, respectively, beginning with postmen, and of cancer incidence in coking plant workers. Minor epidemiological studies of communicable diseases fitted into the general orientation towards dangers in the work place: of colds among office workers, of attempts to reduce illness among schoolchildren by air disinfection, and of incidence of tuberculosis among workers in medical laboratories. But perhaps Reid will be remembered most of all for his influence at administrative level on School policies and, with Geoffrey Rose, for inspired teaching of hundreds of cardiovascular epidemiologists from more than eighty countries; and for always generous guidance of research students from at home and abroad.[75]

Formal incorporation of tropical epidemiology into the department came about with outside help in 1970. This development was made possible by a contribution from the Wellcome Trust. It was one of several ways in which the School benefited from the legacy of Henry Wellcome (1853–1936), whose institutions at home and abroad had, in the early years of the century, shaped the scientific and administrative outlook of Andrew Balfour.[76] Now more than fifty years later, the department could announce in its annual report:

> Thanks to a generous grant from the Wellcome Trust, a special section[1] [[1]Dr.P.J.S.Hamilton and Dr.R.Keenlyside, ODA Technical Assistant Lecturer] devoted to the application of epidemiological methods in the tropics has been established. ...

It was an event that effectively removed any gap which might still exist between the tropical side of the School and its epidemiology and public health. Patrick Hamilton (1934-88) had served in the RAMC with the Brigade of Gurkhas in Nepal, and lectured at Makerere Medical School in Uganda before coming to the School's epidemiology department in 1967. He had acquired a lasting interest in tropical diseases, which now served him well as the head of what became the School's Tropical Epidemiology Unit. His successes here were rewarded in 1975 with the post of Director of the Caribbean Epidemiology Centre in Trinidad before, in 1982, he returned to the School as Professor and Director of the Department of Community Health in the Division of Community Health, one of the three major Divisions in the 1980s' reorganisation of the LSHTM. His contributions there over the six years left before his too early death, while travelling on behalf of the WHO in West Africa, will be considered in the chapter on Social and Community Medicine.[77]

By the beginning of the 1970s, the department had a total of four professors; in addition to Reid and Armitage, and the still 'visiting' Rose, there was now also a Professor of Medical Demography: William Brass. An Edinburgh graduate in mathematics and natural philosophy, Brass had served the war in the Royal Naval Scientific Service, and lectured in statistics at Aberdeen before coming to the LSHTM as Reader in 1965. In the 1962-3 Report, Reid announced that the department was running, for the first time, a combined course in Epidemiology and Medical Statistics, essentially offering instruction to both the DPH class and the special subject class, plus a short course in Medical Statistics. Now Medical Demography was added under Brass, who eventually also became Director of a new Centre for Population Studies. The new appointments, the new directions taken, all reflected a general move within the School towards greater emphasis on preventive medicine at home and abroad.[78]

At the same time, Gordon Smith's earliest years as Dean also involved negotiations which could have brought more radical changes to the School's structure and future in the long term. In the spring of 1972, the Board of Management's Policy Committee, with the approval of the School Council, authorised the Dean to explore 'the possibility of moving the School to another site'. Initially three sites were being considered: Northwick Park with its Clinical Research Centre; The London Hospital; and The Central Middlesex Hospital. Over the next two years there were regular meetings discussing all available possibilities. By July 1973 the School Council had narrowed the choice of sites and teaching associations to another three: still Northwick Park; the UCH/Royal Free/UCL complex; and the London/Bart's/Queen Mary College complex. An alternative suggestion of amalgamation with the Liverpool School on a 'neutral' site such as Oxford was given little consideration. By the end of 1973 and the beginning of 1974 it was becoming clear that the School Council was in favour of remaining in Keppel Street; and on March 27th the Board of Management approved the School Council's recommendations, resolving that the School should stay on the Keppel Street site and in future work towards closer association with the UCL/UCH/UCHMS/RFHMS complex. It was a decision which caused some staff members, in favour of association with Northwick Park's Clinical Research Centre to resign; but the School has stayed in Keppel Street.[79]

The academic year of 1976–7 brought unforeseen changes in the department. Peter Armitage left for a Chair at Oxford; and sadly, Donald Reid died suddenly in the same year.[80] M.J.R.Healy was appointed to the Chair of Medical Statistics from March 1977; Brass took over as Head of Department; and Geoffrey Rose finally accepted the inevitable and became a full Professor of Epidemiology.[81] These events took place at the end of the first decade of Gordon Smith's long tenure as Dean of the School, and at the time when courses in the department were affected by a change in diploma courses, which became instead courses leading to MSc degrees.[82] Greater changes were to come in the 1980s. At the beginning of that decade, a major reorganisation grouped the existing thirteen departments in three Divisions:

Division I. Medical Statistics and Epidemiology
Division II. Communicable and Tropical Diseases
Division III. Community Health

This reorganisation was put into place with high hopes for the School's future. Unfortunately, it was not a great success in the eyes of some who were then younger staff, and who today, with hindsight, are in a position to evaluate the interdepartmental difficulties which ensued. Within the new system, Epidemiology, Medical Demography, and Medical Statistics each had its own Head of Department. For Epidemiology, Geoffrey Rose continued as head; in Medical Demography, W.Brass continued as Director of the Centre for Population Studies; and Medical Statistics remained under M.J.R.Healy. The Tropical Epidemiology Unit was run jointly with the Department of Tropical Hygiene, under P.G.Smith, who in the penultimate 1990s reorganisation of the School headed one of the four main departments, that of 'Epidemiology and Population Sciences', which in addition to the Centre for Population Studies and the Medical Statistics Unit, comprised no less than five separate Units covering different aspects of epidemiology.[83] The logistics of these new arrangements, with three new Divisions on separate floors, was an unfortunate development which only served to underline a lack of understanding and cooperation between disciplines and departments which should, but did not, collaborate in their common interests within the School and its policies. In the event a situation existed, where staff members from the Division of Medical Statistics and Epidemiology, and those from the Division of Communicable and Tropical Diseases, located on separate floors, were hardly 'on speakers', and certainly never attempted mutual coordination of what should have been common problems.

It can be argued, and is being argued by some of those concerned, who are also gifted with a sense of historical perspective, that the state of non-communication which existed at the time between the 'third floor' and the 'second floor' at the LSHTM, was a reflection of a much wider phenomenon, affecting relations between the disciplines of medical microbiology and epidemiology to the cost of both, not just within the School, but in the country as a whole, for most of the twentieth century. This unfortunate situation, the argument goes, can be traced back over the years to the 'battle of the giants' in the early part of the century: the complete lack of any understanding between Almroth Wright (1861–1947), the autocratic bacteriologist at St.Mary's, preoccupied with vaccine and immunisation work, and champion of Alexander Fleming as the 'onlie begetter' of penicillin, and Karl Pearson (1857–1936), whose forceful cerebral approach to Galton's eugenics and his own biometry left little room for patience with those who held other views. Both were strong characters, and both made enemies. Their mutual dislike was in no way modified when Major Greenwood, a favourite and devoted disciple of Pearson's, and no mean controversialist himself, entered the fray with criticism of Wright's work on anti-typhoid vaccine and immunisation and the so-called 'opsonic index'. The resulting very public controversy developed into a celebrated three-way dispute between clinicians, bacteriologists, and statisticians in Edwardian Britain; a dispute which certainly was to cast long shadows into the future of the disciplines concerned.[84] A similarly unproductive division existed between the disciplines of tropical epidemiology at the Ross Institute under George Macdonald, and parasitology in P.C.C.Garnham's department, in the 1960s (Chapter 11).

On the other hand, the case for the suggested unbroken continuity in poor relations between UK epidemiologists and medical microbiologists for the better part of the twentieth century is not entirely easy to justify with regard to the LSHTM. In its early years, between 1927 and the outbreak of World War II, working relations between Epidemiology and Medical Statistics under Greenwood and Bradford Hill, and Bacteriology under Topley and Wilson, were exemplary, especially in their MRC sponsored collaboration on experimental epidemiology. Only later on in the second half of the century, after the end of World War II, and following the deaths of Topley and of Greenwood, and the departure of Graham Wilson for the Public Health Laboratory Service, did cracks begin to appear in the relationship between the two departments, gradually widening and finally growing to unmanageable proportions in the 1970s and 1980s, when relations deteriorated further by physical separation and unsurmountable personality clashes. Only with the radical reorganisation at the beginning of the 1990s, in the wake of expansion and diversification of both disciplines, have good relations and mutually beneficial cooperation been restored within a network of proliferating and highly specialised 'Units'; units which receive outside support from national and international bodies such as the WHO, the World Bank, ODA, the Save the Children Fund, LEPRA, ILEP, the Commission of the European Communities, the Wellcome Trust, Glaxo Pharmaceuticals, the British Council, the Nuffield Foundation, and many others.[85] These developments in the most recent decades have finally bridged the gap which had existed between research into communicable disease on the one hand, and 'chronic disease' on the other. The situation in the mid-1970s has been described by one observer within the School as a 'sharp division' between departments and individuals: the 'purists' under Donald Reid, focused on chronic disease statistical epidemiology, to the exclusion of communicable diseases; J.N.Morris's Social Disease epidemiology; George Macdonald's school intent on the mathematical background to communicable disease; and Paul Fine's focus on modelling and mathematics.[86] In the 1990s, the new order has changed for the better such isolationist preoccupations, and returned a spirit of interdisciplinary cooperation so badly needed in an era when the global perspective is becoming ever more urgently required, and professors of epidemiology –

of seven different kinds of epidemiology – are distributed among the two departments of, respectively, Epidemiology and Population, and Infectious and Tropical Diseases.

It has also emphasised and enhanced a tradition within the LSHTM which can be traced back to Greenwood, Bradford Hill, and the LSHTM/MRC long lasting collaboration. In the words of Richard Feachem, Dean of the School 1989–95, it is a sense of mutual respect and unqualified cooperation between epidemiologists, of whatever persuasion, whether physicians or mathematicians, regardless of individual epidemiological preference. It was initiated by Greenwood, who forged the link between medicine and statistics and legitimised 'Medical Statistics'; it was developed and consolidated under Austin Bradford Hill, the physician *manqué*, by force of circumstance, who fought the good fight to have his department recognised as 'pre-clinical' rather than 'non-clinical'. In his memoirs, Bradford Hill recalled his astonishment, when lecturing in Australia, to find that ' ... the Australian medicos had no concept of the *statistician being the co-equal of the clinicians* in the trials of treatment or in other ways. I was in the hands of the professors of *statistics*'.[87] To-day, this legacy of mutual trust, respect and cooperation among the practitioners of epidemiology, whatever their backgrounds, within the LSHTM, remains a characteristic not easily obtained elsewhere.

NOTES

¹ LSHTM *Annual Report,* 1926-7, pp.11-12.

² L.Wilkinson, 'Epidemiology' *in: Companion Encyclopedia of the History Medicine,* W.F.Bynum and R.Porter (eds), London, Routledge, 1993, pp 1262-82.

³ Developments in the concerns of the societies are reflected in successive volumes of their respective journals, i.e. *Transactions of the Epidemiological Society,* first published in 1860, and the *Journal of the Statistical Society* (from 1887, of the *Royal Statistical Society),* first published in 1838.

⁴ Paul E.M.Fine, 'John Brownlee and the measurement of infectiousness: an historical study in epidemic theory', *J.R.Statist.Soc.* A, 1979, *142,* part 3:347-62.

⁵ W.H.Hamer, 'Epidemic diseases in England – the evidence of variability and of persistency of type', *Lancet,* 1906, *i:*569-74; 655-62; 733-9;
Major Greenwood, 'Sir William Hamer', *Br.med.J.,* 1936, *ii:*154-5.

⁶ R.Ross, *Report on the prevention of malaria in Mauritius,* London, Waterlow and Sons, 1908;
idem, The prevention of malaria, 2nd ed. with an addendum on the theory of happenings, London, John Murray, 1911.

⁷ M.G., 'John Brownlee', *J.R.Stat.Soc.,* 1927, *90:*405-7; Major Greenwood, '"Laws" of mortality from the biological point of view', *J.Hyg.,* 1928, *28:*267-94, p.267.

⁸ Lancelot Hogben, 'Major Greenwood 1880-1949', *Obit.Not.Fell.R.Soc. 1950-1951, 7:*139-54, p.141;
Autobiographical fragment by Greenwood, c1925, in the archives of the American Philosophical Society Library, 'file Greenwood'. We are grateful to Dr.Eileen Magnello who drew our attention to this document.

⁹ M.Greenwood, 'Statistical investigation of plague in the Punjab', 2nd and 3rd reports, *J.Hyg.,* 1911, *11:*47-61; 62-156; M.Greenwood and F.Wood, 'On changes in the recorded mortality from cancer and their possible interpretation', *Proc.R.Soc.Med.,* 1914, *7:*119-70; Section Epid.and State Med.
M.Greenwood and Frances Wood, 'The relation between cancer and diabetes death-rates', *J.Hyg.,* 1914, *14:*83-118.

¹⁰ MRC *Annual Report* 1919-20, p.20 and p.23.

¹¹ W.W.C.Topley, 'The spread of bacterial infection', *Lancet,* 1919, *ii:*1-5; 45-9; 91-6.

¹² MRC *Annual Report* 1922-3, p.115. [authors' italics].

[13] *ibid.* 1924-5, p.42.
[14] M.G., 'John Brownlee, MD., D.Sc', *J.R.Stat.Soc.*, 1927, *90:*405-7.
[15] M.Greenwood, A.Bradford Hill, W.W.C.Topley, and J.Wilson, 'Experimental epidemiology', MRC *Special Report Series*, No.209, London, HMSO, 1936, Preface;
Major Greenwood, *Epidemiology: historical and experimental,* Oxford University Press, 1932 (Herter Lectures, 1931); *idem, Epidemics and crowd-diseases,* London, Williams and Norgate Ltd, 1935.
[16] Hogben, op.cit. note 8;
M.Greenwood, 'William Whiteman Carlton Topley 1886-1944', *Obit.Not.Fell.R.Soc.*, 1944, *4:*699-711.
[17] LSHTM *Annual Report* 1927-8, p.8.
[18] *ibid.*
[19] *ibid.*
[20] In a memoir handwritten in 1988 towards the end of his life, and addressed to the LSHTM's Librarian, Brian Furner (memoir henceforth referred to as A.B.H.), Bradford Hill noted with satisfaction that Greenwood's grandson was working alongside his own son David at Northwick Park.
[21] A.Bradford Hill, 'A pilot in the first world war', *Br.med.J.*, 1983, *ii:*1947-9.
[22] SPL [Stephen Lock], 'Sir Austin Bradford Hill', *ibid.*, 1991, *i:*1017; Sir Richard Doll, 'Austin Bradford Hill', *Biogr.Mem.Fell.Roy.Soc.*, 1994, *40:*129-40;
L.Wilkinson, 'Sir Austin Bradford Hill: Medical Statistics and the quantitative approach to the prevention of disease', *Addiction,* 1997, *92(6):*657-66.
[23] A.B.Hill 'Internal migration and its effects upon the death-rates: with special reference to the county of Essex', MRC Special Report Series No.95, London, HMSO, 1925; also, A.B.H., p.1 of 'My early career'.
[24] The journal *Statistics in Medicine* celebrated Bradford Hill's 85th birthday in 1982 by publishing a collection of essays by his associates, friends and family, which includes a complete bibliography up to 1982, *Stat.Med.*, 1982, *1* (no.4): 369-75; an updated version is attached to Sir Richard Doll's obituary of Bradford Hill in the same journal, 1993, *12:*795-808.
[25] LSHTM, MSS FA: D3:(17) and FA:D1(16);
A.B.H., 'The start of my career', p.2.
[26] LSHTM *Annual Report* 1928-9, p.10.
[27] A.B.H. (Jan.1988), p.3. and personal communication in the last year of his life (1990). Also on p.3: 'Lewis Faning was MG's cousin or some

[28] e.g., LSHTM *Annual Report* 1994-5, p.19; 1945-6, p.17 and p.34.
[29] LSHTM *Annual Report* 1944-5, p.19;
LSHTM *Annual Report* 1975-6, p.27.
[30] Wellcome Contemporary Medical Archives Centre (CMAC), SA/Lis/H9.1.
[31] 'National Health Insurance. First Annual Report of the Medical Research Committee 1914-15'.
[32] *ibid.*, p.9;
Greenwood's autobiographical fragment, op.cit. note 8, gives an insider's unconstrained view of a battle royal between David Bruce and Charles Martin, and also reveals his own resentment at possible subordination to Brownlee, appointed the Committee's statistician.
[33] CMAC, SA/Lis/H.10/f 7-10 and 25-6, JLP to CJM.
[34] CMAC, SA/Lis/H.10/f.11-24 incl.MG to CJM. [authors' italics].
[35] LSHTM *Annual Reports* for the period 1929-39.
[36] LSHTM *Annual Report* 1935-6, p.41.
[37] LSHTM *Annual Report* 1939-40, p.12 and p.23;
Archibald L.Cochrane with Max Blythe, *One man's medicine, Br.med.J.'s* Memoir Club, 1989, p.46 and p.115.
[38] C.M.Clark and J.M.Mackintosh, *The School and the Site*, LSHTM Memoir No.9. London, H.K.Lewis & Co.Ltd., 1954, pp.80-3 and 88-9.
[39] CMAC pp/MEL/B15/3.
[40] Sidney Chave, 'The School, through fifty years', LSHTM, MSS Collection, acc.No. 83461, 1976, pp.11-13.
[41] CMAC, op.cit. note 39.
[42] A.B.H. (Jan.1988), p.5.
[43] CMAC, pp/MEL/B 15/ 4 and 5.
[44] LSHTM *Annual Report* 1944-5, p.10, and 1945-6, p.11, and pp.32-6; and LSHTM MSS op.cit. note 25.
[45] *ibid.*, p.14.
[46] LSHTM *Annual Report* 1949-50, p.12 and pp.57-61.
[47] LSHTM *Annual Report* 1945-6, pp.32-3.
[48] Neville M.Goodman, *Wilson Jameson, Architect of National Health*, London, Allen and Unwin, 1970.
[49] The School Reports and contemporary MRC Reports show evidence of growing collaboration between the three School departments of Epidemiology, Bacteriology, and Public Health, both internally, and externally with MRC Committees.
[50] MRC *Annual Reports* for the post-war years.

[51] A.B.H. (Jan.1988), p.5.

[52] The advent of this system, a corollary of the disappearance of the privately paid GP within the NHS, has been a source of some discontent in some medical schools ever since. Today a similar controversy has arisen among consultants within the EEC.

[53] A.B.H., op.cit. note 51.

[54] *ibid.*, p.6, and LSHTM *Annual Reports;* Sutherland would eventually move to Cambridge, taking the S.R.U. with him, A.B.H. p.15.

[55] LSHTM *Annual Reports* 1946-7, 1947-8, and 1948-9.

[56] LSHTM *Annual Report* 1949-50, p.57.

[57] Richard Schilling, 'Bradford Hill's contribution to Occupational Health', *Stat.Med.*, 1982, *1:*317-24.

[58] After one year, A.B.H. was promoted to 'Dean' – the first non-medical Dean in the School's history – and offered a permanent Dean-ship if he would resign his Chair. The latter he declined. A.B.H. p.9.

[59] John E.Gordon, 'The twentieth century – yesterday, today, and tomorrow (1920–)', in: F.H.Top (ed), *The history of American epidemiology*, St.Louis, C.V.Mosby Co., 1952, pp.115-16.

[60] K.F.Maxcy, *Papers of Wade Hampton Frost. A contribution to epidemiological method*, New York, The Commonwealth Fund, 1941.

[61] W.W.Holland *et al.*, 'Clinical Trials: some reflections', *Stat.Med.*, 1982, *1:*361-8;
J.L.Fleiss, 'Multicentre Clinical Trials: Bradford Hill's contributions and some subsequent developments', *ibid.*:353-9;
Sir Richard Doll, 'Clinical Trials: retrospect and prospect', *ibid.*: 337-44;
P.Armitage, 'The role of randomization in clinical trials', *ibid.*: 345-52.

[62] *Br.med.J.*, 1932, *ii:*1038.

[63] R.Doll and A.B.Hill, 'Smoking and carcinoma of the lung', Preliminary Report, *ibid.*, 1950, *ii:*739-44;
Milton Terris, 'Epidemiology and the public health movement', *J.Chron.Dis.*, 1986, *39:*953-61.

[64] A.B.H. p.28.

[65] MRC *Annual Reports* 1955-6, pp.5-9; 1957-8, pp.4-5; 1958-9, pp.6-14; 1962-3, pp.21-5;
Terris, op.cit. note 63.

[66] Although the discovery of streptomycin came in the wake of the development of penicillin between 1941 and 1943, Waksman had been searching for 'useful antibiotics' produced by soil microbes for decades. S.A.Waksman, *My life with the microbes,* New York, Simon and Shuster, 1954;
T.L.Sourkes, 'Selman Abraham Waksman', in: *Nobel Prize Winners in*

Medicine and Physiology 1901-1965, London etc., Abelard Schuman, 1967;
Milton Wainwright, 'Streptomycin: discovery and resultant controversy', *Hist.Philos.Life Sci.,* 1991, *13:*97-124.
[67] Marc Daniels and A.Bradford Hill, 'Chemotherapy of pulmonary tuberculosis in young adults. An analysis of the combined results of three Medical Research Council trials', *Br.med.J.,* 1952, *ii:*1162-8.
[68] A.B.H., pp.15-16;
A.B.Hill, 'Medical ethics and controlled trials' (Marc Daniels lecture), *Br.med.J.,* 1963, *i:*1043-9;
A.B.Hill, 'Principles of medical statistics', articles I-XVII, *Lancet,* 1937, *i:* between pages 41 and 1003, January to April;
A.B.Hill, *Principles of Medical Statistics,* 1st edition 1937, and ten subsequent editions; in the year of his death was published a revised 12th edition, prepared with his son: A.B.Hill and I.D.Hill, *Bradford Hill's Principles of Medical Statistics,* London, Edward Arnold, 1991.
[69] R.Doll, op.cit. note 61, pp.342-3.
[70] P.Armitage, op.cit. note 61, p.350.
[71] LSHTM *Annual Report* 1960-1, p.16;
R.Doll *et al.,* 'Mortality in relation to smoking: 40 years' observations on male British doctors' *Br.med.J.,* 1994, *309:*901-11;
R.Doll *et al.,* 'Mortality in relation to consumption of alcohol: 13 years' observations on male British doctors', *ibid.,:* 911-18;
R.Peto, 'Smoking and death: the past 40 years and the next 40', *ibid., :* 937-9
[72] G.A.Rose, personal communication;
D.J.P.Barker, 'G.A.Rose', *Br.med.J.,* 1993, *307:*1418.
[73] 'Bibliography' following Geoffrey Rose, 'Professor D.D.Reid', *J.Epid.Comm.Hlth,* 19, *32:*229-30, 231-4.
[74] *ibid.,* pp.229-30; *Lancet,* 1977, *i:763; Br.med.J.,* 1977, *i:*981. ABH, 'Memoir', January 1988, p.7.
[75] Personal communications, Mrs.Barbara Hunt and other former and present members of the department.
[76] E.M.Tansey and R.C.E.Milligan, 'The early history of the Wellcome Research Laboratories, 1894-1914', *in: Pill Pedlars: Essays on the history of the pharmaceutical industry,* J.Liebenau, symposium organiser and chairman; G.J.Higby and E.C.Stroud (eds), Madison, Wis., American Institute of the History of Pharmacy, 1990, pp.91-106.
[77] Obituaries of P.J.S.Hamilton, *Lancet* 1988, *i:*1469; *Br.med.J. 1988, ii*:550; *Annual Report* 1987-8.
[78] LSHTM *Annual Report* 1975-6, p.24.

[79] Board of Management Minutes 28th June, 1972 to 27th March 1974, including Appendix 4, 18th December, 1973.
School Council Minutes 17th July 1973.
[80] A.B.Hill, 'Obituary of Donald Darnley Reid', *J.R.Stat.Soc.*, Ser.A., 1977, *140*:569–70.
[81] LSHTM *Annual Reports* 1976–7 and 1977–8.
[82] LSHTM *Annual Report* 1979–80, p.47.
[83] LSHTM *Annual Reports* 1980–1; 1983–4; and LSHTM *Research Report,* 1992, 'Department of Epidemiology and Population Sciences', pp.20–46.
[84] Lancelot Hogben, op.cit. note 8, p.141;
J.Rosser Matthews, 'Major Greenwood versus Almroth Wright: contrasting visions of "scientific" medicine in Edwardian Britain', *Bull.Hist.Med.,* 1995, *69*:30–43;
L.Colebrook, 'Almroth Edward Wright 1861–1947', *Obit.Not.Fell.R.Soc.,* 1948–9, *6:*298–314;
G.Udny Yule and L.N.G.Filon, 'Karl Pearson 1857–1936', *ibid.,* 1936–38, *2:*73–110.
[85] LSHTM *Annual Reports* 1990–4.
[86] J.P.Vaughan, personal communication, February, 1991.
[87] A.B.H., p.20. [authors' italics].

5

BACTERIOLOGY AND IMMUNOLOGY, AND THE PUBLIC HEALTH LABORATORY SERVICE

The simultaneous appointments in 1927 of Major Greenwood and W.W.C.Topley to the first of the newly established chairs in the LSHTM[1] guaranteed the continuation of a fruitful partnership begun, as it now was to continue at the School, under the aegis of the MRC. Its subject was experimental epidemiology, and the study had been initiated by Topley, in his post-war quest for new approaches to the problems of epidemics and variations in herd immunity.[2]

THE TOPLEY YEARS

Like many others of his generation, Topley had been profoundly affected by experiences in the Great War. Having graduated B.A. at Cambridge, with a First in the Natural Sciences tripos in 1907, he had become assistant director of the pathology department at St.Thomas' Hospital already the year before he obtained the MB, B.Ch. in 1911. From 1911 to 1922 he was Director of the Institute of Pathology at Charing Cross Hospital, moving in 1922 to the chair of bacteriology in the University of Manchester.[3] Twenty-eight years old in 1914, he spent the early years of the war as a Temporary Captain in the Royal Army Medical Corps, attached to the bacteriological laboratory of the British Military Sanitary Expedition to the Serbian forces. In Kragujevatz in March, 1915, he was called upon to examine specimens from patients during a severe outbreak of typhus. He later wrote: ' ... it was my lot to be witness [to] what was, I suppose, ... one of the most terrible epidemics of recent times'. Returned to his own laboratory in London, the exigencies of war 'kept constantly before us the bacteriological aspects of preventive medicine',[4] and reinforced his resolve to study experimentally the mode of spread of bacterial infections.

The Serbian experience had been for Topley a moment of truth, which turned his thoughts from routine hospital pathology to a resolution to study in depth the circumstances attendant on the spread of epidemics. The 1918–19 influenza pandemic was another strong influence on the thinking of not only Topley, but bacteriologists and epidemiologists everywhere, including Major Greenwood. Topley's study of bacterial infections developed into the initiation and determined pursuit of the discipline of experimental epidemiology, which throughout the 1920s became a focal point for close collaboration between Greenwood and Topley, first at the MRC, and after 1927 at the LSHTM. For right from the beginning, Topley had been acutely aware that his own approach, anchored in the bacteriological hospital laboratory, could hope to advance only in partnership with the recently developed techniques of the biometrically informed epidemiologists. In London, in 1919, he did not have far to look for the expert help he needed. In November, 1918, Major Greenwood, then still at the Lister Institute and the Ministry of Munitions, had published a paper on the 'numerical side of the epidemiology' of recent influenza epidemics. It concluded: 'The recent researches of Sir Ronald Ross and of Dr.Brownlee illustrate the importance of numerical epidemiology, and the final solution of the influenza problem will only be obtained by the harmonious co-operation of epidemiologists and bacteriologists'.[5]

The lasting alliance between Topley and Greenwood, forged in the early days of the post-war MRC, firmly established experimental epidemiology as an essential constituent in the framework of ideas on preventive medicine and public health, which provided the inspiration and the *raison d'être* for the new LSHTM. As already noted in the previous chapter, the MRC sponsored collaboration between Topley and Greenwood, and their respective co-workers, was to last for most of their remaining working lives, both before and after they became colleagues at the LSHTM. Their work also provided inspiration for studies in experimental epidemiology elsewhere. Simon Flexner at the Rockefeller Institute for Medical Research had a flair for carrying on promising lines of research where others had left, and sometimes before they had left. In 1908, Flexner had taken up Landsteiner's research on the transmissibility of the virus of poliomyelitis; in 1920, having been shown the work of Topley and his team on a visit to London, he began a study on the experimental epidemiology of mouse typhoid on his return to New York.[6]

When, in 1927, Topley was appointed to the chair of bacteriology and immunology at the LSHTM, bacteriology as an academic discipline, with its roots in the late nineteenth century, was well established as essential for preventive medicine. In time, after developments during World War II and after, virology was to become a separate discipline in its own right, and immunology took its place as an integral part of work in a number of other departments as well. As a consequence, in the 1970s, restructuring took place, from which the department of bacteriology and immunology emerged as one of 'microbiology'.[7] Immunology on the other hand was in the 1920s without the complexities it later acquired. Concerned largely with host resistance, natural and acquired immunity, vaccines, etc., the subject was as yet innocent of the intricacies and genetic insights to be added in the era of molecular biology.

At the time when Greenwood was still working at the MRC, building his position initially in a half-way house between Leonard Hill's experimental physiology and Brownlee's statistical methodology, and taking on added responsibilities at the new Ministry of Health (cf. Chap.4), Topley held a secure position in hospital pathology. From such different backgrounds they managed an almost seamless collaboration in their work on herd and crowd diseases, as summarised in a Special Report to the MRC in 1936.[8] In such exemplary cooperation between bacteriologists and epidemiologists lies a comment on current fashion for assessing differences in 'research styles' between scientists of different backgrounds and training. In the case of experimental epidemiology, the two disciplines involved came together with no thought of competition or desire to exhibit individual 'styles', but in a deliberate move to integrate their methodological knowledge and pool their intellectual resources in the interests of a common goal. It also showed long-term policies of the MRC at their best, in the continued support of research which could never show immediate results. When Topley died, Greenwood wrote in his obituary of the discipline his friend and collaborator had initiated:

> ... experimental epidemiology is *not* a path of research to be *recommended* to those who *pant for quick and dramatic results*. I am not even sure that the results already attained have been fully applied, for instance in the interpretation and possible control of *epidemics in farm stock*. Had Topley been spared to serve the Agricultural Research Council longer this would have been changed.[9]

Topley had been appointed Secretary to the ARC during the darkest days of World War II, three years before his death. Greenwood professed himself 'surprised' that his colleague should have accepted the appointment which effectively ended 'the studies which for twenty years had been his greatest intellectual interest'; but he reflected that, in view of the fact that 'few of [Topley's] family lived much beyond sixty', he had decided to devote his remaining years to 'encouraging younger men in an administrative post'.[10] He did not survive the strain of his wartime duties.

TEACHING

Between 1927 and 1929, when the new building in Keppel Street finally opened, the Division functioned in borrowed premises at 6 Gordon Square. The house belonged to the University of London, and was otherwise occupied by the Institute of Historical Research. The School Report for 1927-8 called the premises 'rather limited but very suitable and central'. Within these limitations, the number of students accepted for courses was necessarily low; in the first two years a total of nine passed the examination for the Academic Diploma in Bacteriology of the University.[11] Most of the students in the full-time course were attached to the Colonial Medical Service; a couple of Indian students were Rockefeller funded; and others included 'a member of the teaching staff of the Medical School at Cairo, a research worker who is undertaking an investigation into the activated sludge process of sewage disposal, and others who are training for laboratory posts'.[12]

For the first two years, in temporary, limited, accommodation, the teaching activities of the Division were necessarily confined to the full-time course for the University Diploma in Bacteriology. As before and since at the School, it was a postgraduate course. The first syllabus of the 'Advanced Course in Bacteriology and Immunology and their application to Medicine and Hygiene' was issued from 6 Gordon Square in 1927. It contained details of the lectures, tutorials, and practical classes offered in a total of eight subjects:

> General Bacteriology;
> Systematic Bacteriology;
> Immunology;
> Infective Disease, from the bacteriological standpoint;
> Comparative Pathology, from the bacteriological standpoint;
> Mycology, in relation to human and animal disease;
> General bacteriological technique;
> Special bacteriological technique.

The *Syllabus* began:

> This course is intended to provide a training in the principles and practice of bacteriology suitable for those students who desire to qualify themselves for higher teaching and research in bacteriology. ... The entire course lasts for one academic year, and occupies the whole time of the student.[13]

BACTERIOLOGY AND IMMUNOLOGY

The course fee, in 1927-8, was 42 guineas. The Division's contribution to the teaching for the Diploma of Public Health, and of Tropical Medicine and Hygiene was yet to be defined; its final form was under discussion throughout the period leading up to the opening of the new premises in Keppel Street. By the end of July, 1929, the Division was able to announce that ' ... detailed arrangements have now been arrived at, with a view to integrating the bacteriological teaching with that of other Divisions concerned'.[14] By the beginning of term in October, 1929, the new arrangements were in place, and the Division's teaching accommodated both the full-time students for the Academic Diploma, and those working for the integrated diplomas in public health and in tropical medicine and hygiene. A year later, Topley remarked in his report on the 'heavy' load of teaching, a situation aggravated the following year by difficulty in filling a staff vacancy; also, as time went on, it became increasingly obvious that a certain amount of revision was needed in order to improve the effectiveness of teaching in bacteriology for the tropical medicine and hygiene course. With such minor revisions, the teaching arrangements of the Division continued largely unaltered until the outbreak of war in 1939, when the courses for diplomas in public health and in bacteriology were suspended, although the courses in tropical medicine and hygiene were still provided and even improved by the provision of short courses in tropical medicine and parasitology.[15] With Topley's move to the ARC, and his subsequent death in 1944, the war effectively ended his career at the School. His place as Head of Department (the divisions had become departments in 1938) was taken by G.S.Wilson, professor of bacteriology as applied to hygiene since 1930.[16]

Graham Selby Wilson (1895-1987) had been associated with Topley for more than ten years before the move to Keppel Street. But for the 1914-18 war and Topley's influence, he might have become a physiologist instead of an eminent bacteriologist, co-author of that bible of bacteriologists, *Topley and Wilson*,[17] and eventual Director of the Public Health Laboratory Service (PHLS). Wilson had been a student at King's College, London, since 1912. He was influenced there by W.D.Halliburton (1860-1931), a physiologist of distinction, and hence intended to take a degree in physiology. The outbreak of war intervened, and Wilson chose (unlike Bradford Hill) to qualify in medicine as soon as possible by following the clinical course at Charing Cross Hospital Medical School. Here began his long association with Topley, with a research project on typhoid fever.[18] It marked Wilson's conversion from the physiology of Halliburton to the bacteriology of Topley. From 1916 onwards, he rapidly developed into one of the country's foremost exponents of the bacteriology of public health and preventive medicine, equally celebrated throughout a long life for his research work, his administrative abilities at the PHLS, and his contributions to *Topley and Wilson*.

THE PUBLIC HEALTH LABORATORY SERVICE

Public health laboratory services had been in existence in some British cities and counties since the late nineteenth century.[19] The London County Council ran no less than seven group laboratories in addition to the Camberwell laboratory, begun in 1891. London also had private laboratories, and the services of the Lister Institute and the bacteriological laboratories of some of its teaching hospitals. Outside London, at least seven university departments offered bacteriological services; one was in Manchester, where Topley's predecessor, and an early influence on his thinking, Sheridan Delépine (1855–1921), began a profitable public health bacteriological service at the turn of the century. In Liverpool, that indefatigable administrator and innovator, Rubert Boyce, organised public health teaching and bacteriological services in the 'City Laboratory and University School of Hygiene', before becoming involved in the founding of the Liverpool School of Tropical Medicine.[20] There was as yet no central organisation for such services, and practitioners and health authorities alike were charged fees for work requested, except in cases of tuberculosis and venereal disease, for which financial support was available under the National Health Insurance Act of 1911.

In the mid-1930s, fears of another war, with attendant public health problems, were to change official attitudes; for where World War I had struck an ill-prepared nation with little warning, World War II was anything but unexpected. The threat of war was recognised by both the public and the authorities for years before 1939, and attempts to anticipate and, if possible, to some extent deflect potential problems were made. First to be considered was the possibility of bacteriological warfare, drawn to the attention of bacteriologists as early as 1934; the Bacteriological Warfare Subcommittee of the Committee on Imperial Defence was formed in 1936. Although the danger of actual bacteriological warfare was not perceived as acute, the committee did, in response to a memorandum drawn up by Topley, make an important recommendation: the establishment of an emergency public health laboratory service; what Topley himself had termed a 'civilian bacteriological service to operate in time of war'.[21]

Wilson Jameson has been referred to by his biographer as 'Architect of National Health'; if Topley did not live to become the architect of the post-war Public Health Laboratory Service, he certainly played a leading role in establishing its precursor, the wartime Emergency Public Health Laboratory Service (EPHLS). His memorandum to the Bacteriological warfare Subcommittee resulted in the setting up, by the MRC, of yet another committee, the Emergency Bacteriological Services Subcommittee, chaired by Topley.[22] It reported to the Committee of Imperial Defence at the end of June, 1938. Its recommendations ranged from matters of equipment and transport of necessary vaccines and sera to questions of staff. As Sir Robert Williams has pointed out, the main list of senior bacteriologists, all male, was supplemented by a list of 'some well-qualified woman bacteriologists who would be of great assistance in ... relieving a member of the senior staff who had to leave the laboratory while carrying out a field investigation'. Over the intervening more than fifty years, the growth in numbers of women in both junior and senior positions testifies to their ability and suitability in these specialties. Since Sir Joseph Smith's retirement in 1992 (Sir Joseph, who had been Senior Lecturer at the School from 1960 to 1965, became Chairman of its Board of Management in July, 1995, sealing the continuing links between the School and the PHLS), the Director of the PHLS is Dr.Diana Walford, who is also a member of the School's Board of Management, and who took an M.Sc. in Epidemiology at the LSHTM in 1987.[23]

Throughout the summer of 1938, efforts to finalise plans for the provisional service accelerated. The MRC accepted responsibility for administration of the Service, and Mellanby, then Secretary of the MRC, suggested a change of name to the 'Emergency Public Health Laboratory Service' to avoid the use of 'bacteriological', thought to have unfortunate associations with 'bacteriological warfare' in the public mind. The Munich crisis in September, 1938, emphasised the need for full contingency plans; the already existing network of consultation and cooperation to this end between the Ministry of Health, the MRC, the Air Raid Precautions Department of the Home Office, and the Department of Health for Scotland, under the umbrella of the Committee of Imperial Defence, was strengthened, and its activities accelerated.[24]

From October, 1938, until war was declared on September 3rd, 1939, the country existed in what the MRC Report called a 'continuous state of war expectancy' and a greatly 'disturbed political atmosphere', reflected at the MRC in special provisions for the protection of the NIMR and its staff. At the same time, fears were expressed that promising research might be interrupted and derailed in an all-out effort to concentrate on 'subjects of immediate war interest'; although it was remembered that the 1914–18 war had, for all its difficulties and tragedies, inspired remarkable research work within a framework of policies being constructed for the then fledgling Medical Research Committee.[25] In the autumn of 1939, the MRC perceived war as 'in one sense, largely a race between the development of instruments of physical destruction and the advancement of medical knowledge for saving the life of wounded and sick men'.[26] The first step in the race must be the consolidation of the war emergency services so carefully prepared during the mounting anxieties of the past two years. At the MRC and the LSHTM, the Emergency Public Health Laboratory Service (EPHLS) was regarded as of prime importance among their war-time duties.

In the final months leading up to the outbreak of war, Topley had emerged as the natural choice to head the EPHLS; and Graham Wilson had been co-opted to the Service early in July, 1939.[27] Topley, who had worked hard to ensure the appointment of Wilson to join himself at the LSHTM even before his own appointment was made official early in 1927,[28] was now adamant that his friend and co-worker must also play his part in the Service. On the last day of August, 1939, Topley wrote to Wilson, posted to temporary accommodation in Florey's laboratories at Oxford: 'It would in many ways be easier if you and I could arrange the scientific side of the organisation – which really means *you and me in the background in London*, just as Chalmers and Thomson [Landsborough Thomson, Principal Assistant Secretary, MRC] run the administrative and supply side. ...'[29] [our italics]. Five days later, after war had been declared, there was a short, soothing note from Topley: 'If you dislike Hitler as much as I do, don't overdo things. It wont matter if subsidiary labs start a day late, but we simply can't do without you at Oxford. I am going to arrange to move Joyce [Wilson's wife] from Horsham to Oxford ... you *must* have *restful evenings* ...'.[30] Before the end of September there were three more letters, long letters full of details regarding the organisation of personnel and laboratories. Wilson was warned that 'You will need many thicknesses of velvet glove, but I think there will have to be the iron inside it for very occasional use'; but on a positive note, Topley informed Wilson: 'I am delighted that you like the young man Fulton [Forrest Fulton, 1913–71]. I took to him greatly, enthusiasm is a wonderful thing ...'.[31] Two days later, Topley wrote from Keppel Street: 'I think that ... my main job from now on ... will be to smooth the difficulties that are arising everywhere between our laboratories and *existing vested interests* in this neighbourhood. ...'.[32] [our italics]

BACTERIOLOGY AND IMMUNOLOGY

The MRC, charged at the outbreak of war with administration of the EPHLS by the Ministry of Health, had no financial obligations in the running of the Service; all costs of war-time emergency were met by appropriate Government Departments. Hence the Council could concentrate on 'scientific control from the centre',[33] without in any way compromising their research funds. This scientific control rested initially with Topley, as chief adviser in pathology at the Council's London Headquarters. When, in 1941, Topley accepted the Secretaryship of the ARC, his central position at the London headquarters passed to W.M.Scott of the Ministry of Health's Bacteriological Laboratory; but even before Topley's final move, Scott, together with fellow Ministry of Health pathologist Frederick Griffith, was killed by a bomb in their Gower Street laboratory, on the night of 16/17 April.[34] Graham Wilson became Director of the EPHLS and principal adviser. It was the beginning of his twenty-two years of running, with A.Landsborough Thomson [1890–1977] of the MRC, what at the end of the war became the Public Health Laboratory Service.[35] The plans developed during the eighteen month's period leading up to the outbreak of war were then perfected to reveal a Service consisting of a network of laboratories throughout England and Wales. Arrangements in Scotland were developed separately, on the basis of already existing bacteriological facilities in the four university cities, Edinburgh, Glasgow, Dundee, and Aberdeen, and a fifth regional centre at Inverness.[36] When the Service emerged as the peacetime PHLS on October 1st, 1945, it was with Graham Wilson as Director and, in addition to the Central Public Health Laboratory at Colindale, thirty-five 'Constituent Laboratories' throughout England and Wales – arrangements in Scotland remained separate – and ten 'Reference Laboratories', each dealing with separate, specific, problems.[37] The majority of the latter were on the premises of the Central Laboratory at Colindale, and only four were located elsewhere: the Dysentery Reference Laboratory at Oxford; the VD Reference Laboratory at St.Peter's Hospital in London's Whitechapel; and the Mycology and the Leptospirosis Reference Laboratories at the LSHTM.

From October 1st, 1945, Wilson was, in name and in deed, head of the PHLS, the man responsible for the successful planning and execution of the developing, efficient service as laid down in the National Health Service Act, which became law on November 6th, 1946.[38] In spite of Wilson's modest assertion that he quite simply carried out the realisation of plans envisaged by Topley, others saw his contribution as much more important. Sir Robert Williams, with his insider's knowledge gained from service as a member of the staff of the PHLS from 1946 to

1960, and as its Director from 1973 to 1981, wrote that ' ... the Service in its developed state, say in 1960, was undoubtedly Wilson's creation'.[39]

For Wilson himself, it meant a break in his links with the LSHTM when he accepted what Mackintosh, the School's new Dean, called 'the key appointment of Director of the National Laboratory Service'. Although he had come to the rescue of his old School department in the autumn of 1944, when hopes for an end to the war in the foreseeable future made resumption of the teaching of bacteriology once again a realistic possibility, he finally left for the full-time activities at the PHLS at the end of September, 1947, to be succeeded by E.T.C.Spooner, who was to run the department from 1947 to 1960, when he became full-time Dean of the School for the next ten years.[40]

Wilson's achievement in the field he had built up during his tenure at the School, since the department's creation in 1927, were outstanding. He had been an inspired teacher, who with Topley had made the department a favourite training ground for microbiologists from home and abroad; his research, initially with Topley in the epic work on the spread of salmonella infections in herds of mice, had made fundamental contributions in the field of public health bacteriology; he went on to take a particular interest in variations, over time, in virulence of cultures of *Salmonella typhimurium*, a subject which led to a controversy with L.T.Webster of the Rockefeller Institute.[41] Very much his own was Wilson's crusade for improvements in the standards of safety for milk. It began already in the Manchester years. In 1926, he published, with M.M.Nutt, a paper recording the high percentage of *Brucella abortus* and of *Mycobacterium tuberculosis* found in cows' milk intended for human consumption. Wilson found this quite unacceptable, and over a period of more than twenty years, the problem engaged his attention in parallel studies of brucellosis, tuberculosis, and milk hygiene. The ramifications of this extensive research included a determined campaign for compulsory pasteurisation of milk, and his careful and prolonged studies on the efficacy, and the *pros* and *cons* of, BCG vaccination.[42] Much of Wilson's bacteriological research in the 1920s and 1930s, especially on milk hygiene, could be seen as the inspiration for the department of nutrition which was finally set up at the School after World War II.

It was above all the precision and meticulous approach to laboratory techniques which marked out Wilson as a bacteriologist *par excellence*, and a teacher who instilled the need for accuracy in all laboratory activities in his students. Before his departure for the PHLS in 1947, his influence had to a considerable extent defined the role of bacteriology and the bacteriological laboratory within the curriculum of the School, and also in its relations with clinical medicine; relations which elsewhere had often presented problems.[43] Indeed, mutual affection and loyalty between Wilson and the School was emphasised when, after leaving the PHLS at normal retirement age in 1963, he returned to the School as 'honorary lecturer' in his old department until final retirement at the age of 75, the year the department changed its title to the more comprehensive 'Microbiology' rather than 'Bacteriology and Immunology' as before.[44]

THE POST-WAR, POST-TOPLEY AND WILSON, YEARS

When Wilson left for the PHLS at the end of September, 1947, E.C.T.Spooner (1904–95) succeeded to Topley's Chair of Bacteriology and Immunology, and took over as Director of the department. A Cambridge man, with a career in pathology behind him, he came to the School facing the arduous task of rebuilding the bacteriology department after its wartime hiatus. In the early days of the war, Spooner had served as bacteriologist with the RAMC's Medical Research Section in the Middle East; in 1943 he became Director of the Cambridge EPHL. Wilson's personal title – it was never an established chair – was conferred on J.C.Cruickshank (1899–1956), and the personal title of Reader in Medical Mycology was created for J.T.Duncan.[45] For Cruickshank, it was a continuation of the task he had undertaken under the part-time direction of Graham Wilson between 1945 and 1946. Educated at Edinburgh, graduating MB, Ch.B. there in 1921 after wartime interruptions of service with the Gordon Highlanders, he had first come to the School as a student in the Dip.Bact. course in 1932. Between 1923 and 1930, he had been MO on West African Medical Staff in The Gambia, and worked for a short time in general practice in a mining area. A dedicated research scientist, he became demonstrator in the department after gaining his Diploma, and remained until the outbreak of war in 1939, when he joined the EPHLS. In 1945 he returned as Reader; and with G.S.Wilson spending much time at the PHLS, it was Cruickshank who shouldered a major part of the practical work involved in restructuring the department, collecting staff and equipment, and organising the teaching for three diploma courses. He was himself a gifted and popular teacher and was, as Professor of Bacteriology as Applied to Hygiene, a major influence on students and the department as a whole during the nine years left to him until his too early death in October, 1956.

In 1947, the new staff members were faced with a considerable workload. In the first post-war years, classes were heavily oversubscribed, both the ones given to DPH and DTM students, and even more those for the full-time University Diploma in Bacteriology. The department considered a maximum of twelve students the limit of its supervising capacity; yet applicants for the course due to begin in October, 1947, numbered more than fifty.[46] When, in the same year, Manchester University announced its intention to resume its course of instruction for the Diploma in Bacteriology, the decision was greeted with relief in London, as removing some of the pressure on the department.

The heavy commitment to teaching in an as yet understaffed department meant less time for research. Topley's team from the experimental epidemiology study had been dispersed during the war, and so had others concerned with immunological aspects of nutrition and antigenic bacterial fractions. For the newly appointed Professor Spooner and the staff he was assembling, the principal aim must lie in a search for excellence, in fundamental research and in teaching, to match the achievements of the department before 1939. It was a challenge intensified by the rapid post-war developments in microbiology, with its multiplying sub-divisions in virology and the many aspects of molecular biology. Throughout the late 1940s, staff continued to increase in numbers and in strength; and in the summer of 1949 Forrest Fulton, noted by Topley for his enthusiasm in the EPHLS in its early days, was appointed Reader in Bacteriology. He came to the School from the NIMR, where he had been working on rickettsiae and virus diseases. Virology as a separate discipline was then still in its infancy everywhere; at the School it was recognised as a subject in its own right when the UK's first Chair of Virology was created for Fulton in 1959; it became a separate department with the major reorganisation of the School at the beginning of the 1970s. By then several members of staff had been involved in virus research since the late 1940s.[47] Sadly Forrest Fulton did not live to take part in the reorganisation when he died unexpectedly in December 1971. It was a loss not only to the School and Virology, but very much to his students, who regarded him as a friend as well as trusted teacher, who always had time for them.

Research and teaching in any department, and especially at the postgraduate level, inevitably reflects the concerns of its director and his associates. Up until 1939, life in the Bacteriology Division had been heavily influenced by Topley's experimental epidemiology and Wilson's 'safe milk' policies. During the 1950s, Spooner's interest in the mumps virus coincided with the rapid growth of virology as a scientific discipline, and the appointment of Forrest Fulton in 1949 emphasised a growing concern with virus diseases. This tendency took another turn in 1957, with the appointment of C.E.Gordon Smith (1924–91). In the 1970s and 1980s, he was to influence developments and policy making at the School as its Dean; from 1957 to 1964, his presence in the department led to its closer involvement with the tropical side of the School. Born in Fife, Gordon Smith, MD, FRCP, F.R.C.Path., was Scots by descent, by birth, and by education; and like many early pioneers, in tropical medicine and at the old LSTM, he had no postgraduate training in tropical medicine when, in 1948, he joined the Colonial Medical Service after qualifying at St.Andrews University. In his own words, he went into the CMS because he 'had just married and needed the job, and the opportunity was there'. For nearly ten years, he served in the Far East, learning on the job like the early pioneers, and never looking back, from 1952–7 as virologist at the Institute for Medical Research at Kuala Lumpur.[48] His interest in arboviruses dated from those years in Kuala Lumpur, and was continued at the School, reflected in collaborative work with Fulton and others.[49]

The appointments of Forrest Fulton as Professor in 1959, and of Gordon Smith as Reader in 1961, in Virology, marked the arrival of the subject as a separate discipline at the School. In his first three years there, the department had, unbeknown to itself, two future Deans under its roof. The practice of recruiting Deans from the department of Public Health, begun with Wilson Jameson and continued after the war with James Mackintosh, changed with the recruitment of Andrew Topping (1890–1955) as the first full-time Dean in 1950. Topping had little academic background, but plenty of experience in the field of general public health and preventive medicine. Twenty years earlier he had shown his flair for public health planning as MOH in Rochdale, before becoming Deputy MOH and School MO to the London County Council. Also full of enthusiasm for international relief and public health work after the war, he renounced his London position to take up a post with UNRRA (United Nations Relief and Rehabilitation Administration). He answered the call to become dean of the School after a short period in the Chair of Social and Preventive Medicine in Manchester.[50]

The promise held out by the prospect of a permanent Dean devoting all his time to furthering the School's role nationally and internationally in promoting public health and preventive medicine in the post–war world, came to an abrupt end when Topping, a member of the Colonial Medical Advisory Service, met with a road accident in Africa in early 1954. He never fully recovered, and died in August, 1955. After an interim period, when Bradford Hill temporarily filled the post for two years, and Sir James Kilpatrick (1902–60) died in office after only three years, E.C.T.Spooner left the department of bacteriology to become full-time Dean at the end of September, 1960.[51]

The growing importance of virology as an independent discipline, and of the study of 'tropical viruses', in particular the arthropod-borne ones, had to some extent changed the direction of the department's research during the 1950s and the 1960s. Staff members visited laboratories abroad, and in turn distinguished visitors from the Americas, the Middle and Far East, African countries, and the WHO in Geneva called in on the department. Teaching continued in its overall pattern; the bacteriological input into the DPH and the DTMH courses, and the course in 'Environmental Control'[52] remained largely unaltered, and the number of students accepted for the popular Diploma in Bacteriology never exceeded twelve, in spite of the much larger numbers applying. The following decades were to see changes, moderate at first, and subsequently accelerating as virology and molecular biology made their inevitable impact.

Although E.C.T.Spooner had been director for one year during the war of the Cambridge Emergency Public Health Laboratory, and had served as a member of the MRC for four years in the mid-1950s, the department's close connection with the MRC established in its early years was somewhat in abeyance during Spooner's tenure. With the arrival of David Gwynne Evans (1909–84) in 1961, the ties with the MRC were once again to the fore. Moreover, Evans was the first director of the department who had never qualified in medicine. In fact, as a scientist he could be described as a late developer. He had graduated B.Sc. in chemistry and physics at Manchester only at the age of 25, having decided to join his younger brother at university.[53] When the assistance of a chemist was needed in the public health laboratory of the Department of Bacteriology there, Evans was appointed, and began a long association with H.B.Maitland (1895–1972). From this introduction to bacteriology and immunology he never looked back. His early work with Maitland in Manchester on whooping cough toxins and their neutralisation, and studies on active immunisation, set the pattern for his future research.[54] At Manchester, at the Department of Biological Standards at the NIMR at Hampstead, and from 1961 at the LSHTM, the development and field trials of vaccines were of absorbing interest to Evans; in addition to pertussis vaccine, over the years he chaired MRC Committees and international symposia on measles and BCG vaccines. On the veterinary front he was involved in the control of equine influenza and foot-and-mouth diseases.

BACTERIOLOGY AND IMMUNOLOGY

At the NIMR during World War II, emphasis was on antitoxins and immunisation against tetanus and the gas gangrene *Clostridia,* and chemotherapy.[55] In the dark days of April, 1940, when Norway and Denmark were invaded and occupied by German forces, the League of Nations requested help from the MRC with the provision of the International Standards for antitoxins and antisera to laboratories previously supplied by Copenhagen's State Serum Institute, a demand readily met by the MRC through the work of Evans and Percival Hartley.[56]

With this background in many aspects of immunisation and vaccine production trials Evans arrived in Keppel Street, where his talents and experience enriched the work of the department during a decade of expansion, of the subsequent creation of new M.Sc. courses (among them later, in 1975, one in Medical Microbiology), and of increasing emphasis on those preventive aspects of public health which so preoccupied David Evans.[57] During the years immediately preceding his move to the LSHTM, Evans was particularly involved with testing the Salk vaccine against poliomyelitis for the Biological Standards Control Laboratory at the NIMR. At a crucial time for vaccine production, and for the public perception of vaccines, with mishaps and tragic accidents causing public anxiety and a certain amount of resistance to their use, he was tireless in his campaign for their acceptance. In a leading article in the *British Medical Journal* in 1963, David Evans wrote that ' ... with proper safeguards in its manufacture and use oral poliomyelitis vaccine offers the greatest possibility of completely eliminating poliovirus as a human pathogen': a prophecy which only now, decades later, is beginning to take shape as an attainable goal.[58]

When David Evans resigned his Chair of Bacteriology at the LSHTM in 1971, it was not with thoughts of retirement, but in a bid to save the Lister Institute's Chelsea laboratory from closure. A year later, it was sadly evident that it was an impossible task; but yet another challenge was left for Evans. He was appointed Director of the newly formed National Institute of Biological Standards and Control. For the next three years his time was fully occupied with major reorganisation and planning of scientific departments and new laboratories. In July, 1976, the Biological Standards Act came into force, and the National Biological Standards Board relieved the MRC of responsibility for the Institute.[59] Even then, Evans had no intention of retiring. Moving to the Sir William Dunn School of Pathology at Oxford, he was happy to return to his erstwhile position of Demonstrator, teaching second year medical students and reorganising their practical course. Not until 1980 did he allow himself final retirement.

By the time Evans left the department, it was becoming obvious that a major change to its structure was advisable. The School Report for 1970–1 announced:

> *Bacteriology and Immunology*
> This will henceforth be called the Department of Microbiology because of its wide interests in virology and mycology as well as in bacteriology and because immunology is now an important element in other departments such as medical helminthology and medical protozoology. The department houses two reference laboratories of the Public Health Laboratory Service – in mycology and leptospirosis.[60]

It was a year marked by change. The department's erstwhile director, E.C.T.Spooner, retired as Dean, to be succeeded by its former Reader in Virology, C.E.Gordon Smith. Forrest Fulton died suddenly and unexpectedly at the end of 1971, following which a number of his papers were removed by Government departments as classified papers covered by the Official Secrets Act; the rest remain for potential inclusion in the LSHTM Archives.[61] Now the new Department of Microbiology had as its director a Professor of Microbiology, Geoffrey Edsall (1908–80), who in an apparent reversal of the brain drain (although this happy situation was not to last long) came to the School from Massachusetts, where he had been Director of the State Public Health Laboratories and Professor of Applied Microbiology at the Harvard School of Public Health. Having taken office on February 1st, 1972, Edsall had already retired by the time the 1974–5 School Report was published, and been 'appointed an Emeritus Professor of the University'.[62] The appointment, and willingness to come to London, of Edsall, seems in retrospect less than easy to understand. He had passed his 64th birthday by the time he took up his appointment on February 1st, 1972, and he had been eminently well established in Massachusetts. Sources within the department felt that possibly personal friendship between Edsall and D.G.Evans might have explained the choice. Unforeseen circumstances would soon prove that Edsall could hardly have chosen a worse time to head the LSHTM Department of Microbiology.

Little more than a year after Edsall took up his duties, a young technician in the department – employed by the PHLS in the Mycological Reference Laboratory, but also on duty in the department generally – fell ill. At first her illness was thought to be no more than influenza. Even when she deteriorated and was admitted to St.Mary's, Paddington, febrile and with an (uncharacteristic) rash, she was placed in a general ward. D.W.R.MacKenzie, Director of the Mycological Reference Laboratory, at first suspected a fungal infection. Only after a specimen, obtained by MacKenzie by somewhat unorthodox means, was examined in the School's Electron Microscopy Unit by David Ellis, was smallpox suspected and notified, amid a certain amount of professional controversy between the Unit and clinical staff at St.Mary's. The diagnosis was confirmed two weeks after her admission. By the time the full seriousness of the situation was realised, two visitors to a patient in a bed adjacent to that of the female technician had become infected. Unlike her, they had not been recently revaccinated. They both died of smallpox. Although the bulk of the work of David Ellis and others in the Electron Microscopy Unit was initially done in the area of parasitology, in the case of Ellis and D.A.Evans notably their work on the development of tsetse-flies (Chapter 9), Ellis's involvement with viruses neither began nor ended with the smallpox diagnosis. In 1978-9 he was, with D.I.H.Simpson, among the early observers of the Ebola virus, which had then only recently been added to the list of emerging viruses making themselves felt in Africa.[63]

The unfortunate and alarming smallpox incident had wide repercussions; not only for the School and the Department, but for several other Public Health institutions named as 'third parties' in the resulting inquiry, and the suit brought by the administrators of the estates of the victims, a married couple with a young family. In addition to the School, the third parties included the Board of Governors of St.Mary's Hospital, the Westminster City Council, the London Borough of Camden, the Department of Health and Social Security, and the Public Health Laboratory Service, none of whom had escaped criticism in the *Inquiry*. Among the more than 90 'witnesses' giving evidence were, in addition to Drs.MacKenzie and Ellis, Miss A.E.Algeo, who was the infected technician, Dr.Rondle in whose laboratory she had become infected during 'harvesting' of the virus (he was aware that she had been revaccinated the previous year), Professor Edsall, and A.J.Zuckerman, then the School's Professor of Virology. It was an episode which led to thorough revision of safety procedures both at the School and elsewhere. Nevertheless, five years later, on the eve of the announcement of total global eradication of the disease in 1979, smallpox virus escaped from a Birmingham laboratory, with tragic consequences. The School's, and the country's, last brush with smallpox, well after the official eradication date, began in December 1985, when examination of a malfunctioning refrigerator revealed among its contents a cardboard box containing seven ampoules labelled 'smallpox SP 22 16.12.52'. Full safety procedures were immediately put into effect; but although in this case there were no serious consequences, the incident served as a timely reminder of potential problems in keeping samples of dangerous viruses after their supposed eradication.[64]

Within the School, another incident with less serious consequences had preceded the smallpox tragedy. A technician in the protozoology department had become infected with a strain of *Trypanosoma brucei rhodiense,* isolated from an African bushman, and studied in rats in the department. In an accident involving a dropped cage, Miss Cornish was bitten by an infected rat, and subsequently developed trypanosomiasis. Treated at the Hospital for Tropical Diseases, she made an uninterrupted recovery and continued to work in the laboratory for several years. The incident was noted in the Minutes of the School's Finance and General Purposes Committee in July, 1972; but with the smallpox inquiry under way a few months later, Gordon Smith asked the department not to publish its account until 'the smallpox wind has blown over'. Buried in the Minutes until today, this rare example of rat-bite transmission is only now, more than twenty years later, being reported by W.E.Ormerod in a letter to the *Transactions of the Royal Society of Tropical Medicine and Hygiene.*

When Geoffrey Edsall left the Department of Microbiology to return to the United States, A.J.Zuckerman took over as Director in 1975 of what then became the Department of Medical Microbiology. In Zuckerman's time research in the department was focused to a considerable extent on his own particular interest in viral hepatitis. He had been in the department since 1965, from 1972 as Professor of Virology. Even before 1965, Forrest Fulton had been working with hepatitis viruses in tissue culture, attempting to 'isolate a virus from acute cases of infective hepatitis', in an age when clinical and laboratory sciences complemented each other as never before. With Zuckerman heading the department, the work was intensified during a period when in any case viral hepatitis was emerging as a public health problem on a global scale; and when initial identification of the viruses of the two major types, (infectious) hepatitis A and (serum) hepatitis B, was followed by the detection of other, previously unrecognised, viral agents. Today there is increasing interest in a still growing number of known hepatitis viruses.[65]

Zuckerman's first year as director of the department was also the first year of the new M.Sc. course in Medical Microbiology. It was accompanied by important changes in teaching in the department, notably the inclusion of a two weeks' course in parasitology. This was no isolated development. Throughout the School, the old diploma courses changed to M.Sc. degree courses during the 1970s, following the replacement of the Diploma in Public Health with a Master of Science degree in Social Medicine in September, 1969.[66] A new M.Sc. in Virology was added in 1987.

In addition to the intense interest in viral hepatitis in the 1970s and 1980s, research in the department went ahead on a wide variety of fronts. The old ally, immunology, was back in the fold, with M.W.Steward as Professor of Immunology; and B.S.Drasar who today heads the Bacterial Molecular Genetics Unit, was Reader in Bacteriology, jointly with the Department of Tropical Hygiene. Other members of the department held their appointments jointly with such other departments as Entomology, Clinical Tropical Medicine, and Human Nutrition. There began to be signs that restructuring would be advisable.[67]

Internal structural reorganisation of the School finally became reality towards the end of the 1980s. When A.J.Zuckerman, after more than twenty years, left the School for the Royal Free Hospital Medical School in 1988, to become its Dean in 1989, major restructuring of departments and courses throughout the School was under way. In October, 1986, the Board of Management had set up a working party under Sir John Reid to consider the options, and to recommend a plan for future developments. Its recommendations were made in time for Gordon Smith to supervise the initial moves in the process of reorganisation, which in the event covered his last year as Dean before retirement; and the first year in office of his successor, Richard Feachem, who took over on September 4th, 1989.[68]

In his first *Annual Report*, the new Dean wrote of the need to prepare for a changing world in the 1990s. Gordon Smith, in his last year at the helm, had worked hard to begin implementing the recommendations of the working party. The revised structure, with four new, large, departments, accommodating between them all essential aspects of the subjects taught in a total of twenty-three 'units', had been put in place, ready for development, by September, 1989.[69]

The changing world and the restructuring are now, in the 1990s, reflected in not just the contents, but also in the changed format of the School Reports. In an increasingly image conscious world, they are 'glossy', highly coloured, and high-profile, with a separate Research Report setting out the aims and achievements as well as the publications of each of the units in each department. In this changed world, the 'Bacteriology' and 'Immunology' of old now exist largely at the molecular

PREVENTION AND CURE

level, in the age of Molecular Biology: B.S.Drasar's 'Bacterial Molecular Genetics', and M.W.Steward's 'Molecular Immunology', were units within Clinical Sciences until the reorganisation in 1987; they now come under the new large Department of Infectious and Tropical Diseases. At the same time, Dorothy Crawford's 'Viral Pathogenesis' disappeared when she left for a Chair of Medical Microbiology at Edinburgh in June 1997. The very names of all three units reflected the increasing preoccupation with research at the molecular level. As far as 'Bacteriology' of old is concerned its progress, via 'Medical Microbiology' to 'Bacterial Molecular Genetics', and its consequent need for closer links, within the School with 'Tropical Hygiene', and outside with laboratories abroad, on an extended environmental front, are well illustrated by papers published, between 1981 and 1993, by Drasar with colleagues from the Ross Institute/Department of Tropical Hygiene and from overseas.[70] At the same time, immunology has branched out into other units in the Department of Medical Parasitology: 'Immunology of Parasitic Diseases', and 'Immunology and Vaccine Design'. Last but not least, echoes of the close links between bacteriology and epidemiology in the days of Topley and Greenwood can be found in Paul Fine's 'Communicable Disease Epidemiology' unit in what is, as of 1997, the Department of Infectious and Tropical Diseases.

If the Department of Bacteriology and Immunology, in the more than sixty years since its inception in 1927, has developed beyond recognition, and far beyond what was then its natural framework, it has done so in time with overall scientific development in the twentieth century. The old order has exhausted itself; the future lies increasingly at the molecular level, aided and abetted by rapid advances now informing such techniques as electron microscopy and DNA sequencing.

BACTERIOLOGY AND IMMUNOLOGY
NOTES

[1] LSHTM *Annual Report*, 1926-7, pp.11-12.
[2] W.W.C.Topley, 'The spread of bacterial infection', *Lancet*, 1919, *ii*, 1-5; 45-9; 91-6; idem, 'A report on a bacterial investigation of typhus fever during the Serbian epidemic of 1915', *JRAMC,* 1915, *25:*215-88.
[3] M.Greenwood, 'William Whiteman Carlton Topley 1886-1944', *Obit.Not.Fell.Roy.Soc.*, 1944, *4:*699-711.
[4] Topley, *Lancet 1919,* op.cit. note 2, p.1.
[5] M.Greenwood, 'The epidemiology of influenza', *Br.med.J.*, 1918, *ii:*563-6, p.566.
[6] S.Flexner, 'Experimental epidemiology', *J.exp.Med.*, 1922, *36:*9-14; S.Flexner and Harold L.Amoss, 'Experimental epidemiology. I. An artificially induced epidemic of mouse typhoid', *ibid.:*25-69.
[7] LSHTM *Annual Report* 1970-1, p.24.
[8] M.Greenwood, A.Bradford Hill, W.W.C.Topley, and J.Wilson, 'Experimental epidemiology', MRC Special Report Series, No.209, London, HMSO, 1936.
[9] Greenwood, op.cit. note 3, p.707 [authors' italics].
[10] *ibid.*, p.708.
[11] LSHTM *Annual Report,* 1927-8, p.3 and p.10; 1928-9, p.11.
[12] *ibid.* 1927-8, p.10.
[13] LSHTM, Division of Bacteriology and Immunology, 'Syllabus of Advanced Course', 1927, p.3.
[14] LSHTM *Annual Report* 1928-9, p.11.
[15] *ibid.* 1941-2, p.10.
[16] Appointed Reader at Topley's insistence by U.L.Senate Resolution of 18 May, 1927, the Senate, again after intervention by Topley, recommended conferment of the title of 'Professor of Bacteriology as applied to Hygiene' on Wilson on 17 July, 1930. Uncatalogued letters in GSW 'Personal File', LSHTM Archives.
[17] In a letter to Balfour dated 29th July, 1926 (*ibid.*), Topley wrote 5 pages of strong recommendations urging the case for immediate appointment of Wilson to his new department at the School. Among the many reasons for the importance of continuing his association with Wilson within the new School was that '... we are writing a textbook of bacteriology which will, I hope be published within the next two years'. The first edition of *The Principles of bacteriology and immunity* was published in 1929; with changes of editors and authors it has since gone through several editions and is now titled *The principles of bacteriology,*

virology and immunity.

[18] G.S.Wilson, 'A short note on the effect on pyrexia of inoculation agglutinins', *Lancet*, 1917, *i*:263–4.

[19] R.E.O.Williams, *Microbiology for the Public Health. The evolution of the Public Health Laboratory Service 1939–80,* London, Public Health Laboratory Service, 1985. In this volume Sir Robert acknowledges his debt to Sir Graham's unpublished 'Some historical notes on the formation and development of the Public Health Laboratory Service, 1938–63', the notes for which are now in the Contemporary Medical Archives Collection (CMAC) at the Wellcome Institute Library: CMAC, pp/GSW, C/29, C/30. We are indebted to both.

[20] Anon., 'Obituary. Sir Rubert William Boyce', *Lancet,* 1911, *ii:* 59–60;
C.S.S. [Sherrington], 'Sir Rubert Boyce' (1863–1911), *Obit.Not.Fell.Roy.Soc.* (September 1911), pp.iii–ix.

[21] Williams, op.cit. note 19, p.4.

[22] *ibid.,* and MRC *Report* 1938–9, p.17, and 1939–45, pp.164–83.

[23] Williams, op.cit. note 19, p.6;
LSHTM *Annual Report* 1991–2, p.26.

[24] MRC *Report* 1937–8, pp.25–6; MRC *Report* 1938–9, pp.15–21.

[25] MRC *Report* 1938–9, p.10.

[26] *ibid.,* p.14.

[27] Letter to Wilson from A.Landsborough Thomson, Principal Asst. Secretary to the MRC, dated 6 July 1939, CMAC, pp/GSW, C.21.

[28] Topley to Balfour, op.cit. note 17 above.

[29] Topley to Wilson, 31.8.39, CMAC, pp/GSW, C.21.

[30] Topley to Wilson, 5.9.39, *ibid.*

[31] Topley to Wilson, 27.9.39, *ibid.*

[32] Topley to Wilson, 29.9.39, *ibid.*

[33] MRC *Report* 1939–45, p.161.

[34] E.S.Anderson and Sir Robert Williams, 'Graham Selby Wilson 10 September 1895–5 April 1987', *Biogr.Mem.Fell.Roy.Soc.,* 1988, *34*:889–919, p.902;
'Death of W.M.Scott and F.Griffith', *Lancet*, 1941, *ii*:584; 588; *Br.med.J.,* 1941, *i*:691.

[35] Anderson and Williams as above, p.904.

[36] MRC *Report* 1939–45, p.169.

[37] MRC *Report* 1945–8, pp.222–39.

[38] *ibid.,* p.224.

[39] Anderson and Williams op.cit. note 34, p.902.

[40] LSHTM *Annual Reports* 1946–7, and 1959–60.

BACTERIOLOGY AND IMMUNOLOGY

[41] Anderson and Williams, op.cit. note 34, pp.892–3;
L.T.Webster in *J.exp.Med.*, 1923, *37:* 231–74; and *38:*33–4, and 45–54;
G.S.Wilson, 'Discontinuous variation in the virulence of *Bact.aertrycke* Mutton', *J.Hyg.*, 1928, *30:*40–54.

[42] G.S.Wilson and M.M.Nutt, 'The occurrence of *Brucella abortus* and *Mycobacterium tuberculosis* in cows' milk', *J.Path.Bact.*, 1926, *29:*141–8;
G.S.Wilson, 'Pasteurisation of milk', *Nature,* 1938, *141:*579–81;
G.S.Wilson, *Pasteurisation of milk*, London, Edward Arnold, 1942;
G.S.Wilson, 'The value of BCG vaccination in the control of tuberculosis', *Br.med.J.*, 1947, *ii:*855–9.

[43] Anderson and Williams, op.cit. note 34, p.891. Because of the School's initial integration with the Hospital for Tropical Diseases, it had always enjoyed special relations between clinical medicine and the bacteriological laboratory, cf. Chapter 1.

[44] Anderson and Williams, note 34 above, and School Reports between 1964 and 1970, and 1986–7.

[45] LSHTM *Annual Report* 1947–8; Duncan left the School the following year;
'John Cecil Cruickshank', *Lancet*, 1956, *ii:*1001–2;
'J.C.Cruickshank', *Br.med.J.*, 1956, *ii,*1061; 1121–2;
'The Late Professor J.C.Cruickshank', LSHTM AR 1956–7, p.15;
LSHTM *Annual Report* 1948–9, p.21;
'Dr Edward Spooner', *The Times* obituary, 15 September, 1995.

[46] LSHTM *Annual Report* 1947–8, pp.52–5;
LSHTM *Annual Report* 1946–7, p.64.

[47] LSHTM *Reports* between 1949 and 1970–1.

[48] Obituary, LSHTM *Annual Report* 1990–1; personal information in interviews kindly given between 1988 and 1990.

[49] Publications listed in School Reports between 1957 and 1964.

[50] LSHTM *Annual Report* 1954–5, p.15.

[51] LSHTM *Annual Report* 1959–60, p.30;
ABH, pp. 9–10;
'James MacConnel Kilpatrick', *Lancet,* 1960, *i:*884–5.

[52] LSHTM *Annual Reports* 1957–8, 1958–9, 1959–60, etc.

[53] A.W.Downie, C.E.Gordon Smith and J.O'H.Tobin, 'David Gwynne Evans 6 September 1909–13 June 1984', *Biogr.Mem.Fell.Roy.Soc.*, 1985, *31:*173–96.

[54] H.B.Maitland and D.G.Evans, 'The preparation of the toxin of *H.pertussis:* its properties and relation to immunity', *J.Path.Bact.*, 1937, *45:*715–31;

idem, 'The failure of whooping cough sera to neutralise pertussis toxin', *ibid*., 1939, *48*:465–7.
⁵⁵ Downie *et al.*, note 53 above, pp.182–3.
⁵⁶ D.G.Evans, 'The protective properties of the alpha antitoxin and theta antihaemolysin occurring in *Cl.welchii* type A antiserum', *Br.J.exp.Path.*, 1943, *24*:81–8;
idem, 'Persistence of tetanus antitoxin in man following active immunization', *Lancet*, 1943, *ii*:316–17.
⁵⁷ Downie *et al.*, op.cit. note 53, *passim*.
⁵⁸ 'Immunization against poliomyelitis', Leader, *Br.med.J.*, 1963, *i*:623–4.
⁵⁹ Downie *et al.*, op.cit. note 53, p.176.
⁶⁰ LSHTM *Annual Report* 1970-1, p.24.
⁶¹ Janet Foster, School Archives Pilot Survey, 1992.
⁶² LSHTM *School Reports* 1971–2 and 1974–5.
⁶³ LSHTM Minutes of the Finance and General Purposes Committee, 11 April, 1973;
'Smallpox in London', *Br.med.J.*, 1973, *ii*:126;
'Questions in Commons', *Br.med.J.*, 1973, *ii*:317;
'Confinement of the poxvirus', *Lancet*, 1974, *ii*:561–2;
Report of the Committee of Inquiry into the Smallpox Outbreak in London in March and April 1973, London, HMSO, 1974;
D.S.Ellis, D.I.H.Simpson, *et al.*, 'Ultrastructure of Ebola virus particles in human liver', *J.Clin.Path.*, 1978, *31*:201–8;
D.S.Ellis, Susan Stamford, G.Lloyd, E.T.Bowen, G.S.Platt, Hilary Way, and D.I.H.Simpson, 'Ebola and Marburg viruses: I. Some ultrastructural differences between strains when grown in Vero cells', *J.Med.Virol.*, 1979, *4*:201–11.
D.I.H.Simpson, Marburg and Ebola virus infections: a guide for their diagnosis, management and control, WHO Offset Publications No.36.
⁶⁴ *Investigation into the cause of the 1978 Birmingham Smallpox occurrence. Report* [Chairman R.A.Shooter] London, 1980. Both outbreaks are described in 'Laboratory-associated outbreaks in the United Kingdom', *in:* F.Fenner, D.A.Henderson, *et al.*, *Smallpox and its eradication,* Geneva, WHO, 1988, pp.1095–1101;
LSHTM Board of Man.Minutes, March 1986, Appendix 2.
⁶⁵ Francis L.Black, 'Infectious hepatitis', *in:* Kenneth F.Kiple (ed), *The Cambridge World History of Human Disease,* Cambridge University Press, 1993, pp.794–9;
A.J.Zuckerman (ed), *Selected abstracts submitted for the 1987 International Symposium on Viral hepatitis and Liver Disease,* London,

1987;

J.Stanton, 'What shapes vaccine policy? The case of hepatitis B in the UK', *Social History of Medicine*, 1994, 7:427–46;

J.Stanton, 'Health policy and medical research: hepatitis B in the UK since the 1940', Ph.D. thesis, University of London, 1995.

[66] LSHTM *Annual Reports* 1969–70 to 1975–6.

[67] LSHTM *Annual Reports* 1975–6 to 1987–8.

[68] LSHTM *Annual Reports* 1987–8, 1988–9, and 1989–90.

[69] LSHTM *Annual Report* 1989–90, p.2.

[70] LSHTM *Research Reports* 1990 and 1992;

Six papers on aspects of the occurrence and survival of *Vibrio cholerae* in the environment, especially in aquatic reservoirs during inter-epidemic seasons, were published in *Tropical Diseases Bulletin, Journal of Hygiene, Journal of Tropical Medicine and Hygiene, and Journal of Diarrhoeal Disease Research,* between 1981 and 1993;

A.Gebre-Yohannes and B.S.Drasar, 'Molecular epidemiology of plasmid patterns in *Shigella flexneri* types 1–6';

B.S.Drasar and P.G.S.Cook, 'Intestinal bacteria and the initiation of cancer', *GANN Monograph on Cancer Research* 31, 1985.

6

PUBLIC HEALTH AND ITS COMING OF AGE: FROM MOH AND DPH TO 'SOCIAL MEDICINE' AND 'COMMUNITY MEDICINE'

When the new Division of Public Health opened its doors at the beginning of the autumn term in 1929, and began to prepare postgraduate candidates for the Diploma in Public Health (DPH), that diploma already had a long history behind it. In the wake of the acceleration of the public health movement in the mid-nineteenth century, itself a corollary of the great cholera epidemics,[1] it had been furthered by the work of Edwin Chadwick and of William Farr, and of the pioneering Medical Officers of Health led by Duncan of Liverpool and John Simon in London.[2] It first became established in Dublin and soon afterwards in Cambridge in the 1870s. The London School of Tropical Medicine, as represented by Patrick Manson, had cooperated with G.H.F.Nuttall at Cambridge to establish a Diploma in Tropical Medicine and Hygiene (DTMH) at Cambridge in 1904, where it continued until 1933, when teaching for the diploma revolved to the LSHTM.[3] The University of London, under whose umbrella the then still new LSHTM operated, had been running a part-time DPH course, as had the independent Royal Institute of Public Health, since early in the century.[4]

In Henry Kenwood's department at University College, London, the young William Wilson Jameson (1885-1962) obtained the DPH in 1914. Kenwood, who had by then been building up the UCL department as Professor of Hygiene for a decade, immediately recruited Jameson as assistant lecturer. Between them, they shared academic and wartime duties for the duration of the Great War. Jameson served in France and Italy – and at Aldershot – as a Specialist Sanitary Officer in the RAMC; in between he deputised for Kenwood, who was frequently absent on duty with the Army Medical Advisory Board, in the teaching and running of the department. His duties also included those of MOH for Stoke Newington (after the war he became MOH for Finchley, a post Kenwood had held between 1893 and 1904), and of Assistant Medical Officer with the Metropolitan Asylums Board.[5]

For Jameson, his multiple wartime activities represented a precipitate introduction to the wider implications of public health, the subject which was to occupy his mind and his very considerable administrative abilities for the rest of his life. Kenwood was what Goodman has called 'a public health doctor in the original German tradition. That is, he was primarily a chemist'.[6] The students who became Jameson's temporary responsibility included both postgraduate physicians preparing for the DPH, and medical and engineering undergraduates to be instructed in hygiene and sanitation. It was invaluable training for his as yet unthought-of future as the first Professor of Public Health and Dean of the LSHTM, and for his role in the development of the National Health Service (NHS) after World War II.

WILSON JAMESON: STRATEGY FOR NATIONAL PUBLIC HEALTH 1929-45

After further wartime service, Jameson was demobilised at the beginning of 1919. Not yet thirty-five, he was now in no doubt that his future must lie in the specialty of Public Health. As a result of his experience, both in Kenwood's department at University College, and in the RAMC during the war, he was a natural choice as joint author, with a UC colleague, to write *Synopsis of Hygiene,* which became a standard textbook.[7] In September, 1919, Jameson was appointed MOH and School Medical Officer for Finchley, and shortly afterwards Deputy MOH for St.Marylebone. Seven years later, the fledgling LSHTM was seeking a professor of public health with sufficient background and experience, and enough enthusiasm and administrative ability, to organise a unique new teaching and research department devoted to public health and preventive medicine. Jameson's erstwhile teacher and by now old friend, H.R.Kenwood, wrote at the end of December to express the hope that he would apply, assuring him of his unequivocal support. Jameson did apply, and was duly appointed. Kenwood, in his note of encouragement, had told him that he believed he had '.. convinced Newman that you are the man needed'; and George Newman in turn wrote to Jameson at the beginning of March, 1928, congratulating him on his appointment, and also warning him of the amount of hard work and patience required. He added a rather fulsome remark regarding the rewards of potential success, which '... would bring credit and honour to yourself and to our branch of Medicine, and what is still better a larger life for all men, an extension of the frontiers of life for all men'.[8] Fortunately, Jameson was well up to the challenge. For the next thirty years, first at the LSHTM and later, throughout World War II and after at the Ministry of Health, the Ministry of Education, and the MRC, he contributed substantially to the Nation's public health services. On the eve of war, he was involved in the replacement of the country's sundry county, municipical, university, hospital, and even private, public health bacteriological laboratories, by a central service, i.e., during the war the EPHLS, and at the end of hostilities, the PHLS; and alongside this, the development of the NHS.[9]

Jameson's appointment to the LSHTM, to take effect on January 1st, 1929, was to 'the Chair of Public Health in the University of London and to the directorship of the Division of Public Health in the School [LSHTM], the term Public Health comprising the principles and practice of preventive medicine, general sanitation and administration'. In the circumstances, the Board of Management 'decided not to create a separate division of Physiology as applied to Hygiene, but to regard this important subject as coming within the Division of Public Health'.[10] The position of physiology within the sphere of public health teaching and research in the School underwent a number of changes over the years, with the creation of specialist appointments in applied physiology, in industrial physiology, and eventually in occupational health; and with the modifications to School structure in 1937, when the six major 'divisions' were replaced by eight 'departments'.[11] By 1940, the nomenclature had reverted to 'seven major Divisions'.[12]

The time and effort spent in organising the curriculum for the DPH, a cornerstone in the School's new responsibilities in the teaching of public health and preventive medicine, was a measure of its seriousness of approach; and the affiliations of the main members of the main Sub-Committee concerned with development of the curriculum were an indication of the diversity of interests considered necessary at this stage. It included, in addition to Jameson himself, the professors of chemistry as applied to hygiene (M.E.Delafield), medical zoology and helminthology (R.T.Leiper), bacteriology and immunology (W.W.C.Topley), and epidemiology and vital statistics (M.Greenwood). Grass-roots instruction in public health administration would be provided within the London area at St.Marylebone and at Willesden, and cooperation was also promised by the London County Council, the City of London, and the Port of London.[13]

In organising the Division of Public Health in its first year, Jameson had the, at first part-time, support of G.S.Parkinson (1880–1953), a retired Lt.-Colonel of the RAMC, who had been appointed Assistant Director of the Division. Also appointed were two full time lecturers: H.H.Clay to lecture on domestic sanitary engineering, and G.P.Crowden to lecture on applied physiology. Crowden (1894–1966) came to the LSHTM from neighbouring University College, where he had been assistant in the department of physiology while completing his medical degree – studies first begun at University College

PREVENTION AND CURE

Hospital in 1913, and suspended during service with the King's Own Yorkshire Light Infantry in France throughout the Great War. It was his wartime experience, especially with the Gas Service Brigade, at Ypres in 1915, in the Somme offensive in 1916, and at Passchendale in 1917, which, together with J.S.Haldane's advice on self protection against gas attacks, kindled Crowden's growing interest in the physiology of work and of stress. It also identified an area of study which would stand him in good stead in his later positions as Reader in Industrial Physiology (1934) and Professor of Applied Physiology (1946–62) in the School.[14] It further accounted for his wide-ranging research interests, from fatigue and recovery in muscular work, to effects of cold and of heat in nutrition. In his second year at the School, the *Annual Report* mentioned among his equipment an air-conditioning plant for teaching purposes, and investigations carried out jointly with the Industrial Health Research Board; also connections with 'business firms and bodies interested in industrial welfare work of every description'. It was to prove another link in the long progression from Bradford Hill's early work for the MRC, to the eventual creation of a department of occupational health, and the TUC Institute.[15]

Over the ten-year period until the outbreak of World War II in 1939, the Public Health Department developed under Jameson's confident guidance. Essential support for its teaching activities derived from the expanding library, and the teaching aids offered by the Museum. By 1933, the central Library – excluding individual holdings in departmental libraries – had an impressive stock of nearly 20,000 bound volumes, and even more pamphlets. A total of 448 current journals were received, of which more than two-thirds came via the Bureau of Hygiene and Tropical Diseases, in a continuation of the long-standing arrangements between Manson's School and the Bureau since the latter's inception in the days of the Sleeping Sickness Commissions. Six years later, before war curtailed developments, the holdings included more than 800 bound sets of periodicals. As several of these were journals which had been discontinued, such figures in no way reflect the intake of current journals, which in 1939 stood at 438. In the 1990s, with the reciprocal arrangement between the School Library and the Bureau of Hygiene and Tropical Disease ceased, the number of current periodicals received lies between seven and eight hundred.[16]

At the same time, the Museum could report notable changes and improvements. In addition to the tropical collections, there was now a growing display in the public health sections, with posters and exhibits relating to public health propaganda, to the activities of the Port Sanitary

Authorities, and to the important subject of maternity and child welfare, both at home and in 'native races'.[17] It was the Public Health collection, situated in the basement, which took the full force of the bomb that hit the School on a Saturday night in May, 1943, and from which it never recovered.[18] In 1938, the Museum's then retiring curator, H.B.Newham, had looked back with satisfaction on the growth of the collections during his nine years in the job. The care of the museum was then in the hands of a small committee, which at the outbreak of war had decided to place the most valuable models and exhibits in the basement for safe custody. Ironically, this led to their total destruction when the German bomb fell on the Malet Street wing. The damage was all but irreversible; and apart from entomological exhibits, the permanent displays were replaced after the war by temporary exhibitions related to topical subjects. The Wellcome Museum came to the rescue as a replacement for the Parasitology exhibits. A few charts and illustrations were salvaged by William Cooper, and were still in use for protozoology demonstrations in the 1960s.[19]

Teaching, the main activity of the department of public health in the pre-war years, relied strongly on cooperation with other departments, as laid down in the initial plan of October, 1929. The plan stipulated coordination of the different subjects necessary to cover the diverse theoretical and practical aspects of public health which then constituted the required qualifications for the DPH. From its earliest days, the Public Health Division had also prided itself on the inclusion of seminars and tutorials as an essential part of its programme. Its formal lectures on the other hand, included special talks given by recognised experts in various fields within public health and preventive medicine. The department's association with the Industrial Health Research Board continued to develop, and not only through G.P.Crowden's teaching of physiological aspects of public health and industrial hygiene to the Diploma course, and special lectures to the DTMH classes; but even more when, in 1931, Millais Culpin (1874–1952) had been appointed University Professor of Medical Industrial Psychology in the School. For Culpin, as for Crowden, his research interests had developed in response to experiences in World War I. In 1915, he had published, with E.G.Fearnsides, a paper on frost-bite in patients on active service abroad, and possible psychological implications; and after the war, his *Psychoneuroses of War and Peace* showed the development of his thoughts while lecturing on psychoneuroses at the London Hospital, and as neurological specialist to the Ministry of Pensions. When Culpin died in 1952, one obituarist recalled how his keen pursuit of his subject affected his teaching: 'Many old students of the School will remember the *rather intense* half-hour they spent *alone with Professor Culpin* while he sought for neurotic traits in them and explained the significance of his findings' [authors' italics]. The activities of Crowden and of Culpin strengthened the School's bonds with industry, and led eventually to the establishment of an intensive course given jointly by Crowden's section of Industrial Physiology and Culpin's department of Medical Industrial Psychology. It became a course much appreciated by a number of industrial concerns, some of whom in turn supported work in the department.[20]

By 1938, the Nation, and the School, were bracing themselves for the threat of war. Air Raid Precautions rated high in the national consciousness; arrangements for emergency shelters became a subject for consideration in the public health department. The *Annual Report* issued in October, 1938, emphasised the importance of 'provision of sanitary appliances suitable for use in temporary buildings of all kinds'. It also referred to 'the modern development of camping as a form of recreation'. The sanitary problems presented by both these developments were given close attention in the department, where possible improvements to the 'chemical closet', and its adaption '... for both European and native use in the tropics', were high on the agenda. The Museum dutifully added '... modern examples of the apparatus' to its collections.[21]

Before teaching activities were suspended by force of circumstance between 1940 and 1945, the course of study for the DPH was a full one. It included instruction in public health administration, sanitary law, sanitary engineering, hospital management, medical industrial psychology, and physiology as applied to hygiene and industry. Departments and divisions outside of the Public Health Division also involved in course work for the Diploma were the Division of Bacteriology and Immunology; the Department of Chemistry as applied to Hygiene; and the Division of Epidemiology and Vital Statistics. When course work was resumed after the end of the war, an attempt was made to analyse the results of course attendance on the subsequent careers and choice of posts by the students, as a means of evaluating the effectiveness of the DPH curriculum in the teaching of preventive medicine. The results of the analysis may be seen in the table below; most striking is the marked increase in the early post–war years in numbers of students intending to pursue careers in research, whereas the majority, destined for the Public Health service in the United Kingdom, showed little or no significant variation over the years from 1930 to 1947.[22]

PUBLIC HEALTH

Courses	1 Public Health Service in UK	2 Colonial Medical Service etc.	3 Hopsital Consultant G.P. Forces	4 Academic Research Industrial etc	No Information	Did not complete DPH	Dominion Students	Indian and other Foreign Students	Total
1930-31 1931-32 1932-33	35	20	10	3	2	2	5	24	101
1933-34 1934-35 1935-36	45	8	7	6	5	2	9	28	110
1936-37 1937-38 1938-39	45	13	13	2	14	5	4	35	131
1945-46 1946-47 (extra) 1946-47	41	11	7	24	23	25	7	8	146

Wilson Jameson's relations with the School's Court of Governors, the Board of Management, and the School Council, during his years as Dean, have been described in detail by his biographer.[23] The thirty-four members of the Court were '... so distinguished that [they] could hardly be expected to do any real work'. That was undertaken by the Board of Management, which included the by no means undistinguished Sir Cooper Perry, Vice-Chancellor of the University of London, Sir Holburt Waring (1866-1953), Sir George Newman (1870-1948) from the Ministry of Health, Sir Walter Fletcher (1873-1933), and later Sir Edward Mellanby, from the MRC, and Sir Thomas Stanton, Chief Medical Adviser to the Colonial Office, with the assistance of the School Council, composed of senior staff. It was a potentially explosive mixture, which needed all of Jameson's fortunately consummate tact and diplomacy to keep its disparate personalities and their individual interests in order and working together to 'solve common problems amicably'.[24] Clark and Mackintosh wrote in 1954: 'So far as one can ascertain, no woman has ever been a member of the Court of Governors, the Board of Management, or the School Council.' Now, forty years later, the situation has changed, but perhaps not in proportion to the increased ratio of women involved in teaching and research in the School. The first woman elected to the Court of Governors was Katharine G.Lloyd-Williams (1896-1973), who served from 1960 to 1962, and was succeeded by Dame Frances Gardner (1913-89), from 1962 to 1982. They were both prominent physicians with Royal Free connections, and both were appointed by the Senate of the University of London. The Board of Management first included women representatives between 1974 and 1976, Eva D.Alberman 'under special arrangement', and Occupational Health's Muriel L.Newhouse.

The latter also served repeatedly between 1965 and 1976 on the School Council, where she had been preceded by Elinor Meynell (Bacteriology) in 1960–1, and by Margot Jefferys (Sociology) in 1963–4.[25]

Wilson Jameson himself, in his annual reports, repeatedly emphasised the indivisibility of his two offices, as Dean and as Professor and head of the Public Health Division.[26] It was a balancing act which again required all his inherent tact and commonsensical mediating skills in order to keep the peace and good working relations between the older established staff of the original tropical school – what Goodman called the 'glittering products of colonialism'[27] – and the rising stars of the rapidly developing public health disciplines. To his eternal credit, Jameson managed; and the importance of his leadership was reflected in the problems of succession when in 1940, in the first year of the war, he left the School to become Chief Medical Officer to the Ministry of Health. In one sense he kept his connection with the School. Working long hours, and often unable to return to his home in war-torn London, he slept in the School's basement, until even that refuge was denied him by enemy bombs. In 1940, the Chair of Public Health and the office of the Dean had passed briefly to G.S.Parkinson; and when Brigadier Parkinson in turn moved on to direct the Public Health Subcommission, Allied Control Commission, Italy, the LSHTM had for a short period as acting dean a senior professor from outside the department of public health. The difficulties experienced in solving that particular problem have been described above (Chapter 4).

Jameson's further and very distinguished career has been documented in detail elsewhere.[28] His influence at the Ministry of Health and the Ministry of Education was considerable; his impact on the creation of the National Health Service was decisive and lasting, setting a seal on the busy years spent establishing academic public health as an integral part of a unique institution, the LSHTM.

In the spring of 1944, at the height of discussions on the government White Paper on the National Health Service, it fell to Wilson Jameson to defend the government's plans in public. In a measured statement, he made a special effort to consider the possible responses of both the public and the medical profession, and to assure both parties that the proposed scheme would be in the best interests of everybody: that patients would be served by their doctors backed by 'good specialists, good hospitals, good pathology, and x-rays ...'; and that for his part the doctor would enjoy an improved career structure, with 'enough financial assurance ... to free him from being harassed and restricted in the work he is doing ...'.[29] He did not succeed in convincing everybody. The policy was not flawless, and the debate was destined to rumble on, however subdued for long periods, until it has erupted again with full force, fuelled by party-political arguments, in the latter decades of the twentieth century.

MACKINTOSH AND AFTER: 1945-67

By the end of the war, stability returned to the Department of Public Health. Major Greenwood had been relieved of the yoke of the deanship (cf. Chapter 4) when James Macalister Mackintosh, Professor of Public Health from October, 1944, took over as Dean in January, 1945. Mackintosh (1891–1966), who came to the School after a distinguished career in the RAMC during World War I, and after obtaining the DPH after demobilisation, as MOH in various counties until he returned to his native Scotland in 1937 as Chief Medical Officer of Health for Scotland. Four years later, he was appointed Professor of Public Health in the University of Glasgow, leaving in 1944 for the LSHTM. He was to be the last dean to combine the office with that of the Chair of Public Health.[30]

At the end of his first year at the School, J.M.Mackintosh took stock of the activities in his department. With teaching suspended during the war, staff members away on active service, and no member of the teaching staff remaining at the School, the department in that first year functioned mainly in an advisory capacity for former students and public health departments throughout the country. The main concern was preparation for an anticipated heavy influx of students following the period of demobilisation. Thirty ex-servicemen were enrolled for the first diploma course which began in November, 1945; with the accelerating pace of demobilisation over the next three months, and applications from serving men and women returning from overseas, a duplicate course was organised to begin in April, 1946. At the same time the Rockefeller Foundation, whose European Office had enjoyed the School's hospitality with an office in the Keppel Street building during the war, offered fellowships to a number of students. The Chairman of the Board of Management announced in March, 1946:

> Perhaps the outstanding event of the year was the gift of over £20,000 from the Rockefeller Foundation to the Public Health Department for the training of picked men who may afterwards reinforce the teaching staff of the School and fill important

vacancies in the Public Health Service. This benefaction is especially welcome at a time when it is urgently necessary to renew recruitment for health appointments which has been suspended for the long period of the war.[31]

On the part of the Rockefeller Foundation it was a gesture of renewed assistance in the post-war revival of the School's Public Health side which it had so generously brought into being in the 1920s. One of the fellowship students was A.L.Cochrane who, influenced by the teaching of Bradford Hill and Donald Reid in Medical Statistics, made good use of the experience in his later work in the Welsh valleys. The Public Health Department then emerged from its wartime hiatus with an unprecedented intake of students, never matched before or since, and a full complement of teaching and research activities for staff and students, for the academic year 1946–7.[32]

The post-war diploma course combined lectures with seminars and discussion groups run by the students of the DPH class themselves. Practical work and fieldwork were carried out with the generous help of local authority health services and health departments. Cooperation with other Schools of the University also grew in the immediate post-war years, especially with the Institute of Child Health and the Postgraduate Medical School at Hammersmith. Significantly, there also began an exchange with the London School of Economics (LSE), which was to influence developments in the department over the next twenty years and more: initially, T.H.Marshall lectured on sociology to the DPH students at the LSHTM; and Mackintosh in turn gave a course of lectures on social medicine at the LSE.[33] The perceived importance of this new approach was reflected in the appointment of J.H.F.Brotherston as lecturer in preventive and social medicine at the School jointly with Guy's Hospital Medical School which, the Dean noted in his report, 'brings together in the School the two streams of postgraduate and undergraduate teaching'.[34] Two years later, Brotherston was Senior Lecturer, and in 1953 Reader, with T.McL.Galloway as Lecturer in the same subject, in his case jointly with the Royal Free Hospital Medical School. These developments formed part of a much broader based post-war move towards emphasis on preventive aspects of medicine, which had been brought on by the necessities and exigencies of war, as well as by the creation of the NHS – all forceful reminders of Manson's original policy statement on the essential need for prevention as well as cures (Chapter 1).

Overall, the department's staff had increased very considerably, and now included appointments in Public Health Engineering and Hospital

Administration, as well as the existing, outside and part-time, lecturers (London MOsH and others) in Public Health Administration and Practice, and in Industrial Health. The diploma course in Public Health Engineering was run on an inter-collegiate basis, with Imperial College in South Kensington.[35]

During the five years in the early 1950s, when Mackintosh was finally allowed to concentrate on the Public Health Department while Andrew Topping took over as full-time Dean, the School continued, especially in its DPH and DTM&H course, to adapt to new perspectives in public health made necessary by the introduction of the NHS at home, and by an increasing awareness of the potential importance of global health policies as introduced in the post-war world by organisations such as the WHO, the Rockefeller Foundation, and various American aid plans. Other factors affecting general attitudes to public health and preventive medicine on a global scale were the early successes of campaigns against certain tropical diseases using newly developed insecticides which will be discussed below.[36]

When James Mackintosh reached retirement age in 1956, the department had recovered well from the forced inactivity of wartime. If there had been no radical changes in teaching and course work for the Academic Diploma in Public Health, there had at least been steady development towards an approach reflecting social and academic changes in the post-war world. The year 1956 also saw the end of the Certificate in Public Health (CPH), which had up until then been awarded at the end of the three months' preliminary course, or first part of, the Academic Postgraduate Diploma in Public Health according to the rules issued by the General Medical Council.[37]

The 1950s and 1960s were above all the decades when emerging 'medical sociology' made its mark in the Public Health movement. Margot Jefferys, who came to the School in 1952 at the instigation of Brotherston, to lecture on Public Health from an economist's point of view, has described at some length her own and others' struggles in their attempts to legitimise 'medical sociology' as an accepted and necessary component, on equal terms with 'social medicine' as defined by the medical profession, in academic teaching and research on public health.[38] This battle for academic acceptance can also be seen as part of a much wider effort on behalf of sociology in general, during its years of growth in popularity reflected in rapid increases in numbers of students, and in the unprecedented student riots of the late 1960s.

During the few years Brotherston spent at the School – he left for a Chair at Edinburgh in 1955 – he began the reshaping of the department of public health which was to continue for subsequent decades. The appointment of Margot Jefferys was one of a number of innovations, which included the gradual introduction of new methods of teaching, involving students from other London Schools and Colleges such as the LSE and the Royal College of Nursing, in joint study groups with LSHTM students. These developments helped to broaden the outlook of teachers and students at a time of rapid expansion, in both relative and absolute terms, in the numbers of foreign and Commonwealth students from developing nations attending the DPH and other more specialised courses. From the late 1940s to the mid-1950s, the ratios of foreign and Commonwealth students at the School jumped from c.45 per cent to c.68 per cent, compared to a fall from c.55 per cent to c.33 per cent for UK citizens, of the total. At the beginning of the 1970s, at the beginning of a new era with a new Dean (Gordon Smith) and new dynamic head of the public health department (J.N.Morris), when the old style MOH was in the process of being replaced by the 'community physician', the ratios had stabilised: 50 per cent of the total number of the School's students came from Britain, 23 per cent from Commonwealth countries, and 27 per cent from foreign countries.[39] India's achievement of independence in 1947 had no significant effect on the numbers of Indian students attending the School. Only later did misguided government guidelines raising fees for overseas students in universities divert significant numbers to American institutions.

According to Margot Jefferys, Brotherston during his short stay at the School was the catalyst necessary to effect the changes to a broader outlook, which acknowledged the importance of cultural factors in health problems in the Western world as well as, and perhaps even more so, in developing countries. The support he received from J.M.Mackintosh she has described as 'willing if passive'.[40] A more positive appreciation of Mackintosh during his last five years as head of the department is recorded by Michael D.Warren, who was a DPH student at the beginning of the 1950s, and was subsequently involved in the department's teaching and research for more than twenty years, until he decided to devote all his time to his Chair in Social Medicine and the Health Services Research Unit at the University of Kent. Warren remembers Mackintosh's lectures – including a course, open to the public, on trends of opinion about public health – as 'outstanding'. Also commendable was the 'considerable choice and flexibility' in elective special subjects – Warren chose industrial health – and the encouragement of student initiative and originality.[41]

Research in the department, between the end of the war and

Mackintosh's departure in the mid-1950s, focused mainly on 'operational', i.e. health services, subjects, exemplified by Brotherston and Cartwright's studies on primary health care, and later Jefferys and Cartwright's study of the health of working mothers and their children. By the time Brotherston and Cartwright left for Edinburgh in 1955, a number of more specialised studies were under way.[42]

The year 1955 did in fact signal a certain amount of upheaval, both in the department and elsewhere in the School. Andrew Topping died, and was followed by one temporary (Bradford Hill) and one short-lived (Sir James Kilpatrick) Dean; neither had the time to make a lasting impact on the running of the School. Within the department, Mackintosh's imminent departure was followed by the appointment of W.S.Walton (1901-79) to the Chair of Public Health. Walton came to the LSHTM from the department of public health at Newcastle. A kindly man, with special interests in medical administration and child health, he was increasingly unhappy in his new position, and the department came to lack the enthusiasm and optimistic taste for change and improvement which had characterised the Mackintosh years. One teaching innovation straddling the years of change-over may be regarded by some as trivial in the context of public health, but it was very relevant to the increase in numbers of overseas students and the broadening of outlook from local to global concerns. In 1953, M.D.Warren was asked to act as tutor to groups of foreign students who, in their first term, had difficulties following the English of their lecturers and course directors, and perhaps also had personal problems adjusting to life in a strange city away from family and familiar surroundings. It was a successful, although not lasting, attempt to deal with a problem which had been in evidence since the early days of the LSHTM, as Major Greenwood had observed in an early Report more than twenty years before.[43]

By all accounts, relations within the department during Walton's tenure were not helped by the presence of Stuart Hinds (1916-83), who had been appointed Reader in Public Health in the year of Mackintosh's retirement. In the words of M.D.Warren:

> Hinds' special interest was in child health and at that time as many of the English doctors started their career in public health as "clinic" doctors this was seen as an important development. However it was to cause difficulty as Stanley Walton ... had been associated with Pence's studies of child health in Newcastle and considered child health to be one of his special areas; he was also critical of the appointment of the reader before his arrival at the

School. Furthermore Hinds did not have the DPH [but he *did* have the DTM&H] and had no experience in public health; he became a rather solitary figure in the department.

This unfortunate rift between the Head of Department and his Reader may also have short-circuited a potentially important initiative by Hinds following his arrival at the School. With Dr.A.S.Watts, who had been a colleague at Hammersmith Hospital after they both left the forces at the end of World War II, Hinds arranged for a party of students on the DPH course to spend a day at Mortimer, near Reading, to observe a new health centre at work: the Mortimer was one of the very early joint practices which incorporated district nurses and health visitors, and which also had its own pharmacy with a resident pharmacist. The project was perceived at the time as a considerable success by all involved, but was never repeated – perhaps because of the prevailing tensions within the department.[44]

The presence of Hinds, who was to remain in the department as a lone and increasingly isolated figure until the change-over to J.N.Morris's 'social medicine' in 1967, contributed to what appears to have been for Walton a growing state of paranoia, a feeling that both staff within his own department, and senior staff in other departments were 'turning against' him, and comparing the performance of the department unfavourably with achievements in Mackintosh's time. Matters were brought to a head by criticism of the DPH course voiced by two former students in the pages of the *Lancet* in January, 1961. It contained an objective analysis of the School's DPH course, factual information concerning the curriculum, numbers of students and their backgrounds, the variety and commitment of teachers, and a critical assessment of the subjects taught and methods of instruction.[45]

Today, the article seems mild enough, and largely justified; Walton chose to see it as 'unforgivable treachery', and even suspected staff members of complicity, although this seems unlikely.[46] Its publication certainly further soured what were already difficult relations in the department, although on a number of the points raised concerning the course, changes were already being considered.

The School's Development Policy documents for the two quinquennia covering the period 1957–67 reflect the search for lasting and definitive changes, which would enable public health education to meet the demands of increased expectations in the network of health services developing rapidly on a number of levels throughout the world. As did the School's Annual Reports, the policy statements sought to identify areas in particular need of development. One obvious one was occupational health, with its core of industrial health and training for examination for the Diploma of Industrial Health of the Conjoint Board and the Society of Apothecaries.

Already in 1955, developments in occupational health at the School had been given realistic and important help by the Rockefeller Foundation, the benefactor which had made the creation of the LSHTM possible in the 1920s, and which had continued to give support to the School, and its students and staff, in a number of ways over the years. With an initial Rockefeller grant of £15,000 over five years, the Rockefeller Unit of Occupational Health was established with R.S.F.Schilling (1911–97) as University Reader (Professor, 1959) and Director in September, 1956. It replaced a previous 'Sub-unit', run jointly with Applied Physiology and Public Health and linked with the Slough Industrial Health Service.[47] The same Quinquennium forecast emphasised the need for expansion of the existing elective courses in tropical hygiene and child health, given jointly by the department with the Department of Tropical Hygiene and the Institute of Child Health, respectively. Also singled out for expansion of teaching capacity was the subject of mental health.

Five years later, another Development Policy Statement for the Quinquennium 1962–7 was prepared in response to a request from the University Grants Committee after a visit to the School in early 1960.[48] It was a policy statement which defined in general terms the developments in the School's objectives over the years, and put in perspective the relationship between the tropical side and its public health counterpart, both within the School, and in the wider context of global concerns:

> As countries develop, their health problems change in kind and in magnitude; and advances in medicine and science create new methods of study and prevention of disease. In tropical countries, control of the physical environment is still the chief problem in preventive medicine, whereas in temperate and more developed countries, where the worst defects of the physical environment have been rectified, social and occupational environments have become more important. There is, however, *no sharp line between tropical and other countries in these matters;* all Departments of the School are concerned in one way or another with both. ....[49]

After summing up the teaching needs and objectives of the DPH and DTM&H courses and their students in a changing world, the policy statement looked to the future, and to the growth areas which would require increased attention:

> As the acute killing diseases come under control, chronic diseases and the diseases of older people will need more intensive study. Changes in social patterns are changing the emphasis of preventive medicine. *Epidemiology* (in the new sense of the word which no longer relates only to infectious diseases) is growing fast. It requires *men with clinical training for medical survey work, and also experts in the advanced statistical methods now used in both laboratory and field research.* The developing countries are recognising the value of vital statistics and of field surveys.[50]

Finally, the statement also pointed to practical problems. One was of space: with growing numbers of students and research activities, costly rebuilding must be considered. Another problem shared by all schools within the University of London, and indeed by most redbrick universities, was student welfare, above all housing. It is a problem which still shows no sign of being within sight of a satisfactory solution.

The report's attempt at clarification of the teaching policies of the School was also reflected in the School Council's response to the recommendations of the Royal Commission on Medical Education 1965-8 (Todd Committee).[51] The Council not surprisingly endorsed the Report's support for continuing British involvement in research in tropical medicine. It also declared a particular interest in the stress laid on the need for more extensive training in epidemiology and community medicine, and on the development of community and administrative medicine as specialties, areas already under scrutiny within the DPH curriculum. On the other hand, the Council was obviously disappointed to note that

> The Royal Commission (para.52) does not appear to have appreciated the scope or potentialities of occupational medicine in which the School is playing a leading role.

J.N.MORRIS AND SOCIAL MEDICINE

However, all the cautious recommendations of the later 1960s were soon to be overtaken by vigorous sweepings of new brooms when Stanley Walton retired and was succeeded by Jeremy N.Morris on October 1st,

1967. It was an event which marked the end of an era, for the School and for the department, and for its DPH. At the end of Walton's last year in the department, the Annual Report had detailed the DPH course arrangements in full. When J.N.Morris joined the department, he brought with him the MRC's Social Medicine Research Unit of which he remained Director. Following his appointment, the Dean, at a special staff meeting, made the surprise announcement that the School had agreed that all of the present academic staff would leave the department to make way for the MRC Unit. Only Sidney Chave (1914–85) remained and, until 1971, M.D.Warren, who eased the transition from DPH to M.Sc. course and taught the last batch of DPH students during 1967–8, since 'Morris insisted that he would not be associated with any DPH course', but wanted a year free of students in order to plan and negotiate a completely new degree.[52] In his first annual report from the department, Professor Morris wrote:

> The major concern ... has been the design of the course for the M.Sc. in social medicine recently instituted by the University. During recent years the School has tried to adapt the DPH to meet changing needs, but it became clear that an entirely new and longer course is necessary: this was the stage at which Professor Morris was invited to become head of the department. The M.Sc.in social medicine will aim to provide professional training for doctors wishing to specialise in social medicine and to follow careers either in medical administration or in teaching and research. With common training it will be possible for medical administrators to move from one part of the Health Service to another and easier for them to interchange with academic appointments.

and further:

> .... The course will ... include nine to twelve months of project work in an academic or service unit under the supervision of a local preceptor and the School tutor. ... To accommodate this period of fieldwork the course will last *two calendar years*. The course was planned before we had any idea of the Todd proposals; it turned out that the M.Sc. course closely resembled the Royal Commission's recommendations for a *minimum period of two years' specialist training*. ...

> The new M.Sc. represents a considerable act of faith; ...[53]

It was Morris's credo for teaching in his new department. Over the following decade, the new M.Sc. in social medicine was established as an integral part of the School's public health education, with its first year devoted to theoretical teaching, and the second to epidemiological fieldwork, completed by the preparation of a final dissertation. Morris had studied a large sample of MOH's and RMO's Reports, and met many of them individually and in groups. He had been struck by the virtual absence in their work of reference to epidemiology, which he considered the basic science of Public Health. A year's practical experience under guidance was regarded by him as an essential part of basic training. The Ministry of Health and the Regional Authorities agreed, and readily provided the necessary financial backing; Spooner, Dean at the time, supported the plans enthusiastically. At the same time, relationships were re-established with the London School of Economics, involving both its Department of Sociology (Professors Macrae and Glass), and of Social Administration (Professors Titmuss and Abel-Smith). The new M.Sc. course then was designed to meet the needs of a new breed of community physicians and medical administrators with much wider terms of reference than the old style MOH. The need for such a change in approach was felt at the time not only in Britain, but also in a number of other countries.

Morris felt equally strongly about research in his new department, where R.F.L.Logan was brought in to head a team (initially funded by the Ministry of Health in the absence of university grants) in the 'Organisation of Medical Care Unit'. Here also epidemiology had to be a critical input. The knowledge which was lacking, and which an increasingly well-informed public was now beginning to demand, reflected population needs for health and social care, and the impact on communities of such services.

The 'Chronic Disease Control Unit' of the Ministry of Health, also housed in the department, was carrying out two studies both concerned with screening practices, yet very different in their aims and focus. One study aimed at evaluating the relative acceptabilities to women of three different methods used in screening for pre-cancerous and early cancerous lesions of the uterus. The second study involved comparisons of a number of screening tests for remediable defects of vision, heating, and mobility, and of income support in the elderly. In the 'Human Genetics Unit' J.H.Renwick (1926–94) reassembled in London a research team concerned with location of gene loci on chromosomes, similar to the team he had headed in Glasgow before coming to London. He had arrived at the

School in the same year as J.N.Morris, when the University of London established a Readership in human genetics within the Department of Public Health. In common with many other disciplines at the School, Renwick's received MRC support. A Captain in the RAMC during the Korean War (1950–3), he had begun his research career studying genetically expressed effects of the atomic bomb in Hiroshima in the early 1950s. When, after ten years, his unit was re-styled the 'Preventive Teratology Unit', Renwick became Professor of Genetics and Teratology.

Finally, Morris's original MRC 'Social Medicine Unit' continued its long-term studies on the epidemiology and prevention of cardiovascular diseases, on lifestyle and health in middle age, on social conditions and population health; and a different, if cognate, study of juvenile delinquency, its causes and predictability, in London's East End, based at the London Hospital, the Unit's previous home.[54] One long-term study of particular importance was representative of the department's research ethos and its continuing emphasis on the epidemiology of cardiovascular disease: the pioneering studies on the role of exercise in protection against heart-attack. The Unit first demonstrated this in studies of physically active workers (e.g. London bus conductors and postmen) as opposed to their sedentary counterparts. At the School this was extended to an examination of the effects of leisure-time activities in sedentary workers: executive-grade civil servants engaging in aerobic exercise of moderate intensity such as swimming, brisk walking, cycling, were protected in the same way as men physically active in their jobs. Yet another aspect of cardiovascular disease research in the Unit involved studies of effects of levels of mineral content in drinking water in 'hard' and 'soft' water areas of the country. People living in 'hard' water areas were found to be substantially protected by comparison with those in the 'soft' water areas of the North and of Scotland – intriguing observations which as yet have proved impossible to explain – or indeed disprove.[55]

At the time Morris set out his aims, hopes and objectives in his early annual reports, he also found the time to deliver a seminal lecture at the School's American counterpart, the Johns Hopkins School of Hygiene and Public Health. Here John Brotherston had, in a sense, cut his public health teeth, taking a doctorate in public health; now Morris, venting his strong socialist belief in adequate health care for all, introduced the concept of the 'community physician' as an 'administrator of local services, epidemiologist, and community counsellor', with much wider points of reference than the old style MOH, and ready to respond to his patients in a world of changes in medical needs, clinical practice, and prevention policies. He pointed to the need for an 'effective intelligence system' to underpin the local medical services. It was essentially an introduction to an American audience of a British view of the impact of the National Health Service since its initiation more than twenty years earlier. Morris concluded by expressing his own faith in the new style community physician and his potential for 'reducing suffering and improving the quality of life'; he also rejoiced in 'our good fortune to be able in this field to combine medicine and social science in public service'.[56]

The community physician, and community health care in a broader context as developed over the years within and without the School, set the seal on work by a long line of physicians, whose social conscience had led them into public health work and the development of the discipline of 'Social Medicine'. From John Ryle (1889–1950) and Wilson Jameson to Brotherston and Morris, they had worked unceasingly to educate the public, the politicians, and the medical profession, in order to increase general awareness of the social context of health and disease. The new two-year M.Sc. course, designed by Morris and his staff, was introduced in 1969. M.D.Warren has described it as in a way 'a combination of a one-year taught Master's degree and a one-year research Master's degree'. Intended to train a new breed of community physicians in preparation also for the changes at home to the National Health Service structure discussed in two Green Papers, a consultative document, and a White Paper, between 1968 and 1972, the M.Sc. course also heralded a gradual replacement, in departments throughout the School, of academic diplomas by M.Sc. degrees, although at the time only that in Social Medicine required a course lasting two academic years.[57]

As had been the case with the old DPH course, other departments in the School contributed to the Social Medicine course; not only Medical Statistics and Epidemiology, which by now included Medical Demography, and Medical Microbiology, but also Human Nutrition. It was no coincidence that B.S.Platt (1903–69), the chemist who became the first Professor of Human Nutrition at the LSHTM when that department was created after the war, had made observations on his subject which echoed J.N.Morris's closing remarks in his Johns Hopkins lecture, and in the same year, 1969. In what became Platt's last lecture to students in the Nutrition department, he emphasised the need to see 'the science and logistics of nutrition as inseparable from economics and sociology as well as from medicine and health'.[58]

For ten years the course, and other teaching and research in the department, flourished under the dedicated leadership of Morris. The department continued to expand. At the beginning of the 1970s, it acquired a Professor of Social Psychiatry, with junior positions added over the next few years; and in 1972 the Centre for Extension Training in Community Medicine, with Roy Acheson as Director and Professor of Public Health, was set up following negotiations with the DHSS, for the continuing education of health professionals in the field. After Acheson left for Cambridge in 1976, the Centre carried on under an 'Acting Director', R.J.Donaldson, until Morris retired in 1978.

During his last five years as Director, Morris's Chair became the Chair of Community Health, in the Department of Community Health, in keeping with national nomenclature. At the end of the 1970s, with Morris retiring, his MRC unit being disbanded, and restructuring of the NHS causing uncertainties with regard to the DHSS funding, which was of major importance for the financing of the department, there were also difficulties concerning the choice of the successor to the Chair.[59] M.D.Warren, who had by then been at Kent since 1971, was approached by the Dean, Gordon Smith, to fill the gap. Warren was reluctant; he was happy with his position at Kent, and was reluctant to take on what was seen as a 'caretaker' appointment in a department which was, for financial and other reasons, in some difficulty.[60] When Warren did after all acquiesce, he soon found that he had made the wrong decision, and left the following year to return to a new post at Kent. With Dame Rosemary Rue as part-time Director on secondment from the Oxford Regional Health Authority the department survived another year until finally settling down, in 1982, with Patrick Hamilton as Director and Professor of Community Medicine.[61]

At the end of the Morris years, the two-year M.Sc. course which he had championed tirelessly was changed back to its former one-year duration. Morris, who as Emeritus Professor still takes a lively interest in School matters, and is active in the Health Promotion Sciences Unit, has never ceased regretting this return to a one-year course, a development he considers to be an unfortunate backwards step and a deviation from the standards he had worked so hard to create, and which he has seen vindicated in many noteworthy career achievements by former graduate students across the world.[62] Others saw those developments as not only inevitable, but 'necessary and desirable' in view of other circumstances: the DHSS funded bursaries for students on two-year courses were withdrawn in 1978, and the new regional health authorities preferred to second newly appointed registrars on courses for one year only. At the same time, the second year's 'fieldwork' requirement could be met, it was hoped, by the specialist training programme instituted by the newly created Faculty of Community Medicine as part II of its membership examination.[63]

When Patrick Hamilton returned to the School in 1982 (he had been a senior lecturer in the Department of Medical Statistics and Epidemiology from 1967 to 1974), he had spent the intervening years as Director of the WHO Caribbean Epidemiology Centre in Trinidad, pursuing the tropical epidemiology which was his main interest. Back at the School, he threw himself into the major and much needed reorganisation which was then in progress not only in the Department of Community Medicine, but throughout the LSHTM. Because of the short-sighted Government policy on overseas students' fees and its effect on the School's financial support from the UGC and other government sources, there had been reductions in numbers of permanent staff, and even inability to fill no less than five vacant Chairs. In response to recommendations of a Working Party, the School emerged in 1982 with an entirely new structure, its formerly more or less autonomous departments and units accommodated within three Divisions under Divisional Chairmen.[64] Division III, 'Community Health', with Hamilton as Chairman, comprised the departments of Community Health, Human Nutrition, Occupational Health, the Evaluation and Planning Centre from the Ross Institute, and Renwick's Preventive Teratology Unit, which had first appeared as a separate unit in the year of Morris's retirement, 1978.

In six short years, before his much too early death in Africa at the age of 53, Patrick Hamilton rebuilt the Department of Community Health and improved both teaching and research by establishing links with the NHS regions and districts, and opening up wider connections with developing schools of public health in Europe as well as with the Overseas Development Administration. It was his dedication to tropical medicine which indirectly led to his death in Ougadougou in June, 1988. He had gone there, in spite of medical advice to the contrary, to fulfil obligations to the WHO Onchocerciasis Control Programme.[65]

In the year of Hamilton's death, and Gordon Smith's last year as Dean – and after little more than six years of the Divisional system, there was another radical change to the School's structure. The three Divisions formed in 1981–2 now became four Departments of a very different complexion, with far-reaching changes to both research and teaching programmes, and a revised Institutional Plan approved by the Board of Management in June, 1989. In this later development, 'Community Health' again disappeared from the terminology describing the activities of the LSHTM's departments. Until 1996 there were four major departments, with no less than twenty-one separate units between them; and 'Community Health' has reverted to a major 'Department of Public

Health and Policy', consisting of five units: 'Environmental Epidemiology'; 'Health Policy'; 'Health Promotion Sciences'; 'Health Services Research'; and 'Human Nutrition'. The very latest restructuring in 1996–7 (Chapter 12), with three major departments replacing the previous four, saw the 'Health Promotion Sceinces' become 'Health Promotion Research' and 'Human Nutrition' (Professor P.S.Shetty) moved to the Department of Epidemiology and Population Health. Within such a framework, students are able, throughout the School and its M.Sc. courses, to exercise a degree of choice in creating their programmes within the fifteen named M.Sc. courses offered at present.[66] In addition to the last remaining diploma course, in Tropical Medicine and Hygiene, there are also shorter courses throughout the four departments, ranging in duration from 1 to 6 weeks.

In this form, the department, in the decade leading up to the School's centenary, has been developing the restructuring which began when Patrick Vaughan, Professor of Health Care Epidemiology, was its head between 1989 and 1993 and continued under Charles Normand, Professor of Health Policy, and from 1997 under Professor N.A.Black, Professor of Health Services Research. With an ever growing number of chairs, several occupied by women, in old and particularly in new aspects of epidemiology, public health and nutrition, which would have surprised staff members in early days of the School, the department hopes to maintain a definitive influence in the developing world by applying research methodology successfully used in the developed world decades earlier; at the same time, it is realised that data there will be more difficult to obtain.

In its efforts to coordinate its many diverse interests, and provide support for its many research units, and with an economist at its head, the department is placing increasing emphasis on building up its strength in economics. It is also obtaining large research grants for many projects from an impressive range of national and international bodies: e.g., the UK Departments of Health and of the Environment support a Small Area Health Statistics Unit; the NW Thames Regional Health Authority and the Health Education Authority support projects in a Health Promotion Sciences Unit, and the ODA (now DfiD) supports work in a number of units.[67]

As the School moves towards its centenary, and the world towards another millennium, public health problems are as acute as ever, and the department's research and teaching continues to expand in its many areas of interest in global health care and policy studies, although the vitally important Centre for Population Studies is a unit in the Department of

PREVENTION AND CURE

Epidemiology and Population Sciences. The Policy studies so central to planning for the future, have been exemplified in recent years by the major historical study, with outside funding over the past five years, on the development of policies designed to counter the threat of AIDS.[68] Such studies, using the School resources and experience in the field, will become increasingly important in the future, especially in the context of, and against the background of, Medical Demography and family and population planning. In all these areas, students and library users in general can refer to a growing volume of information technology available in the LSHTM Library, where the latest additions the databases include the compact disc *Popline* with bibliographic information on population and family planning.[69] Hence the Library joins with all the units of the four major Departments of the LSHTM in the 1990s, to demonstrate the basic indivisibility of, and the continuing importance of successful interrelations between, all the subjects representing the rich diversity of a School concerned with teaching and research in Public Health on a global scale.

NOTES

[1] From the extensive literature on cholera and the public health in the nineteenth century may be cited:
Asa Briggs, 'Cholera and society in the nineteenth century', *Past and Present,* 1961, *19:*76–96;
Margaret Pelling, *Cholera, fever and English medicine 1825–65*, Oxford University Press, 1978;
Anne Hardy, 'Cholera, quarantine and the English preventive system, 1850–95', *Medical History,* 1993, *37:*250–69;
and on the Diploma in Public Health:
Dorothy Watkins, The English revolution in social medicine, 1889–1911, Ph.D.thesis, University of London, 1984;
Roy Acheson, 'The British Diploma in Public Health: birth and adolescence', in: *A history of education in public health,* E.Fee and R.Acheson (eds), Oxford University Press, 1991;
idem, 'The British Diploma in Public Health: heyday and decline', *ibid.*

[2] W.M.Frazer, *Duncan of Liverpool,* London, Hamilton Medical, 1947; Royston Lambert, *Sir John Simon 1816–1904 and English Social Administration,* London, MacGibbon and Kee, 1963.

[3] G.S.Graham-Smith, 'George Henry Falkiner Nuttall', *J.Hyg.,* 1938, *38:*129–40.

[4] C.D.Lycett, *The Royal Institute of Public Health and Hygiene,* London, The Institute, c1986.

[5] Neville M.Goodman, *Wilson Jameson, Architect of National Health*, London, Allen and Unwin, 1970.

[6] *ibid.,* p.41; Kenwood obituaries, *Lancet,* 1945, *i:*804; and *Br.med.J.,* 1945, *i:*890.

[7] The first edition, written with F.T.Merchant, was published in 1920; in later editions Jameson collaborated with G.S.Parkinson.

[8] Letter from Kenwood, dated London 29.12.1927, LSHTM archives, MSS FA: D1 (4);
Newman quoted by Goodman, op.cit. note 5, p.57.

[9] R.E.O.Williams, *Microbiology for the Public Health. The evolution of the Public Health Laboratory Service 1939–80,* London PHLS, 1985.

[10] LSHTM *Annual Report* 1937–8, pp.3–4.

[11] LSHTM *Annual Report* 1937–8; C.M.Clark and J.M.Mackintosh, *The School and the Site,* London, H.K.Lewis & Co.Ltd., 1954, pp.73–4.

[12] LSHTM *Annual Report* 1939–40, p.9.

[13] LSHTM *Annual Report* 1928–9, pp.9–10.

[14] We are grateful to Crowden's son, Captain G.Crowden, for the

manuscript of his 'First Class Return – Ossett to London via Ypres', article for Koyli Regimental Magazine, September 1990, and other personal information;
The Times obituary, 5 August, 1966.
[15] A 'Sub-unit' of occupational health had been established as early as 1950, see below.
[16] LSHTM *Annual Reports* 1932-3, pp.10-13, and 1939-40, p.13;
Cyril C.Barnard, 'History of the Library', LSHTM pamphlet, 1947; Barnard was School Librarian from 1921 until 1959; Brian Furner, present School Librarian, personal communication, February 1994.
[17] *ibid.*, pp.13-15.
[18] *The School and the Site*, op.cit. note 11, pp.88-93.
[19] LSHTM *Annual Reports* 1937-8 and 1938-9;
The School and the Site, pp.80-3;
W.E.Ormerod, personal communication.
[20] LSHTM *Annual Reports* between 1930 and 1938;
Culpin obituaries, Lancet, 1952, *ii:*543; and *Br.med.J., 1952, ii:*727-8; ABH, p.5.
[21] LSHTM *Annual Report* 1937-8, p.39.
[22] LSHTM *Annual Report* 1946-7, pp.94-8, and Table p.96.
[23] Goodman, op.cit. note 5, pp.61-71;
The School and the Site, op.cit note 11, pp.65-72.
[24] Goodman, p.70.
[25] *The School and the Site,* p.67;
LSHTM *Annual Reports* between 1960 and 1985.
[26] LSHTM *Annual Reports* between 1930 and 1940.
[27] Goodman, op.cit. note 5, p.71.
[28] *ibid.;*
Sir George Godber's article on Jameson in the DNB, 1961-70.
[29] *Lancet,* 1944, *i:*513-14;
for the development of the NHS see Frank Honigsbaum, *Health, Happiness, and Security. The creation of the National Health Service,* London and New York, Routledge, 1989.
[30] Mackintosh obituaries, *Lancet,* 1966, *i:*988-90; and *Br.med.J.* 1966, *i:*1118-19.
[31] LSHTM *Annual Reports* 1944-5, p.9 and pp.20-1, and 1945-6, p.42.
[32] For Cochrane cf. Chapter 4, p.15 and note 37;
LSHTM *Annual Reports* between 1946 and 1951.
[33] LSHTM *Annual Reports* 1946-7, p.63, and 1947-8, p.51.
[34] *ibid.* 1947-8, p.50.
[35] LSHTM *Annual Reports* 1951-2, Appendix 2, p.93, and 1960-1,

Appendix 3, p.128.

[36] James R.Busvine, *Disease Transmission by Insects. Its discovery and 90 years of effort to prevent it,* Berlin etc., Springer-Verlag, 1993.

[37] LSHTM *Annual Report*s 1955–6, pp.10–11, and 1956–7, pp.20–1.

[38] M.Jefferys, 'Serendipity: an autobiographical account of the career of a medical sociologist in Britain', in: *Medical sociologists at work,* R.H.Elling and M.Sokolowska (eds), New Brunswick, New Jersey, Transaction Press, 1978, pp.135–61;

idem, 'Medical sociology and public health: inter-disciplinary relationships, 1950–90' *Public Health,* 1991, *109:*15–21; also personal communication, December, 1993.

[39] LSHTM *Annual Report*s 1950–1, pp.90 and 91; 1960–1, pp.132–3; and 1971–2, p.17.

[40] M.Jefferys, MSS 'Social medicine and medical sociology 1950–1970: the testimony of a partisan participant', p.3.

[41] We are indebted to Professor Warren for personal comments and unpublished 'Reminiscences' of his long connection with the School, which in addition to his appointments included the award of one of five travel scholarships for recent past DPH students, given to the School in memory of Wilson Jameson by his widow, LSHTM *Annual Report* 1965–6, p.17.

The 'open course' was published as the 1951 Heath Clark Lectures: J.M.Mackintosh, 'Trends of opinion about the public health 1901–51', University of London Heath Clark Lectures, London and New York, Oxford University Press, 1953.

[42] *Br.J.Prev.Soc.Med.,* 1958, *12:*159–71, and LSHTM *Annual Report*s.

[43] M.D.Warren, 'Reminiscences', p.1; cf. Major Greenwood in LSHTM *Annual Report* 1928–9, Chapter 4 above, p.11.

[44] Warren as above, p.2;

Hinds obituary, *Lancet,* 1983, *i:*136;

W.E.Ormerod, personal communication.

[45] J.Cohen and A.M.Robertson, 'A postgraduate public-health course from the students' point of view', *Lancet,* 1961, *i:*102–5.

[46] Warren, op.cit. note 43, p.3.

[47] LSHTM *Annual Report* 1955–6, p.19, and LSHTM undated internal document of comments on the quinquennium policy 1957–62, p.8. We are grateful to Professor Warren for the loan of quinquennium policy and related documents.

[48] LSHTM Development Policy, Quinquennium 1962–7, D.P.S.29, p.319.

[49] *ibid..* (authors' italics)

[50] *ibid.,* p.320. (authors' italics)
[51] LSHTM internal comments, prepared for the School Council, on the Report of the Royal Commission on Medical Education 1965-8 (Todd).
[52] Warren, op.cit. note 43, p.4;
On Sidney Chave see: Sidney Chave, *Recalling the Medical Officer of Health,* Writings by Sidney Chave, M.Warren and Huw Francis (eds), King Edward's Hospital Fund for London, 1987, especially *Prologue* by Michael Warren, pp.15-18.
[53] LSHTM *Annual Report* 1967-8, p.79; (authors' italics)
J.N.Morris, personal communications gratefully acknowledged.
[54] LSHTM *Annual Reports* between 1967 and 1977;
LSHTM *Annual Report* 1967-8, p.20;
LSHTM *Annual Report* 1993-4, p.26;
'Professor James Renwick', *The Times* obituary, October 18th 1994;
'James Renwick', *Br.med.J.,* 1995: *310:*187.
M.J.Power, R.T.Benn, and J.N.Morris, 'Neighbourhood, school and juveniles before the courts', *Br.J.Criminol.,* 1972, *13:*111-32;
J.N.Morris's views on the place of epidemiology in public health are represented in his classic textbook, *Uses of epidemiology,* first published in 1957 and running through a number of editions (including Japanese and Spanish translations) and reprints over nearly thirty years, the last in 1985. In 1992 Morris was one of many contributors to *Coronary heart disease epidemiology,* edited by Michael Marmot, Professor of Epidemiology and Public Health at University College, London, and Paul Elliott, Reader, and head of the Environmental Epidemiology Unit in the School's Department of Public Health and Policy.
[55] J.N.Morris, J.A.Heady, P.A.B.Raffle, C.G.Roberts, J.W.Parks, 'Coronary heart disease and physical activity of work', *Lancet,* 1953, *ii:*1053-7, and 1111-20;
J.N.Morris, D.G.Clayton, M.G.Everitt, A.M.Semmence, E.H.Burgess, 'Exercise in leisure-time: coronary heart attack and death rates', *Br.Heart.J.,* 1990, *63:*325-34;
M.D.Crawford, M.J.Gardner, and J.N.Morris, 'Cardiovascular disease and the mineral content of drinking water', *Br.med.Bull.,* 1971, *27:*21-4. The late Margaret Crawford (Lady Crawford at the time of her death in 1973) was the mother of Dorothy Crawford, Professor of Microbiology, and head of the Viral Pathogenesis Unit in the School, 1990-96.
[56] J.N.Morris, 'Tomorrow's community physician', *Lancet,* 1969, *ii:*811-16.
M.D.Warren quotes two more influential papers, i.e.
J.J.A.Reid, 'Future of Public Health', *Br.med.J.,*1964, *ii:*1483-6; and

J.H.F.Brotherston, 'Change and the National Health Service', *Scottish Medical Journal,* 1969, *14:*130-44, and points out that together the three papers reflect '... what we, in the Department of Public Health, were reacting to and were trying to achieve during that decade'.
[57] Warren, op.cit. note 43, pp.4-5;
LSHTM 'Student's Handbook, M.Sc. Social Medicine' between 1970 and 1980, copies kindly supplied by Professor Morris and Professor Warren; LSHTM *Annual Report*s 1970-1 (p.20) to 1977-8, when the Diploma in Tropical Health was also replaced by an M.Sc. degree in Community Health of developing countries; LSHTM *Annual Report* 1973-4, p.25, on implications of NHS reorganisation;
For John Ryle, see
D.Porter, 'Changing disciplines: John Ryle and the making of social medicine in Britain in the 1940s', *Hist.Sci.*, 1992, *30:*137-64;
idem, 'John Ryle: doctor of revolution?', in: *Doctors, politics and society: historical essays,* D.and R.Porter eds, Amsterdam, Rodopi, 1993, pp.247-74.
[58] LSHTM *Annual Report* 1945-6, p.18;
LSHTM *Annual Report* 1968-9, p.18;
Anne Hardy, 'Beriberi, Vitamin B1, and World Food Policy, 1925-1970' *Medical History,* 1995, *39:*61-77.
[59] Warren, op.cit. note 43, pp.5-7.
[60] *ibid.,* p.5.
[61] LSHTM *Annual Report* 1981-2, pp.14-15, and p.20.
[62] Warren, op.cit. note 43, p.7.
[63] *ibid.*
[64] LSHTM *Annual Report* 1981-2, pp.8-21.
[65] LSHTM *Annual Report*s between 1981 and 1988; Hamilton obituary, LSHTM *Annual Report* 1987-8, p.8.
[66] LSHTM *Annual Report*s between 1988 and 1992; Research Reports 1990 and 1992. Course descriptions in LSHTM *Annual Report* 1991-2, p.27 and p.30.
[67] Charles Normand, personal communication;
LSHTM *Annual Report*s and Research Reports, 1990-5.
[68] Virginia Berridge, 'AIDS, the media and health policy', *Health educ.J.,* 1991, *50:*179-85;
AIDS and Contemporary History, Virginia Berridge and Philip Strong (eds), Cambridge History of Medicine Series, CUP, 1993.
[69] 'Academic services offered by the Library', LSHTM *Annual Report* 1991-2, p.30.

7

THE WIDER SPECTRUM OF PUBLIC HEALTH: BASIC RESEARCH IN DEVELOPING BIOCHEMISTRY; AND APPLIED SCIENCE AND STATISTICS IN OCCUPATIONAL HEALTH

When the LSHTM opened its doors in Keppel Street in 1929, one of its six divisions represented the one basic science which had been an integral and necessary part of the public health movement back in the nineteenth century: chemistry. In those days, the old science of chemistry and the new science of bacteriology had gone hand in hand in the primary quest for pure and safe water supplies. In Keppel Street in 1929, chemistry shared a division with its rapidly growing offspring, biochemistry; and before long, when 'divisions' were replaced by 'departments', '... the Department of Chemistry as Applied to Hygiene [was] merged in the Department of Biochemistry'.[1] By then on the other hand, chemistry was back in the spotlight of concern with pure water supplies, both in teaching and research.

Nevertheless, it was clear from the beginning that within the LSHTM biochemistry had not only caught up with, but had overtaken in importance for public health, its parent discipline of pure chemistry. The University Professor and Director of the Department of Biochemistry and Chemistry as Applied to Hygiene at the new School, appointed in 1929, was Harold Raistrick (1890–1971), who in the development of his career had reflected the complex changes affecting relationships between chemistry, biochemistry, and public health, in the early decades of the twentieth century.

Already at school Raistrick had shown marked interest in, and ability for, the subject of chemistry. At Leeds University he was particularly influenced by J.B.Cohen (1859–1935), whose enthusiasm for natural products chemistry turned many a student in the direction of the emerging discipline of biochemistry. On the other hand, inorganic and analytical chemistry were by no means neglected; and Harold Raistrick, alone in his year, decided to train for the post of Public Analyst, the statutory requirement being a Diploma in the Chemistry (including Microscopy) of Food, Drugs and Water (Branch E) of the Institute (later Royal Institute) of Chemistry.[2] With this qualification, and having obtained his honours degree and spent an additional year as a research student at Cambridge, Raistrick was all set to go to Emil Fischer's laboratory at Berlin with a Board of Agriculture and Fisheries Research

Scholarship when World War I broke out in 1914. Prevented from active service by a physical disability, he stayed in the School of Agriculture at Cambridge. Then, in 1915, the newly established Medical Research Committee awarded him a grant for work under the direction of Gowland Hopkins (1861–1947) who was a Committee member, on products of bacterial action. It was work which came to define Raistrick's research interests for the rest of his life; and incidentally, the main study in Gowland Hopkins's laboratory at this time, on breakdown products of tryptophan and other amino-acids by bacteria, was closely related to the work, denied him by the war, in Emil Fischer's laboratory in Berlin.[3]

At the end of World War I, the continued need to keep abreast of developments in Germany's explosives industry led Nobel's Explosives Company, in Ayrshire, to create a new research department of applied biochemistry. On the recommendation of Gowland Hopkins, Raistrick was put in charge of this department in January, 1921. Here he embarked on the study of new organic compounds produced by fermentation of moulds.[4] Building on earlier German industrial research, he and his co-workers began commercially important studies on production of citric and oxalic acids by micro-fungi, and on glycerol production by fermentation, important for the explosives industry. When Raistrick resigned from ICI (Nobel's Explosives Company had in 1926 become part of the newly formed Imperial Chemical Industries) in 1929 in order to accept the University of London Chair of Biochemistry tenable at the LSHTM, it was understood that the main function of his Division would be the research into the biochemistry of microorganisms which he had so successfully begun. Formal teaching commitments were restricted to instruction in bacteriological chemistry for the few postgraduate students preparing for the academic Diploma in Bacteriology. These specifications with regard to both research and teaching placed not only Raistrick, but also the very subject 'biochemistry' in an anomalous and isolated position within the departmental structure of the developing School. 'Biochemistry' came to be viewed with suspicion in other departments; one unfortunate result was the difficulties experienced by staff elsewhere, who legitimately wanted to use a biochemical approach in other work: W.E.Ormerod in Medical Protozoology, with a degree in chemistry in addition to his medical qualifications, can comment with hindsight on the unique – and difficult – part played by Raistrick and his Biochemistry Department within the School. He still laments the 'gulf in understanding' between Raistrick's department and the rest of the School, caused largely by his difficult personality as well as misunderstandings surrounding the term 'biochemistry' at the time, when Raistrick's subject would have been better described as 'natural product chemistry'. Ormerod's own efforts to introduce biochemistry into the curriculum for the Diploma in Applied Parasitology and Entomology (DAP&E, later to become a M.Sc. in Medical Parasitology) were hampered by the existence of 'an active department of so-called Biochemistry in the School' which would have nothing to do with the diploma course.[5]

The teaching of chemistry to the DPH students was the responsibility of Max Everard Delafield (1886–1974), Professor of Chemistry as Applied to Hygiene. Raistrick had not in fact been the first choice for the Chair and the Division. Percival Hartley, ten years' his senior and Henry Dale's collaborator both at the Wellcome Physiological Research Laboratories and at the MRC's NIMR at Mill Hill, had initially been selected for the post, but immediately fell ill and resigned. Although his health was 'restored after a [short] period of rest and quiet', he did not offer to return, and Raistrick was appointed. Bradford Hill put it more bluntly: '... it was Percival Hartley who withdrew and stayed with Dale at the NIMR'.[6]

Once installed, Raistrick ran the Division – later the Department – for the better part of thirty years, until he retired in 1956. The School thus became the setting for the best of his mature work, and for fruitful collaboration with other Fellows of the Royal Society (Raistrick became an FRS in 1934): with Robert Robinson and Alexander Todd, and within the School with W.W.C.Topley and Graham Wilson on immunological chemistry. On the other hand, during the 1930s Raistrick also suffered what more than one observer have called the disappointments of his career. Bradford Hill wrote: ' [He] was I think a disappointed man – he missed out on the biochemistry of penicillin ... and introduced some drug for the common cold which was useless. ...'[7]

In the case of penicillin, Raistrick's successor in the Chair, J.H.Birkinshaw (1894–1995), later wrote: 'In 1932, an investigation on the production of Fleming's antibiotic penicillin showed that the substance was produced on a synthetic culture medium and that it was extractable from the aqueous medium by ether. Raistrick's decision not to proceed further with this investigation was due to several factors: (a) the extreme instability of penicillin in aqueous solution to acid, alkali and bacterial decomposition compared with the recently discovered prontosil, (b) its unsuitability as a research subject for Ph.D. students, (c) the advice of medical friends that penicillin *could never be of practical use in clinical medicine* because of its instability.'[8] Sir Edward Abraham, who during the war became closely involved in Florey's successful efforts to produce and purify penicillin, and later developed cephalosporin, points to another limiting factor in Raistrick's research. He was, according to Sir Edward, always preoccupied with the production of crystals and their analysis and, as Ronald Hare also noted, as a chemist was 'primarily interested in the products produced by moulds that could be isolated by the *ordinary chemical processes,* purified and if possible crystallised.' Although he and his co-workers at the School learned much about the properties of penicillin, they ' ... got no nearer to the evolution of a method for its purification than Ridley and Craddock. It may well be asked why they stopped when they did'. Frederick Ridley and Stuart Craddock, both recently qualified, had worked with Fleming at St.Mary's on lysozyme in tears, and were called upon to help with the chemical problem of purification, concentration and stabilisation of penicillin in 1929–30. Hare discussed the reasons why their work never became generally known: 'Both of them worked hard and made many significant advances, most of which were neither published nor referred to by Fleming. ...' Even two years later, when the chemist Lewis B.Holt joined the inoculation department and was asked by Fleming, in the words of Hare, to 'add his name to the rapidly lengthening list of those who had attempted to purify and concentrate penicillin', Fleming failed to inform him in any way of the work of Ridley and Craddock, in his own laboratory, two years earlier. In 1975 Ridley (1903–77) wrote down his own version of the sorry sequence of events in a letter to N.G.Heatley. In it he quotes Holt as saying: 'It is quite incredible, if I had known what you had done, I would have had Pen[icillin] out in a few weeks.'[9] The solution to the problems of producing pure and stable penicillin was finally achieved in Florey's laboratories in Oxford only in response to the exigencies of war in the early 1940s.

The second 'disappointment' of Raistrick's career involved the work of a number of colleagues, and could and should have been avoided were it not for the urge to publish prematurely results which had not been checked and double-checked as rigorously and carefully as might have been expected of scientists of the calibre of Raistrick, Gye, and Greenwood.[10] In the *Lancet* in 1943, it was boldly headlined: 'Patulin in the Common Cold'; it is probably no coincidence that when Birkinshaw wrote Raistrick's 'Biographical Memoir' for the Royal Society in 1972, he gave only the subtitle of 'Collaborative research on patulin, a derivative of *Penicillium patulum* Bainier' for the paper in the accompanying bibliography.[11] If W.E.Gye, supplied with a quantity of patulin by Raistrick, for chemotherapeutic tests in cancer, had not been suffering from a severe cold at the time, and decided to douche his nasal passages with a watery solution of the substance, all concerned would have been saved a good deal of embarrassment. But he did, and recovered, which he would undoubtedly have done anyway. The ensuing 'preliminary trials in the common cold' gave mixed results, although Gye chose to refer to them as 'strikingly successful'. His co-authors were rather more careful, and after that initial paper, no more was ever heard of the putative value of patulin treatment in the common cold. Unfortunately, in the wake of the early penicillin successes in Oxford, it was widely read and is still remembered by contemporaries as a resounding and embarrassing fiasco.[12]

Fortunately research in the department also yielded many successes. The work of Raistrick and his staff on griseofulvin, mould tropolones, tetronic acids, and quinones, defined important structures; some of these, and especially griseofulvin, proved to be of use as fungicides both against plant diseases, and in the treatment of human fungus infections. In an obituary notice in *The Times* in March, 1971, E.B.Chain (1906–79), who could by then afford to be magnanimous, wrote of Raistrick that he was ' ... one of the finest natural products chemists this country has ever produced. He became the internationally acknowledged pioneer and leader in a large and very fertile field of natural products chemistry which is still very far from being exhausted, that of the metabolic products of the lower fungi, of which some of the most important antibiotics form part.'[13]

Raistrick retired in 1956, and was succeeded in the Chair by J.H.Birkinshaw, Reader in the department, who had worked closely with Raistrick since their early days with the Nobel Explosives Company. When Birkinshaw in turn was due to retire in 1962, the School's Development Policy document for the quinquennium 1962–7 said of biochemistry: 'In 1962, the present Professor of Biochemistry retires. Future policy with regard to Biochemistry will have to be defined, bearing in mind the growing complexity of the biochemical needs of other Departments and the overall deployment of the School's resources in space and finance.'[14] Five years later, the next quinquennium policy statement had this to say of *'BIOCHEMISTRY'*:

> The need for research and teaching in biochemistry in the School is no less than it was five years ago; it has indeed grown. Meanwhile, the Biochemistry Department has been absorbed into other departments with biochemical needs. In a School with such diverse biochemical interests, and in which accommodation and resources are strictly limited, it now seems impossible to recreate a Department of Biochemistry big enough to meet all the School's

needs, and also to attract a professor of adequate standing who would need to be free to follow his own interests.[15]

It was decided to integrate biochemical activities in individual departments with major biochemical interests, i.e. Human Nutrition, Bacteriology, Entomology, Parasitology, Tropical Hygiene, and Environmental Physiology, 'until the School contains a community of biochemists with complementary interests. ... The Department of Clinical Tropical Medicine needs a chemical pathologist with supporting technical staff, and he would naturally fall into the biochemical consortium.' These developments were clear indications of the growing complexity of not only biochemical research, but of all the subjects taught in a School with a need to widen its horizons in Public Health in the post-war world.

The separate department of 'Chemistry as applied to Hygiene' had disappeared long before, with Delafield's retirement in 1950. Over the years, its teaching commitments had been primarily to candidates for the Diploma in Public Health, with a special course in chemistry for the never very large class for the academic Diploma in Bacteriology. In the 1930s, a short course of lectures on the chemistry of water and of sewage purification was added for the benefit of students of Tropical Hygiene. Research in the department was largely done in collaboration with the Division of Bacteriology, where A.F.B.Standfast collaborated with Chemistry's W.R.Woolridge in a study of the mechanism of sewage purification with special regard to the 'activated sludge' process; work which was supported by a grant from the Water Pollution Research Board. Other collaborations with the Division of Bacteriology included MRC supported work on bacterial metabolism, and aspects of Graham Wilson's milk research, where R.S.Twigg studied electrode potential drifts caused by raw whole and skim milks.[16]

With the outbreak of war in 1939, the departments of chemistry and biochemistry were, like most of the School, forced to suspend many of their activities, although Raistrick initially came down on the side of 'business as usual'. The direct hit on the School buildings in May, 1941, interfered with such noble intentions, and in any case Raistrick was involved in the wartime efforts to produce sufficient quantities of penicillin as adviser to the Ministry of Supply, while Delafield had been seconded to the MRC from the beginning of the war.[17]

At the end of the war, Raistrick's department began the slow recovery; the chemistry department never did. Delafield's staff had dispersed; he continued giving a few lectures until he retired in 1949 (*not* 1959, as the *Annual Report* had it when recording his death in 1974).[18]

The post-war reports only intermittently listed even the existence of the Department of Chemistry as Applied to Hygiene and its few activities. Bradford Hill, always ready with the occasional sarcastic remark, wrote years later: 'Delafield's job had long gone (his subject was no longer taught in the DPH course and he seemed to me to lounge around with nothing to do – and he did that gracefully)'.[19] Certainly Delafield's retirement marked the end of chemistry as a separate subject at the School.

OCCUPATIONAL HEALTH

The academic disciplines 'occupational health' and 'occupational medicine' presuppose concern with 'occupational diseases'; concern which had been available only as specific advice to particular groups of workers, such as miners, and those exposed to metal fumes, until the publication, at Modena in 1700, of Ramazzini's pioneering treatise, *Diseases of workers*.[20] At that early stage, Ramazzini could do little more than record a number of cases of a variety of diseases which could reasonably be assumed to have been caused by the patient's occupation: a chronicle of specific diseases of individual professions, and not of any wider issues of incidence or patterns of such diseases. Such issues came to be taken into consideration, slowly at first, and later accelerating, in step with the growing industrialisation of Europe in the nineteenth century.

With the growth and diversification of industry, the range of diseases directly attributable to particular industrial tasks expanded. With increasing numbers of physicians turning to the study of occupational diseases, institutes of occupational health, concerned with clinical and preventive aspects and research, were established in several European countries from the early years of the twentieth century. The first such institute was founded by Luigi Devoto (1864–1936), professor of medicine at Pavia, Milan's neighbouring university town. The institute, the *Clinica del Lavoro,* was planned and built between 1904 and 1910 in Milan, where Devoto later became professor of occupational health.[21]

In Britain, it took the outbreak of war in 1914, and the failure of stressed and over-extended munitions workers to meet the demands of the Great War, to initiate the country's first research project in occupational health. As already mentioned in Chapter 4 above, the government established the Health of Munition Workers Committee (HMWC) to report on questions of industrial fatigue, hours of work, suitable diets, etc.; in fact on any factors which might adversely affect the health and efficiency of the workers. At the end of the war, the HMWC was replaced by the Industrial Fatigue Research Board (IFRB), appointed in June, 1918, by the Department of Scientific and Industrial Research jointly with the Medical Research Committee. With wider terms of reference than the HMWC, and on a national scale, the IFRB began peacetime research into health problems associated with environmental factors in the work place.[22]

From such general beginnings grew individual initiatives, which resulted in the establishment of a network of organisations, throughout the country, active in the field of occupational health. By the late 1960s, these included five university departments, from Wales to the North of England; twelve MRC research units; and units associated with the Armed Forces and the National Coal Board. In addition, industrial concerns such as ICI, Shell, and the Institute of Directors, had developed research units of their own. Of these units, whether supported by public or private funds, each was concerned with the relatively narrow horizons of particular local industries, or particular types of hazard. An institute covering a broad range of industrial health problems, with an advisory service to match, had to wait for the exemplary cooperation between the LSHTM and the TUC (Trades Union Congress) on the occasion of the latter's centenary in 1968.[23]

One member of the original HMWC was the physiologist Leonard Hill. By his recruitment of his protégé, Major Greenwood, he ensured a close working relationship between the two developing disciplines of occupational medicine and medical statistics. The links were further strengthened in the 1920s, when Major Greenwood in turn involved Hill's son, Austin Bradford Hill, in epidemiological statistics, first at the MRC, and subsequently at the LSHTM. From the 1920s to the 1950s, it was above all Bradford Hill who played a pivotal role in the development of studies in occupational health and occupational medicine at the London School.[24]

In parallel with these developments in medical statistics, the public health department at the School had also over the years moved in the direction of aspects of occupational health, in teaching and research. In the 1930s, the sections of Applied Physiology under Crowden, and of Medical Industrial Psychology under Culpin, represented new attitudes and concerns which, like the IHRB (Industrial Health Research Board, as the IFRB had been renamed), grew out of the stresses of World War I with clear messages for peacetime industrial health problems. As early as 1931, when Culpin was appointed to a University Chair of Medical Industrial Psychology at the School, Jameson's report on the work of the Public Health Division devoted considerable space to 'Physiology and

Medical Psychology as Applied to Problems of Industry'. Pointing out the close existing relations between these subjects and Greenwood's Division of Epidemiology with its links to the IHRB, Jameson wrote:

> ... the whole problem of the relation of the School to industrial questions, which form a vast and most important part of the field of public health, has engaged the attention of the Board as well as of the staff. It was following the recommendations of a joint committee that the new University Chair was established, and also that the section of work which had been labelled "Applied Physiology"... was renamed the Section of Industrial Physiology ....[25]

Throughout the 1930s, until Culpin retired in 1939, the fruitful relationship between all these disciplines was consolidated at the School in the work of Bradford Hill, Crowden, and Culpin. The hiatus during World War II affected teaching and research in all departments. With regard to Medical Industrial Psychology, the first wartime *Annual Report* announced that

> The war has inevitably modified considerably the work of the Department of Medical Industrial Psychology, particularly ... [as] the normal courses in public health and in industrial psychology have not been held. A certain amount of teaching ... has been given by Dr. May Smith ...[26]

Many years before, May Smith's work had to some extent been responsible for Culpin's introduction to the field of industrial psychology. A report by May Smith and Eric Farmer on 'telegraphists' cramp to the IHRB had prompted Major Greenwood to suggest that Millais Culpin should be asked to evaluate their results by interviewing the subjects tested in the light of possible psychoneurotic findings.[27]

In the post-war reorganisation of the School's departments, Crowden's 'applied physiology' remained a department within the Department of Public Health. The section of 'applied psychology' was incorporated in Public Health, with just one lecturer, H.G.Maule.[28] Five years later, towards the end of the 1950-1 session, there was a development which looked back to the School's pre-war forays into collaborative efforts between applied physiology and medical industrial psychology under the public health umbrella, and forward to new and wider horizons for teaching and research programmes in industrial health.

PREVENTION AND CURE

The establishment of a 'Sub-Unit of Occupational Health' had its roots in the local Industrial Health Service at Slough, with its 'group of small industries which form the Slough society'.[29] It was staffed by one P.H. Nash, Senior Clinical Assistant in the Service, and R.J. Sherwood, the Service's Industrial Health Engineer. For five years, the work of this sub-unit proved the worth of its approach: a linking of practical work in the field with a university department, and based on a policy of prevention, i.e. observation-based elimination of health hazards in local industry.[30]

In early 1955, the LSHTM's initial benefactor, the Rockefeller Foundation, without whose help it might never have become established in the 1920s, made another significant gesture: a grant of £15,000 to the University of London towards the formation of a 'Department of Occupational Health' in the School. As a consequence, the 'Sub-unit' was replaced by the 'Rockefeller Unit of Occupational Health'. This time, there appears to have been no objection on the part of the Foundation to the inclusion of the Rockefeller name (cf. Chapter 3). R.S.F. Schilling became Director of the Unit, and also University Reader in Occupational Health, a position he had held at Manchester from 1947 to 1976. The country's first university department of occupational health had been established there, supported by the Nuffield Foundation, in 1945, with Ronald Lane (1897–1995) as Nuffield Professor of Occupational Health. It was not Schilling's first experience of the School; he had obtained his Academic Postgraduate Diploma in Public Health there in 1947. Of the four 'starred' of fifty-four successful candidates on that year's pass list, Schilling eventually became Professor of Occupational Health; J.N. Morris Professor of Community Health; and John Knowelden a valued member of the Department of Medical Statistics before moving to Sheffield as Professor of Community Medicine in 1960.[31]

After five years of steady development of the Unit's teaching and research, its progress and importance was recognised by additional grants from the Rockefeller Foundation and from the Leverhulme Trust Fund. This outside generosity enabled the unit to become a full department, with R.S.F. Schilling as professor, in 1960. The timing of this development was no coincidence: it took place during the two short years when Bradford Hill was prevailed upon to accept the deanship of the School, after Sir James Kilpatrick had died suddenly in office in 1960. It was a fitting seal on Sir Austin's involvement in the development of the research in occupational medicine and occupational health in the country and in the School.[32]

Throughout the administrative changes, teaching and research continued to develop. The director's own intense interest in byssinosis and chronic bronchitis was reflected in MRC supported research, in collaboration with the Pneumoconiosis Research Unit, on effects of accumulated dust exposure in Lancashire cotton workers and mule spinners. The latter project was undertaken in response to a request from the Ministry of Pensions and National Insurance.[33] In the 1960s, with additions to staff and facilities made possible first by the merging of the department with Applied Physiology in 1962, and more substantially by the creation of the TUC Centenary Institute in 1968, a broader range of studies was undertaken.[34] By 1960, 33 per cent of academic staff members were women. Dr Suzette Gauvain was involved in analyses of sickness absence in collaboration with Industrial Medical Officers in individual factories and organisations such as the British Overseas Airways Corporation; and Muriel L.Newhouse pioneered research into occupational dermatitis in various industries. Later she studied asbestosis and, with Professor Schilling, Dogger Bank itch (an oil allergy) at Lowestoft, at the request of the White Fish Authority. It was a demanding task of painstaking questioning of incoming crews, carried out by Muriel Newhouse. When going to sea with the crews became necessary, Professor Schilling took over: there were strict rules forbidding the presence of women on sea-going vessels (deep-sea fishing ranks prominently among statistics for occupational mortality).[35]

In 1967, negotiations between the School's Board of Management, the University of London, and the Trades Union congress (TUC), led to the establishment of an Institute of Occupational Health within the School, its constitution and administration similar to that of the Ross Institute. The TUC offered an initial £125,000 towards construction and equipment, to mark its coming centenary in 1968. An attempt to obtain similar support from the employers' organisation was unsuccessful.[36]

The new institute – the TUC Centenary Institute of Occupational Health – opened in 1968. The School's request to the University for simultaneous establishment of a chair in occupational health was granted; and Schilling, who since 1960 had been professor by conferment of title, now held the University Chair of Occupational Health. In addition to its initial contribution, the TUC also pledged an annual sum of £20,000, with the stipulation that the Institute should run an information and advisory service encouraging workers, through their Unions and medical advisers, to seek guidance concerning occupational health risks. The service proved to be of great value over the years, both to the TUC and the unions, and to the department itself in identifying areas to be explored in its research. The TUC's medical adviser, Robert Murray, was a forceful influence in the organisation and administration of the Institute, as was also its physician-in-charge, P.J.Taylor.[37]

Over the years, the TUC Institute also established important working relations with the MRC's Environmental Physiology Research Unit under J.S.Weiner (1915–82), Professor of Environmental Physiology since 1965. The Unit had transferred to the School from Oxford in 1963, and remained at the LSHTM until it was disbanded when Weiner retired in September, 1980. Even then, J.S.Weiner continued to serve as consultant in charge of the Industrial Advisory Service of the TUC Institute until his death two years later.[38]

When R.S.F.Schilling retired in 1976, he was succeeded by John Corbett McDonald, who had qualified in London and served with the RAMC during the war before joining the PHLS. In 1964 he moved to McGill University in Montreal as Professor and Head of its Department of Epidemiology and Health until 1976, when he returned to London, and the TUC Institute, for five years. He 'retired' in 1981 to return to McGill to establish there a new School of Occupational Health. McDonald's five years at the School coincided with the period of Gordon Smith's deanship when the School, including the TUC Institute, benefited from growing links established with other London Colleges, Medical Schools, Government Departments and, above all, with neighbouring University College Hospital and its Medical School (UCHMS). The TUC Institute and UCHMS were able to arrange a joint weekly outpatient clinic for patients with known or suspected occupational disease and health problems. Links with industry also steadily increased; and Occupational Health and the MRC Environmental Health Unit cooperated in an advisory capacity on sewage treatment centres as far afield as Cairo and, in Saudi Arabia, along the Mecca pilgrimage route.[39]

In his first departmental report, for the academic year 1976–7, McDonald outlined important changes in the department's approach to teaching. The M.Sc. course in occupational medicine and occupational hygiene, begun in 1969–70, would continue as separately planned one-year programmes; in the autumn term would be offered an additional 3-month course preparing physicians with 'substantial experience' for the Diploma in Industrial Health. For all full-time students there was a 'core' programme of seven obligatory course units; in the spring term, each student could chose from fifteen elective subjects: physicians for the M.Sc. were required to elect five, whereas the hygienists and those preparing for the DIH must elect six.[40]

During the remainder of McDonald's five years in office, the department changed little, except for the relentless advances in computer technology, which facilitated the increasing analytical use of medical statistics. At about the time of McDonald's departure for Canada, the University of London, under financial pressure, requested that a review be made of the role and activities of the School by the Dean of the University's Faculty of Medicine, Professor L.P.LeQuesne. The resulting report placed under consideration possible closure of the institute, with its main functions in occupational health being taken over by the department of medical statistics and epidemiology. The following year's *Annual Report* noted with relief that the 'uncertainty' posed by the LeQuesne Report had been lifted by the University 'confirming its intention to maintain the Institute and fill the vacant Chair of Occupational Health'. It was filled the following year by the appointment of Charles E.Rossiter, a statistician with the MRC, to the Chair and Directorship of the TUC Institute.[41]

However, the appointment did not mark the end of troubles for the department and the Institute. Towards the end of Gordon Smith's period as Dean in the later 1980s, the question of possible closure of the TUC Institute was again brought to the fore. It was a time of upheaval for universities and medical schools throughout Britain; within the LSHTM there were also signs that restructuring and reform of academic departments must be considered. For the School, a working party under Sir John Reid, Chairman of the Board of Governors, reported in 1988, recommending far-reaching changes in departmental structure. A specific proposal was a final closing-down of the Department, and the TUC Institute, of Occupational Health. This recommendation was met with a mixture of despair and disbelief in the department, which received encouraging support in the form of public protest from industry, commerce, and even the Forces. The response from the Board of Management was a decision not to implement the closure; but it was not to last. At a higher level, the UGC was reviewing academic occupational health throughout the UK, and recommended its removal from central London. The following year, the TUC Institute had disappeared altogether from the School Report, and 'Occupational health and hygiene research' appeared as an adjunct to the Department of Public Health and Policy. G.Kazantzis, who had succeeded Rossiter as Professor of Occupational Health, retired; and by 1990-1, Occupational Health as such had disappeared altogether from the School structure as described in the new-style reports. Five years later, an observer from outside the department comments on its demise:

> Occupational Health has always seemed to me to be one of the lost causes of the School. It had some of the best people in it and

clearly did some excellent work. Richard Schilling, Mollie Newhouse and Chris Wood were the tops. I suppose that its funding was too deeply involved in politics to give it a secure base.[42]

With the reorganisation of occupational health studies and services, on a country-wide basis for the 1990s, Birmingham now is recognised as the UK's main centre for occupational medicine. At the LSHTM, 'occupational medicine' is no longer taught. The Occupational Health Unit was closed in September, 1990, to some extent replaced by a new 'Environmental Health Unit' in the Department of Public Health and Policy. The new unit has absorbed some of the activities of occupational hygiene, although with totally different staff members. Closest to the occupational traditions is the work of A.C.Fletcher, who came to the School from Birmingham, and who is involved in European Community studies on health and safety in relation to occupational exposure limits.[43] Such investigations widen the scope, and place in an international context the Unit's major programme of identification of geographical clusters of disease throughout Britain in relation to environmental pollutants. Barely two years after its opening, the Unit was recognised as a WHO Collaborating Centre for Research Training and Co-ordination in Environmental Epidemiology. In line with developments elsewhere in the School, its occupational health tradition has gone European, and global, as part and parcel of a department 'well placed to pursue public health and health policy research in countries at all stages of development'.[44]

THE WIDER SPECTRUM
NOTES

[1] C.M.Clark and J.M.Mackintosh, *The School and the Site*, LSHTM Memoir No.9, London, H.K.Lewis & Co. Ltd., 1954, p.73.
[2] J.H.Birkinshaw, 'Harold Raistrick 1890-1971', *Biogr.Mem.Fell.Roy.Soc.*, 1972, *18:*489-509, p.490.
[3] *ibid.;*
R.Bentley and Robert Thomas, 'Harold Raistrick, 1890-1971 An appreciation', *The Biochemist,* 1990 *12* (6):3-6.
First Annual Report of the Medical Research Committee, 1914-15, London, HMSO.
[4] Bentley and Thomas, op.cit., p.3.
[5] LSHTM *Annual Report* 1947-8, pp. 50 and 59;
Erik Bergengren, *Alfred Nobel: the man and his work,* London etc., Thomas Nelson & Sons Ltd., 1962, pp. 59, 61, 89 and 91;
W.F.L.Dick, *A hundred years of alkali in Cheshire,* Birmingham, Imperial Chemical Industries Mond Division, 1973;
Birkinshaw, op.cit. note 2, p.494;
W.E.Ormerod, personal communication, 1995.
[6] LSHTM *Annual Report* 1928-9, pp.4-5;
ABH 1988, 'Notes on prof.s', p.1.
Sir Henry Dale, 'Percival Hartley 1881-1957', *Biogr.Mem.Fell.Roy.Soc.*, 1957 *3:*81-100.
[7] A.B.H.1988, as above;
Sir Edward Abraham, personal communication February 1994.
[8] Birkinshaw, op.cit. note 2, p.497. [our italics]
P.W.Clutterbuck, R.Lovell and H.Raistrick, 'The formation from glucose by members of the *Penicillium chrysogenum* series of a pigment, an alkali-soluble protein and penicillium – the antibacterial substance of Fleming', *Biochem.J.,* 1932, *26:*1907-18.
[9] Ronald Hare, *The birth of penicillin and the disarming of microbes,* London, George Allen and Unwin Ltd, 1970, pp.93-8, and 100-3; [authors' italics]
E.P.Abraham, 'Howard Walter Florey Baron Florey of Adelaide and Marston 1898-1968' *Biogr.Mem.Fell.Roy.Soc.,* 1971, *17:*255-302, pp.264-5.
Letter from Ridley to Heatley, dated 21/1/75. We are indebted to Professor Heatley and Sir Edward Abraham for providing a copy of this letter.
[10] H.Raistrick, J.H.Birkinshaw, S.E.Michael, A.Bracken. W.E.Gye, W.A.Hopkins, M.Greenwood, 'Patulin in the common cold; collaborative

research on a derivative of *Penicillium patulum* Bainier', *Lancet,* 1943, *ii:*625-35.

[11] Birkinshaw, op.cit. note 2, p.508.

[12] Abraham, as note 7.

[13] *The Times*, 19 March 1971, also quoted by Birkinshaw.

[14] LSHTM Quinquennium 1962-7, D.P.S.29, p.321.

[15] LSHTM Statement of Development Policy for the Quinquennium 1967-72: the work of the School during 1962-7, p.6.

[16] LSHTM *Annual Reports* between 1930 and 1939, e.g. 1931-2, p.23, and 1934-5, p.31.

[17] Birkinshaw op.cit. note 2, p.495;
Bentley and Thomas, op.cit. note 3, p.6;
LSHTM *Annual Report* 1942-3, p.10.

[18] LSHTM *Annual Report* 1974-5, p.33.

[19] LSHTM *Annual Reports* between 1945 and 1950;
A.B.H.March 1988, p.10.

[20] L.Wilkinson, 'Epidemiology', in: *Companion Encyclopedia of the History of Medicine*, W.F.Bynum and Roy Porter, eds, vol.2, pp.1262-82, p.1266, London and New York, Routledge, 1993; Bernardino Ramazzini, *Diseases of Workers*, translated from the Latin text *De morbis artificium* of 1713, by Wilmer Cave Wright, New York and London, Hafner, 1964.

[21] E.C.Vigliani, 'Practice of occupational medicine in the *Clinica del Lavoro "Luigi Devoto"'*, *Arch.Environ.Health,* 1968, *17:*135-42;
R.S.F.Schilling, 'The new TUC Centenary Institute of Occupational Health at the London School of Hygiene and Tropical Medicine', *Indian J.Industr.Med.,* 1969, *15:*199-210;
S.Forssman, 'Occupational Health Institutes: an international survey', *Am.Industr.Hyg.Assoc.J.,* 1967, *28:*197-203.

[22] Report of the Medical Research Committee 1917-18, p.78; *ibid.* 1918-19, p.76-80; Report of the Medical Research Council, 1920-1, pp.97-8.

[23] R.S.F.Schilling, op.cit note 21.

[24] Richard Schilling, 'Bradford Hill's contribution to occupational health', *Stat.s in Med.,* 1982, *1:*317-24;
R.S.F.Schilling and J.C.McDonald, 'Occupational health at the LSHTM', *Br.J.industr.med.,* 1990, *47:*135-7.

[25] LSHTM *Annual Report* 1930-1, pp.33-4.

[26] LSHTM *Annual Report* 1939-40, p.118.

[27] Culpin obituary, *Lancet,* 1952, *ii:*643;
MRC *Reports,* 1922-3, p.124; 1925-6, p.129; 1926-7, pp.130-1;

M.Smith, M.Culpin, and E.Farmer, 'A study of telegraphists' cramp', *Reports of the Industrial Fatigue Research Board,* no.43, 1927.
[28] LSHTM *Annual Report* 1945–6, p.12.
[29] LSHTM *Annual Report* 1950–1, p.72.
[30] LSHTM *Annual Report* 1952–3, p.66.
[31] LSHTM *Annual Reports* 1954–5, p.17; 1955–6, p.13; 1956–7, pp.89–92;
LSHTM DPH Pass List, June 1947;
'Professor Ronald Lane', obituary, *Independent,* 31.3.95, p.20.
[32] LSHTM *Annual Reports* 1957–8, p.99; 1959–60, p.76;
R.S.F.Schilling, 'A brief history of occupational health at the LSH&TM', LSHTM MSS, August 1988;
idem, op.cit. note 24.
[33] LSHTM *Annual Report* 1956–7, pp.89–92.
[34] LSHTM *Annual Reports* 1962–3, p.57; 1967–8, p.57; 1968–9, p.110;
Schilling and McDonald, op.cit. note 24.
[35] R.S.F.Schilling, personal communication, March, 1990;
M.L.Newhouse, 'Dogger Bank itch among Lowestoft trawlermen', *Acta Allerg.,* 1966, *21:*278–84;
idem, 'Dogger Bank itch: a survey of trawlermen', *Br.J.Med.,* 1966, *i:*1142–5;
R.S.F.Schilling, 'Trawler fishing: an extreme occupation', *Proc.R.Soc.Med.,* 1966, *59:*405–10;
idem, 'Hazards of deep-sea fishing', *Br.J.ind.Med.,* 1971, *28:*27–35.
[36] R.S.F.Schilling, op.cit. note 32.
[37] *ibid.;*
LSHTM *Annual Reports* 1966–7, p.19; 1967–8, p.57; 1968–9, 110–11.
[38] LSHTM *Annual Reports* 1966–7, pp.92–3; 1969–70, p.124; 1979–80, p.26; 1981–2, pp.25–6.
[39] LSHTM *Annual Reports* 1973–4, p.26; 1976–7, p.22.
[40] LSHTM *Annual Report* 1976–7, p.42.
[41] LSHTM *Annual Reports* 1982–3, p.71; and 1983–4;
Schilling and McDonald, op.cit. note 24.
[42] LSHTM *Annual Reports* between 1987 and 1991;
W.E.Ormerod, personal communication.
[43] R.Feachem, personal communication, March, 1994;
A.C.Fletcher, 'The use of "real-life" problem-centred learning in multi-disciplinary teaching of occupational health', *Journal of University of Occupational and Environmental Health* [Japanese publication], 1992, *14:*suppl.: 370–5;
M.V.Smillie *et al., Health and Safety; occupational exposure limits.*

Criteria document for monochloroethane. Commission of the European Communities. 1992. (EUR 14241 EN).
[44] LSHTM *Annual Report*s 1989–90, p.9; 1991–2, p.11.

8

FEEDING THE HUNGRY, BALANCING THE DIET: NUTRITION AND PUBLIC HEALTH

The creation of the Department of Human Nutrition in 1946 marked a new departure in the School's research and policy interests, and reflected the growing international concern with nutrition which had emerged in the years just before World War II. It was the first university department of nutrition in Britain, and its professor for many years occupied the only Chair of Human Nutrition in the country.[1] Twenty-five years previously, Robert Leiper had listed 'Dietetics and Deficiency Diseases' as one of the six subjects to be covered by the proposed Imperial Hygiene Institute, but the interests of the new department were less rigorously defined. In the intervening quarter century several distinct styles of nutritional research and concern had developed and several different communities of professional nutrition scientists emerged. A number of these were to be represented in the new department in the years that followed.

Modern nutrition science emerged in the first decades of this century under the stimulus of war, of the study of deficiency diseases and of the discovery of vitamins. During these years, the field was dominated by physiologists and physiological chemists, notably at the Institute of Physiology in Glasgow and the Lister Institute in London. Although human nutrition and dietetics had been an important interest of Queen Elizabeth College, London, where Edward Mellanby had been appointed to the Chair of Physiology in 1913, the first institute specifically for nutrition studies, the Dunn Nutrition Laboratory in Cambridge, was only established in 1927, the year of the LSHTM's birth. (The Rowett Research Institute, founded in 1913 and functional from 1919, was initially for the study of animal nutrition.[2]) The small number of British nutrition scientists, and the physiological and biochemical nature of their research probably lay behind the failure to establish a dietetics department at the LSHTM in 1927. With the Division of Biochemistry itself a relative innovation, and Wilson Jameson's vision of Applied Physiology expanding into the field of nutrition, the grounds for a separate dietetics department are not likely to have been strong.[3] Nutrition in these years was seen very much as a scientific concern; the concept of applied nutrition gathered strength only in the 1930s, with the publication of Boyd Orr's *Food Health and Income* in 1936 and with the realisation of colonial nutrition problems.

The absence of a dietetics department did not, therefore, mean that problems of nutrition were not studied at the LSHTM. All the different divisions of the School were at one time or another engaged in work relating to nutrition in the years up to 1946. Much of this work was concerned with either family diet and nutritional status surveys, or with the nutritional qualities of different foodstuffs. In the 1930s, for example, Graham Wilson was supervising M.P.Cowell's study, in association with Jack Drummond who held the Chair in Biochemistry at University College London, of the nutritive value of raw and pasteurised milk.[4] Both the Bacteriological and the Biochemical divisions were later involved in studies of cheese moulds. In the Department of Industrial Physiology, meanwhile, Mabel Clark's early studies of the relationship between milk consumption and the growth of schoolchildren had given way to dietary and sociological surveys, while G.P.Crowden had become increasingly interested in the adequacy of diets.[5]

Domestic and scientific concerns thus dominated nutrition research at the school in the 1930s. In 1940, however, R.A.Webb began work in the Biochemical Division on the microbiological factors involved in enhancing the nutritional quality of native colonial foodstuffs. Webb joined B.S.Platt (1903–69) and J.C.Waterlow (b.1916) on the staff of the MRC's Human Nutrition Research Unit when it was set up, with Platt at its head, at the beginning of 1944. Platt's early work had been on beriberi in China,[6] and this had developed his interest in the biological enhancement of foods by methods of preparation – a subject of special importance in the prevention of beriberi among poor people subsisting essentially on rice diets – and he was able to extend this interest through his association with Webb. The importance of fermented foodstuffs in providing B-vitamins in traditional colonial diets became a special focus of interest, and investigations into the properties of yeast and Kaffir beer and the nutritive values of rice and maize were among the projects undertaken by the new Unit. Other projects included skin metabolism in wound healing (of significance in tropical ulcer), and the dispatch of Waterlow to Jamaica to investigate malnutrition and oedema in babies and young children.[7]

The activities of the Human Nutrition Research Unit in its first years presaged the interests of the new Department of Human Nutrition at the LSHTM after Platt's appointment to the Chair in 1946. Platt remained Head of the Unit, and it remained closely associated with the Department until it was disbanded on 31 July 1967, when most of its staff transferred to the School.[8] His interests were primarily in tropical nutrition problems, the resolution of which he saw primarily as an interdisciplinary matter, involving both the behavioural sciences and clinical and laboratory research.[9] During the 1930s, he had worked in the clinical division of the Henry Lester Institute in Shanghai, but he returned to England after the Japanese invasion of China and found employment at the MRC. He organised the Nyasaland Survey of 1939-40 for the MRC,[10] and visited Tanzania, Kenya, Uganda and Rhodesia; in 1944 he visited the West Indies, and in 1945 the West African territories. The primary object of the Human Nutrition Research Unit was to coordinate and develop field studies in the colonies, and to this end a Nutrition Field Working Party for 'combined practical work' in an area of the Gambia was set up, followed by the establishment of a Nutrition Field Research Station at Fajara in 1947. The work of both was to be integrated with that of the London Unit, and was intended to involve not only research but education and training: 'A major factor in improving the state of nutrition in colonial territories,' noted the post-war MRC report, 'will be the provision of suitably trained personnel.'[11]

Platt's experience in tropical and colonial nutrition made him an obvious choice for the Chair at the LSHTM in 1946; he was besides highly thought of by Edward Mellanby, at that time both Chairman of the MRC Human Nutrition sub-committee, and the MRC appointed governor at the LSHTM. The new department was initially very small, consisting only of Platt and A.Dean Smith as lecturer, and it remained among the smallest departments of the School – a Cinderella, in the eyes of J.C.Waterlow, and indeed of others.[12] In an institution like the School, with a strong medical science ethos, the interdisciplinary orientation of the Human Nutrition Department, many of whose staff were not medically qualified, inevitably set it somewhat apart.

In the first eight years of its existence, the work of the department was very closely bound up not only with that of the MRC Human Nutrition Unit, but also with that of the MRC's Gambian enterprises. Academic research was focused principally on problems of colonial malnutrition, especially as manifested in the Gambian experiment of improving nutrition in the village of Genieri undertaken by the Nutrition Field Working Party and financed under the Colonial Development and Welfare Act. The Gambian connection offered the opportunity both for working out techniques for practical improvements in agriculture, and for scientific studies of malnutrition. Among the areas investigated were the part played by parasites in ill health, the impact of infectious diseases and malaria on nutritional levels, aspects of protein deficiency and nitrogen metabolism, and the relationship between infant growth and breast milk consumption. Although the experiment at Genieri and the work of the Fajara Field Station were at the local level eminently practical in orientation, they were backed up by activities of the clinical and laboratory researchers in the MRC unit. The implications of much of this research were significant for the science and practice of nutrition in the longer term. Work on food preparation and preservation by Webb was complemented by achievements in basic laboratory research. Using the then very new technique of chromatography, Leslie Fowden and James Done discovered a previously unknown amino-acid in peanuts.[13] Waterlow adapted the Cartesian diver micro-respirometer, which had been developed by Linderstrom-Lang in Copenhagen during the war, for the study of human tissues. In 1948–9, for example, he was using the technique to measure the enzyme contents of the tissues of Gambian infants, especially with a view to protein deficiency.[14] The use of Tritium (radioactive hydrogen) as a 'label' for nutrients, and methods for measuring it in biological tissues, were also pioneered by workers in the MRC unit.[15] After three years, the experiment in village development at Genieri was taken over by the Gambian government, but in those three years the types of problems for continued investigation in the laboratory and the clinical ward as well as in the field, had been defined.[16]

Meanwhile the Gambian research fed back into the teaching of the department in London, and proved valuable in providing practical illustration for visitors and students. While postgraduate training as well as research took place in the Gambia, teaching in London was initially done through the DPH and DTM&H courses. It was not long, however, before numerous short courses were being added for the benefit of specialised groups of workers, such as nurses, domestic science teachers and colonial service personnel.[17] Increasingly, too, the department found itself coping with numbers of overseas visitors of different kinds – a reflection of the upsurge of interest in nutrition which took place in the developing world in the aftermath of the war. In 1952, at the instigation of the Colonial Office, an Applied Nutrition Research Unit was added to the department's strength. Funded by the Colonial Office under the Colonial Development and Welfare Act, but administered by the School, the Unit was to collect and study technical information on nutrition and food technology in the colonial territories, and to provide information to colonial governments on request. It was also to assist in training colonial personnel in nutrition work. By 1954 it had developed a wide-ranging overseas correspondence, as well as a special contact system for colonial service officers on leave in Britain.[18] By the mid-1950s, its services were in increasing demand for the instruction and training of staff from countries which had recently achieved political independence. With the expiry of the Colonial Development Act in 1960, the Unit as such was closed down.[19] The pattern of work and interests evolved in the department during its first eight years, a 'pattern of teaching, field investigations, applied nutrition and research',[20] came to an abrupt halt in 1954. In his annual report for 1954-5, Platt recorded that some activities prominent in the past, such as fieldwork and research overseas, were no longer a major concern. His explanation for this sudden break in the pattern rested on the increased involvement of 'the large foundations' and individual governments in all types of regional planning and development; fieldwork was no longer a matter for 'pioneering and research'. The department's position had shifted accordingly, 'from the front line to the position of "guide, philosopher and friend"' to those in the front line.[21] The reality was rather more prosaic. In 1953, Platt experienced the first manifestations of the illness which was to dog the rest of his career, and which rendered him unfit for fieldwork.[22] In 1954, moreover, there was a disagreement between Platt and Mellanby's successor at the MRC, Sir Harold Himsworth, about the running of the Fajara Field Station, which ended in Platt's withdrawal from the project.

The ending of the Gambian involvement brought an immediate shift in the department's concerns. The broad-ranging approach to nutritional problems which had been evident in the Gambian years gave way to a narrower focus. Although protein malnutrition had featured in Platt's reports and publications before 1955, it had done so in equality with other concerns. For several years in the late 1950s, however, the subject features more prominently in his annual reports. He had been appointed to the WHO's Protein Advisory Group in 1955, and his work as a consultant for both the WHO and the FAO in these years focused his attention on the problem of assessing the nutritional quality of tropical diets, and more especially on the fact that their protein content was often derived mainly from vegetable sources.[23] In June 1956, the Rockefeller Foundation awarded the School £17,000 for a three-year research investigation of the protein value of tropical dietaries and supplementary foodstuffs, which was renewed in 1959. This grant was used to develop a methodology for measuring the nutritional quality of human diets, enabling them to be compared with the recommendations of WHO expert committees, and led to new insights in the understanding of the metabolic interactions between dietary sources of protein and of energy.[24] From 1956 onwards, the research of the Human Nutrition Unit came to focus strongly on protein studies, both in human subjects and in experimental animals.[25]

Although protein deficiency in a sense hijacked the interests of the tropical nutrition community in the 1950s and 1960s, Platt was never wholeheartedly enthused by the problem, or by the technical solutions which were frequently invoked in the attempt to resolve it.[26] It was his belief that because of the metabolic interactions between protein and energy sources, and because of the additional complications of the effects of infectious diseases, it was simplistic to attempt to prove that there were two separate and independent syndromes, one specific to protein deficiency, the other to energy deficiency.[27] Indeed, he considered kwashiorkor to be the outcome of a combination of infection and diet, rather than a nutrient syndrome.[28] In his report for 1955–6, for example, he noted that 'The cheapest and probably the most effective first step in dealing with this problem lies in the control of zymotic disease factors. A complete solution to the problem of securing proper feeding of the peoples of tropical communities requires attention to many matters outside the sphere of science of nutrition and much more information is needed before the nutritionist can give good advice on the best use of foods and the best directions in which to develop food resources.'[29] Indeed Platt questioned the contemporary emphasis on kwashiorkor, arguing that types of malnutrition in which marasmus was a feature were far more prevalent than kwashiorkor itself.[30] It was a view finally endorsed by the Joint FAO/WHO Expert Committee on Nutrition which in 1960 recommended that in the revision of the International Statistical Classification of Disease Injury and Causes of Death, 'marasmic kwashiorkor' should be included with kwashiorkor as the first sub-division under the heading protein-calory deficiency diseases.

    The post-war burgeoning of international agencies and of international concern with the food problems of developing countries increasingly drew Platt away from the LSHTM itself in these years, as he spent much time travelling abroad in the role of international expert and consultant. Within the department at the School, Wallace Ruddell Aykroyd (1899–1979), recently retired as the Director of the FAO's Nutrition Division, who became Senior Lecturer in the department in 1960, and Trewavas Pearce Eddy (1908–92), formerly Director of Medical Services in Sierra Leone, were more closely associated with some of the significant developments of the 1960s. Aykroyd concerned himself largely with teaching overseas students, and played a notable part in establishing the joint London–Ibadan Fellowship Course in Food Science and Applied Nutrition, which was first run in 1963. The project was supported by UNICEF, which in 1960 had broached plans for the training of specialised senior nutrition workers through a series of linked training and research centres in developed and underdeveloped countries. In December 1962, UNICEF's Executive board undertook to provide

£221,000 for five annual courses, with the object of equipping Fellows for applied nutrition work in developing countries. Four months' intensive study in London were to be followed by four months' fieldwork in Nigeria, where nutritional problems in urban and rural areas, and the observation of and participation in, local nutritional improvement programmes were important features. One hundred and five Fellows benefited from the scheme before deteriorating political conditions in Nigeria compromised its future in 1967. In that year, the field training period had to be transferred to Ghana at the last minute. While the training of senior nutrition workers remained an urgent priority for UNICEF, WHO and FAO, plans for the renewal of the scheme had to be shelved.[31]

Meanwhile the University of London had introduced the Academic Postgraduate Diploma in Nutrition, and in July 1964 it was decided that the LSHTM should offer this option.[32] In 1971-2 this was replaced by the M.Sc. in Human Nutrition, a course which combined elements both of the Diploma and the Fellowship scheme, with nine months study in London and a six months' project either in Britain or overseas. The aim of this course was to train overseas nutrition workers for responsible positions in universities or government services in their own countries; British students were to be oriented mainly towards overseas work. In comparison with earlier courses, however, the M.Sc. testified to the increasing integration of nutrition in the wider field of development: the public health and epidemiological aspects of the subject were to be given special emphasis, and the teaching was to involve liaison with the Department of Medical Statistics and Epidemiology.[33]

These developments in teaching continued to be geared to the department's overseas interests and the need for nutrition workers in developing countries: it was expected that most students would come from overseas.[34] Within Britain itself, however, changing social and political conditions, and the expanding concerns of the Welfare State, brought requests for new studies on domestic issues. T.P.Eddy became increasingly identified with these concerns. An important stage in this development was the Hospital Feeding Survey, initiated by the Nuffield Provincial Hospitals' Trust in 1959. This brought six researchers into the department, and Eddy was appointed Medical Officer in charge of the project.

The hospital feeding survey aroused a good deal of comment and indignation when it was eventually published, as *Food in Hospitals,* in 1964.[35] Although King Edward's Fund for London had published a series of memoranda on hospital diet since 1943, this was the first large-scale survey, based on a study of 152 randomly chosen National Health Service hospitals in England and Wales, of what was essentially a new question in hospital management. Up until World War II, hospitals had provided only one full meal a day, and had relied very considerably on contributions brought in by patients' relatives; the National Health Service from its inception had, however, undertaken to make full dietary provision for all patients. The hospital feeding inquiry was initiated by a request from the West Cornwall Hospital Management Committee to the Nuffield Provincial Hospitals Trust for an investigation into the feeding arrangements of their seven Cornish hospitals. They were anxious to establish an economical method of providing a diet adequate for the physical needs of patients in bed which would be appetising and well served, and they were concerned that the project should be carried out with special reference to the therapeutic values of a good dietary, about which little appeared to be known.[36]

The results of this study were so disturbing – it showed not only that there was excessive waste, but that half the meals served were not nutritionally adequate – that the Nuffield Provincial Hospitals Trust undertook to finance the wider survey. This reinforced the early findings, and also revealed widespread defects in hospitals kitchens and food hygiene, problems of distribution and delivery, and ignorance of nutritional values among hospital staff. In an attempt to solve some of these problems, experimental trials of frozen meals were instituted at the Whittington Hospital and the National Hospital for Nervous Diseases, and in 1963 the Trust granted the School a further £332,102 for three years to report on the application of new methods to hospital feeding.[37]

Almost in parallel with the hospital feeding survey, the department began to acquire an interest in the dietary needs of old people. As Platt noted in 1961, problems of gerontology were attracting increasing attention in Western countries, because of the progressive ageing of their populations.[38] In that year a sub-committee of the British Society for Research in Aging concerned with nutrition was centred in the department with Eddy as secretary. This was singularly appropriate, for half the sample patients in the hospital feeding survey were over 60, and it had been found that sound recommendations on their dietary needs could not be made for lack of basic knowledge.[39] In the years that followed, the problem of nutrition in the elderly became established as one of the department's perennial research themes, with projects on the use of pre-cooked frozen meals in old peoples' homes, on the biochemical assessment of nutritional status of old people associated with the DHSS geriatric surveys of the early 1970s, and on X-ray analyses of the mineral content of the bones of the hand in elderly people (in cooperation with St.Pancras Hospital). At this time osteoporosis was just beginning to become a public health concern, and its aetiology was not understood. Some workers emphasised nutritional, others endocrine factors. Statistical analyses performed by Eddy showed that there had been a steady increase in incidence in Britain since 1920, except for a dramatic fall during World War II.[40] As an extension of the earlier studies on bone, R.J.C.Stewart together with A.N.Exton-Smith of UCL, began to make histological and chemical analyses of femoral heads removed from elderly subjects at operation: like Eddy's statistical study, this research demonstrated the relationship which exists between nutrition and general clinical medicine, and which the nutritionists felt needed strengthening.[41]

During the 1960s, the department's research interests diversified. David Morley, who joined the department in July 1961, and who had been studying measles and measles vaccine in West Africa, received a WHO grant for a world-wide inquiry into the incidence and severity of measles, which he conducted jointly with W.J.Martin. There were investigations into the nutritional needs of spastics, and of infants in immigrant Asian families. Eddy and Erica Wheeler (1937–92) collaborated with the MRC's Environmental Physiology Research Unit on the nutritional balance of people travelling on an Esso oil tanker in the Persian Gulf, and Platt completed a study of the nutritional aspects of psycho-social deprivation. Towards the end of the decade a growing interest manifested itself in the diet of pregnant women and the nutrition of foetuses and newborn children.[42]

In July 1969, however, Platt died. He had been due to retire at the end of the next academic year, and there followed something of an interregnum until his successor, J.C.Waterlow, arrived in the autumn of 1970. Waterlow's arrival signalled a decided turn-around in the department's interests and vitality. As Waterlow recalled, 'the challenge was to build up the department in the four areas of metabolism, clinical medicine, public health and policy and planning'.[43] The time was perhaps ripe for such ambitions: in the next decade Waterlow achieved the facilities and funding to enable the continuity of research programmes as well as to support new developments beyond the constraints imposed by the physical limits of space within the Keppel Street building. The Human Nutrition Research Unit at Mill Hill had finally closed at the end of 1969 (the transfer of five senior researchers and their technical assistants from that Unit, successfully negotiated by Platt, ensured the continuity of the unit despite his retirement), and the animal studies then in progress were transferred to the Keppel Street site. Gordon Smith had just taken over as

Dean and was inaugurating a process of reassessment within the School, and at the same time a trend towards growing dependence on government funds for research was becoming manifest, and research funds were becoming increasingly tight. The Wellcome Foundation provided £118,000 for the construction of a new clinical and metabolic unit for Waterlow's department, which was built in the grounds of the Hospital for Tropical Diseases.[44] The building housed chiefly laboratories, but there was some animal accommodation, and it was intended to facilitate clinical research in collaboration with the Hospital staff, as well as 'a great expansion in the experimental work of the department'. The clinical attachment was a new departure, and one to which Waterlow attached great importance.[45] The physical location of the Unit at a distance from the main department (with an 'unrivalled view' of the St.Pancras shunting yards) posed problems of isolation for the scientists working there. Although it was hoped to avoid these by setting up frequent staff meetings and joint seminars, the Unit and the Department remained to a large extent distinct communities.[46]

Although existing research projects continued to their conclusion, Waterlow introduced three new themes into the range of the department's interests: protein turnover under various conditions of nutrition and stress, gastro-intestinal function, and obesity. Each of these themes was to be developed in the following years. At one level, the department's work quickly came to reflect Waterlow's own preoccupation with protein calorie malnutrition – the work on which he had been engaged during his fifteen years at the MRC Tropical Metabolism Unit. Although reinvigorated by Waterlow's arrival, the research on muscle protein turnover and later on protein metabolism nonetheless maintained continuity also with the work on nutritional adaptation undertaken for the MRC and the experimental protein–calorie malnutrition studies which had for so long been fostered by Platt. The protein–calorie work also began to reflect new concern with long-term marginal undernutrition rather than with acute malnutrition which was emerging in the development field, and to this end long-term studies of malnutrition in animals were undertaken: by 1973, rat colonies had been maintained through twelve generations on diets of differing protein values.[47] Within the CNU, moreover, metabolic work began to move in new directions. With a programme grant from the MRC, Waterlow was able to build up a team of researchers, including D.J.Millward, Peter Garlick, Virginia Pain and G.Laurent, who achieved international recognition with their isotopic studies of protein metabolism in man and animals.[48]

The interest in intestinal function found expression primarily in studies of malabsorption, a condition which commonly presented at the Hospital for Tropical Diseases in people who had been living or travelling abroad. In counterbalance to the exotic origins of this problem, the interest in obesity represented another area of late twentieth-century social concern, that of chronic and degenerative diseases. Although the department's contribution to knowledge in this area remained limited, pioneering work in the field included an examination of the energy metabolism of obese children by Philip Payne and Mary Griffiths, and a computer model constructed by Payne and the Australian researcher A.E.Dugdale, of the factors leading to obesity.[50] This recognition of obesity as a clinical problem was reinforced by practical experience: since 1973, the department had operated a weekly out-patient clinic for obesity at University College Hospital. Some 400 cases a year, around sixty of them new, presented themselves for treatment, so that the clinic was 'clearly fulfilling a practical need'.[51]

Obesity and malabsorption research extended the range of the department's public health interests, which, encouraged by DHSS funding from the early 1970s, had a history going back to the Hospital Diet Survey. The focus on policy and planning, however, reflected the most recent developments in nutritional thinking which had grown, in part, out of the perceived failure of the protein supplement programmes to resolve childhood malnutrition in developing countries.[52] In 1977, the creation of the Nutrition Policy Unit, headed by Philip Payne and financed by the Ministry for Overseas Development, spearheaded the department's expansion into the fields of nutrition policy and planning. It was hoped that the Unit would help to elucidate the nature and dynamics of nutrition problems and that its members would be extensively involved in training programmes, workshops, and consultancy exchanges, and in producing teaching materials. More broadly, the Unit picked up on Payne's existing interest in data and information systems for nutrition planning, and sought to establish working relationships with governments, in the hope of instituting nutrition policy analysis as a component of central planning. Techniques for predicting and monitoring the impact of agricultural development projects on the nutritional status of local populations became a special interest. The department as a whole had for some years had a special interest in nutritional surveillance, as the DHSS funded projects on the health of pre-school children and the elderly, and later of pregnant women, demonstrated. Indeed, the DHSS sponsored survey of pre-school children focusing also on the role of welfare milk in their growth and development, which was initiated following the Conservative government's withdrawal of free school milk in 1970–1, resulted in an important long-term surveillance programme, as well as the integration of biochemical analyses by Joan Stephen into surveys being conducted by the Ministry of Health.[53] The Nutrition Policy Unit extended this interest in surveillance overseas. By 1981, there were nutritional surveillance projects going in India, Nepal, Costa Rica and Turkey.

Both in research and teaching, the NPU built on the department's established overseas interests, continuing the tradition initiated by Platt. As a result of his period in Jamaica, Waterlow considered it important that some members of his staff at least should gain solid experience overseas, and three such secondments were arranged, for Michael Golden in Jamaica, for Andrew Tomkins in Nigeria and the Gambia, and for David Nabarro in Nepal. David Nabarro's important work on the assessment of nutritional status among rural communities in Nepal led to the development of the Nabarro Chart, a simple method of assessing nutritional status. He also developed some clear conceptual approaches towards community-based strategies for the improvement of nutrition. These approaches challenged the assumption that severely malnourished children needed to be managed within clinical facilities. As part of a large programme grant awarded by the Wellcome Trust on the interaction between nutrition and infection, collaborative studies between Waterlow, Peter Garlick, Margaret McNurlan and Andrew Tomkins were established between Nigeria and the CNMU. The Mass Spec facilities were crucial for the analysis of protein turnover using stable isotopes. Waterlow himself retained a personal research interest in global health problems, and in the mid-1970s developed the 'Waterlow Index', a system of classifying children with undernutrition and growth failure which was later adopted by the WHO and used throughout the world.[54] Moreover, his work as a consultant for the ODA and for the Research Institute of Health Sciences in Thailand, extended the department's overseas connections. Overseas projects also formed an important part of the M.Sc. course, and student projects in such places as Nepal, Kenya, Brazil and St.Lucia, extended and maintained the department's overseas contacts, sometimes over many years. The connection with Brazil, for example, in both teaching and research was continued into the 1990s by Ann Hill.

The addition of the Nutrition Policy Unit also affected the department's teaching, and the social science content of the M.Sc. and Diploma courses became more extensive, with special emphasis on economics as applied to food. The M.Sc. course originally comprised a one-year study unit at the School followed by a one-year research project, usually in the student's country of origin. As funding for postgraduate courses became ever tighter through the 1970s, the number of two-year courses in the school was steadily reduced, so that by 1980 the M.Sc. in Human Nutrition was the only two-year course remaining. In 1981, this too was converted to a one-year course, and was at the same time restructured: the three options offered besides the core course were nutrition and metabolism; nutrition and health; and applied nutrition and planning: options which reflected the department's long-term research interests.[55] Indeed, the department was at this time, in the early 1980s, developing a lively, innovative teaching style, and an atmosphere which its students and research workers found highly stimulating.[56] Among the novel teaching departures of these years were the development of audio-visual teaching materials in the form of tape/slide packages; of the 'Green revolution' game, a simulation which demonstrated the survival problems of poor farmers, and the absence of simple solutions to problems of nutrition and development; and, at the behest of Save the Children, of packages detailing techniques of assessing nutritional status.[57]

The expansion and consolidation of the department's research and teaching activities during the 1970s was aimed at providing an academic environment in which basic nutritional science could be taught in an integrated way with relevant aspects of social, economic and political science. In this respect, Nutrition in the School evolved in parallel with, and drew inspiration from, several courses in other universities and academic institutions, both in Britain and in other countries. The common objective of these was to train professionals to help the governments of developing countries to plan the course of social and economic development. However, this ethos – that government planning together with the adoption of new technology would accelerate development and so improve nutrition,[58] masked a growing unease within the wider nutrition community about the discipline's academic status and practical relevance. Indeed, the general idea that balanced and equitable development would automatically result from assisting central governments to engage in rational planning, came under increasingly fierce attack.[59] In reviewing the thirty or so years of nutrition work that had passed since the end of World War II, nutritionists found little to celebrate. In 1975, A.H.Boerma, then Director-General of the United Nations Food and Agriculture Organisation, noted that none of the Organisation's efforts had measured up to the dimensions of the world food problem, or of the human poverty which is its chief cause.[60] Four years later, John Rivers (1945–90), then a lecturer in the Human Nutrition Department, launched a sweeping attack on professional nutritionists and both the wartime and post-war policies for which they were responsible.[61] By the early 1980s, John Waterlow was speaking of a crisis in the discipline as a whole. In particular, he noted the problem was a crisis of identity for the nutritionist: 'What is he trying to do?'[62] This internal questioning within the discipline was met by an increasing emphasis, in line with broader School policy, on teaching, and on overseas research. Waterlow retired as Professor of Human Nutrition in September 1982, in which year he was also made a Fellow of the Royal Society, and his chair was frozen in accordance with the current School policy for financial survival. It was not to be filled again until 1992. Philip Payne, Reader in Applied Nutrition, succeeded as head of the department, taking it forward into a difficult decade of both academic expansion and financial stringency. Payne was given a personal chair in Applied Nutrition in 1987, and became head of the amalgamated Department of Public Health and Policy (including Nutrition) in 1988, when headship of the Centre for Human Nutrition passed to Erica Wheeler.

Three significant academic developments had taken place in Waterlow's last years: an advisory association with the Overseas Development Agency; participation in a UNRISD/UNICEF research project on Food Systems and Society in north-east India; and the establishment of the Famine Research Unit, a joint venture with the International Disaster Institute, based in the department. These were integrated into the broader social and political orientation which Payne's leadership brought to the department's activities.[63] The association with the ODA was the result of a review of Britain's overseas aid policy in the mid-1970s, in which both Waterlow and Payne were involved, following which Waterlow was appointed as part-time Nutrition Adviser (one day a week) to the Agency. By 1982, however, the Agency had decided that this level of representation for nutrition was not justified, and it was arranged that the Department (or the Centre for Human Nutrition, as it became) should provide advice on an *ad-hoc* basis. In this fashion, the Centre was linked into the overseas concerns of the British government, with Payne in practice undertaking the role of government representative at United Nations' meetings related to nutrition, and generally acting as consultant on nutrition questions.

Meanwhile, the Food Systems project proved the launching pad for a series of important research projects in India, several of them undertaken by Barbara Harriss, and for an extension of departmental interests overseas on a scale unknown since the mid-1950s. By the end of the decade, projects had been completed or were in progress in several Indian states, and in Bangladesh, Nepal, Sri Lanka, Zaire, Ghana, Kenya, Brazil and South Asia. Many of these projects were directly concerned with the social and economic aspects of food supply and nutrition. Thus much of Harriss's work was concerned with Indian food marketing systems, and with the relationships between producers, merchants and moneylenders, while other studies investigated socio-economic status, nutritional status and seasonality in a Daka slum, and the biological and socio-economic causes and consequences of adult energy malnutrition in a poor rural Indian population.[64] The expansion of research interest in the developing world was complemented by the emergence of the directly practical focus on nutritional problems represented by the Famine Research Unit. Under the directorship of Julius Holt, the Unit's principal concerns were the use of social and economic indicators to improve detection of impending food crises, and the long and short-term effects of international food aid programmes in famine relief. Its success in forecasting the worsening of famine conditions in northern Ethiopia in 1984 attracted the attention of a number of international agencies, including UNICEF and the World Food Programme.[65] The practical work of the Unit thus enhanced the department's positive contribution to the resolution of food problems, while its collection of literature on famine and food aid complemented the existing resources of the departmental library for the purposes of teaching and research.

There were also developments in teaching. The Government imposition of full fees on overseas student in the early 1980s caused some problems, but did not discourage a consistent rise in applications from within the European Community. Financial pressures within the department were mirrored throughout the School. As early as 1974, the School had settled on a policy of developing collaboration in both teaching and research with outside institutions as a means of sustaining the breadth of its interests and requirements,[66] and this policy became very visible in the Human Nutrition Department from the early 1980s. The extension of research links with bodies like Save the Children, to whom D.N.Nabarro was seconded in 1983, and the International Disaster Institute, was complemented by the development of teaching links with, among others, the Liverpool School of Tropical Medicine, the Open University, the Royal Army Medical Corps, and Reading University besides several of the London colleges, including Royal Holloway, King's and the London School of Economics. Overseas teaching links were achieved through participation in course development at universities in China, Brazil and Africa. A new M.Sc. in Food Technology for Development was launched jointly with King's College, and, in a move which represented a step towards resolution of the long-term global problem of the lack of trained nutrition personnel in government posts, the Nutrition Policy Unit, at the request of the FAO's Nutrition Policy Division, developed materials for the FAO's training programme for senior development planners – a programme designed to teach the use of nutrition concepts and technologies in the planning and management of agricultural development programmes.[67]

In the 1980s, therefore, the Human Nutrition Department's interests diversified more broadly into teaching and overseas concerns, while at the same time clinical, metabolic and physiological studies continued along the lines which had become almost traditional within the department. In 1983 the Clinical Nutrition and Metabolism Unit underwent major restructuring, when its clinical facilities were transferred from the Hopital for Tropical Diseases to University College Hospital to form a new Clinical Nutrition Unit, while the metabolic laboratories at St.Pancras were renamed the Nutrition Research Unit. Here, with D.N.Millward, Reader in Nutritional Biochemistry, as Director, research continued on the nutritional regulation of growth, with special emphasis on protein and energy balance, while a major new programme on the coordinated regulation of muscle and bone growth was developed from the mid–1980s. At the Clinical Nutrition Unit, meanwhile, work continued to focus on energy expenditure and protein metabolism.[68]

Politically speaking, however, the 1980s was not a happy decade for the department. In the early 1980s, the Overseas Development Agency, a major source of funding, first instituted biennial reviews resulting in increased preparation and tension among staff, and later introduced a wide-ranging programme of funding cuts. At the same time, London University's Joint Planning Committee indicated the desirability of an amalgamation of the Human Nutrition department with the Food Science department of King's College – a development resisted by Payne in the mid 1980s, until realisation of the likely costs and practical outcomes of amalgamation eventually led to the abandonment of the proposal. In the meantime, the School itself was undergoing reorganisation, following the Reid Report. In 1988 Human Nutrition was submerged in the Public Health and Policy as the nine existing departments were reduced to four, and its Clinical Nutrition Unit was transferred to the department of Clinical and Tropical Medicine. This move was to prove unfortunate for the CNU – D.J.Millward and Andrew Tomkins soon left to pursue their careers elsewhere – while for the department as a whole, the withdrawal of the metabolic and clinical research interest spelt the end of its truly multi-disciplinary character. The School's annual reports testify to the depressing effect which the implementation of the Reid Report had on the department's research productivity, but, largely through the efforts of Ann Hill, Soraiya Ismail and others, its student intake and teaching continued to be well maintained.[69] While the success of Human Nutrition's teaching, consultancy and research work had sustained the department's finances during the 1980s, the prospect of a further reorganisation following Richard Feachem's appointment as Dean in 1989 was unsettling. In that year, Payne chose to take early retirement, with re-employment at two-fifths of his time for two years, specifically with the agreement of the School, as a means of freeing funds for the unfreezing of the Chair in Human Nutrition.[70] Following his final retirement in 1991, Prakash Shetty, formerly Professor of physiology at Bangalore, was appointed to the Chair in Human Nutrition, and took up his post at the School in May 1993.

Despite the financial and organisational clouds which dogged the department in recent decades, it was a rewarding and enjoyable place in which to work. Much valuable research was accomplished not only by the department's staff, but also by its students: a range of Ph.D. students complemented the work of the more senior scientists, especially in the areas of protein metabolism, food microbiology, (including the role of fermented food which showed microbiology and nutritional benefits) and the impact of deficiency of zinc and folate on gut metabolism.[71] Through its training of students and research workers, through the research and consultation work of its staff in Britain and abroad, and for international organisations, the department extended the disciplinary boundaries and the scientific expertise of the discipline of human nutrition not only in Britain, and in other British institutions, but also of the international nutrition community.

NOTES

[1] LSHTM *Annual Report* 1952-3, p.38.
[2] See 'John Boyd Orr', *Biographical Memoirs of Fellows of the Royal Society,* 1971, pp.47-51.
[3] Joyce Doughty, *Nutrition at the London School of Hygiene and Tropical Medicine 1924-45,* Occasional Paper No.6, Department of Human Nutrition, LSHTM, 1987, p.9.
[4] G.S.Wilson and M.P.Cowell, 'Comparison of the nutritive value of raw and pasteurised milk for mice', *J.Soc.Chem.Ind.,* 1993, *52:*402T-6T.
[5] G.Leighton and M.L.Clark, 'Milk consumption and the growth of schoolchildren', *Lancet* 1929, *i:*40-3;
J.B.Orr and M.L.Clark, 'The effects of school milk on the growth of schoolchildren', *ibid.* 1930, *ii:*594;
All these researches are detailed in Doughty, *Nutrition*, op.cit . note 2 above.
[6] See Anne Hardy, 'Beriberi, Vitamin B and World Food Policy, 1925-70', *Medical History,* January 1995.
[7] MRC *Annual Report* 1939-45, p.284.
[8] LSHTM *Annual Report* 1966-7, p.45.
[9] P.R.Payne, personal communication, 10 January 1995. See also J.C.Waterlow, in Elsie Widdowson, *The Nutrition Society* 1941-91, Wallingford, 1991, pp.91-9, p.94.
[10] See Veronica Berry and Celia Petty eds, *The Nyasaland Survey Papers* 1939-40, ...1994.
[11] MRC *Annual Report* 1939-45, pp.103-4. See also Jennifer Beinart, 'The inner world of imperial sickness', in J.Austoker and L.Bryder eds, *Historical perspectives on the role of the MRC*, 1989, pp.120-35. The question of 'suitable training' for government nutrition advisers was, and remains, problematic.
[12] J.C.Waterlow, personal communication, 13 July 1993.
[13] J.Done and L.Fowden, 'A new amino-acid amide in the groundnut plant (*Arachis hypgaea*): evidence of the occurrence of γ-methyleneglutamine and γ-methyleneglutamic acid', *The Biochemical Journal,* 1952, *51:*451-8.
[14] LSHTM *Annual Report* 1948-9, p.40.
[15] D.F.White, I.G.Campbell and P.R.Payne, 'Estimation of radioactive hydrogen (tritium)', *Nature,*1950, *66:* pp.628-30.

[16] *Ibid.*, 1949-50, p.39.
[17] LSHTM *Annual Report* 1950-1, p.38.
[18] LSHTM *Annual Reports* 1951-2, pp.15, *34:*1953-4 p.45.
[19] More detailed information on the unit's activities can be found in Doughty, op.cit., pp.2-4.
[20] LSHTM *Annual Report* 1947-8, p.76.
[21] LSHTM *Annual Report* 1954-5, p.44.
[22] MRC Archives: File no PF 240; P 16/17, vol.2 no.39. See also nos 42, 43 45, 56, 57, 112, 132.
[23] P.R.Payne, personal communication, 10 January 1995.
[24] B.S.Platt, D.S.Miller and P.R.Payne, 'Protein values of human foods', in J.F.Brock ed, *Recent advances in human nutrition, with special reference to clinical medicine,* London: J&A Churchill, 1960, pp.351-74.
[25] LSHTM *Annual Reports* 1955-6, pp.54-5; 1957-8, p.60. An extensive review of the Unit's research work was published as B.S.Platt, C.R.C.Heard and R.J.C.Stewart, 'Experimental protein-calorie deficiency' in H.N.Munro and J.B.Allison eds. *Mammalian Protein Metabolism* vol.2, 1964, chapter 21, pp.446-521.
[26] Donald S.McLaren, 'The great protein fiasco', *Lancet* 1974, *ii:*93. For a review of this whole debate, see Kenneth J.Carpenter, *Protein and Energy. A Study of Changing Ideas in the History of Nutrition,* Cambridge, CUP, 1994, chapters 8-10.
[27] Platt's research in this area, using pigs and dogs as animal models, fuelled controversy for the rest of his life, notably with Nevin S.Scrimshaw of the Massachusetts Institute of Technology, and with R.A.McCance of the Dunn School of Nutrition in Cambridge: P.R.Payne, personal communication, 10 January 1995.
[28] P.R.Payne, personal communication, 13 July 1994.
[29] LSHTM *Annual Report* 1955-6, p.54.
[30] McLaren, op.cit., p.93; LSHTM *Annual Report* 1960-1, pp.61-2.
[31] LSHTM *Annual Reports* 1962-3, pp.40-1; 1966-7. P.46; 1967-8, p.47.
[32] LSHTM *Annual Report* 1963-4, p.46.
[33] LSHTM *Annual Report* 1971-2, p.31.
[34] *ibid.*
[35] B.S.Platt, T.P.Eddy and P.L.Pellet, *Food in hospitals,* Oxford University Press for the Nuffield Provincial Hospitals Trust, 1963. See *Lancet* 1963, *ii:*1152.
[36] *Ibid.*, p.viii, 1.

37 LSHTM *Annual Reports* 1963–4, p.47; 1965–6, p.40.
38 LSHTM *Annual Report*s 1960–1, p.59.
39 *ibid.,* pp.59–61.
40 T.P.Eddy, 'Deaths from domestic falls and fractures', *Br.J.prev.soc.med.,* 1972, *26:*173–9;
idem, 'Deaths from falls and fractures. Comparison of mortality in Scotland and the United States with that in England and Wales', *ibid.,* 1973, *27:*247–54.
41 LSHTM *Annual Report* 1972–3, p.82.
42 LSHTM *Annual Report* 1967–86, pp.49–50.
43 Waterlow, in Widdowson, *The nutrition society,* p.98.
44 LSHTM *Annual Report* 1969–70, p.48. It may be noted that the *Annual Report* ascribes the grant to the Wellcome Foundation; Philip James and Andrew Tomkins pointed out that it came from the Wellcome Trust, a fact confirmed by the Trust's own records, and in its *Annual Report* for 1969–70.
45 LSHTM *Annual Report* 1970–1, p.24.
46 LSHTM *Annual Report* 1976–7, p.28; P.R.Payne, personal communication, 13 July 1994.
47 LSHTM *Annual Report* 1969–70, p.48.
48 LSHTM *Annual Report* 1972–3, p.80.
49 For the theoretical basis of this work see, J.C.Waterlow, P.Garlick and D.J.Millward, *Protein Turnover in Mammalian Tissues and in the Whole Animal,* London: Elsevier, 1978; in 1988, this was recognised as a 'Citation Classic' by the American Institute of Scientific Information.
50 M.Griffiths and P.R.Payne, 'Energy expenditure in small children of obese and non-obese parents', *Nature,* 1976, *260:*698–700; P.R.Payne and A.E.Dugdale, 'A model for the prediction of energy balance and body weight', *Annals of Human Biology,* 1977, *4:*525–35.
51 LSHTM *Annual Report* 1976–7, p.59. See also Report of the Joint DHSS/MRC Working Party, *Research on obesity,* compiled by W.P.T.James, London HMSO, 1976.
52 P.R.Payne and J.C.Waterlow, 'The protein gap', *Nature,* 1975, *259:*114–16.
53 See LSHTM *Annual Reports* 1970–1, p.6; 1971–2, pp.85–6; 1975–6, p.47; 1978–9, p.38; 1982–3, p.67; 1983–4, p.74.

[54] J.C.Waterlow, 'Classification and definition of protein-calorie malnutrition', *Br.Med.J* 1972, *3:* 566-69; *idem,* 'Classification and definition of protein-energy malnutrition', in G.H.Beaton and J.M.Bengoa eds, *Nutrition in preventive medicine* Geneva, WHO, 1976 (Monograph series no.62), Annex 5, pp.530-55.
[55] LSHTM *Annual Report* 1980-1, p.59.
[56] Barbara Harriss, personal communication, 4 July 1994.
[57] LSHTM *Annual Report* 1982-3, p.67.
[58] The emergence of a new development ethos can be charted through the writings of Alan Berg: *The nutrition factor. Its role in national development,* The Brookings Institution, Washington DC, 1973; *idem,* 'Nutrition planning is alive and well, thank you', *Food Policy, 12:*(November 1987), 365-75.
[59] J.O.Field, 'Multisectoral nutrition planning: A post mortem', *ibid.*
[60] A.H.Boerma, 'The 30 years' war against world hunger', *Proceedings of the Nutrition Society,*1975, *34:* 146-57: p.153.
[61] J.P.W.Rivers, 'The profession of nutrition - a historical perspective', *Proc.Nutr.Soc.,* 1979, *38:*225-31.
[62] J.C.Waterlow, 'Crisis for nutrition', *Proc.Nutr.Soc.,* 1981, *40:*195-207, p.197.
[63] Harriss, personal communication, 4 July 1994.
[64] LSHTM *Annual Report* 1982-4, p.73. Refs.
[65] LSHTM *Annual Report* 1981-2, p.84; 1983-4, p.74.
[66] LSHTM *Annual Report* 1973-4, pp.23-4.
[67] LSHTM *Annual Report* 1987-8, Supplement, p.35.
[68] LSHTM *Annual Reports* 1983-4, p.72; 1984-5, pp.83-4.
[69] J.C.Waterlow, personal communication, 11 December 1994.
[70] P.R.Payne, personal communication, 10 January 1995.
[71] We are grateful to Andrew Tomkins for emphasising this point.

9

WINCHES FARM:
FROM AGRICULTURAL COMPARATIVE
PARASITOLOGY TO LSHTM
FIELD STATION

When the major reorganisation of the LSHTM and its departments in the early 1990s resulted in the closing down of Winches Farm Laboratories (WFL) and the sale of the field station, it marked not the end, but the end of an era, for parasitology at the School; the end of a system within which research in parasitology could benefit from complementary facilities: laboratory work in Keppel Street, and hands-on experimental fieldwork at St.Albans. It was also the end for a unique institution first created by Robert Leiper in 1924, the year when building of the new LSHTM on the Keppel Street site began in London. When WFL closed down in 1992, it had existed as a field station for more than 65 years, a monument to Leiper's vision and versatility.[1]

Ironically, it was also an institution whose existence testified to Leiper's concern with wider issues of crop and animal diseases affecting the country's agricultural economy. Ironic because Leiper, perhaps more than anyone at the School, could be perceived as representative of the type of dedicated scientist, cool and remote in his quest for answers to problems in the laboratory, whose detachment allowed few sideways glances at more human implications of his research. But the story of the creation of Winches Farm shows Robert Leiper in a different light. The story began towards the end of Leiper's first two decades at the School, after his early expeditions, when he had been appointed University Professor, when the Great War was over, and when Manson had retired and subsequently died.[2]

From the day he graduated in medicine at Edinburgh, Robert Leiper had indeed been intent on devoting himself to pure research rather than clinical medicine. It has been suggested – in fact, Leiper himself admitted – that this was to some extent a reaction to his father's early death from tuberculosis, in an age when the medical profession was powerless to fight this major nineteenth-century killer as well as other infectious diseases.[3] Looking back at the age of eighty, Leiper said: '... my father had been an invalid for so many years that I didn't care for the prospect of taking up medical practice'. In this spirit he had enthusiastically accepted Manson's offer of a research and teaching appointment at the LSTM in January, 1905, at a time when Manson began his moves to supplement clinical instruction by physicians and surgeons at the Hospital for Tropical Diseases with specialised teaching in laboratories and lecture rooms. This move was in line with developments in other teaching hospitals and medical schools at the turn of the century. Leiper's early work as helminthologist at Manson's School, and his pioneering contributions to schistosomiasis research in Egypt and the Far East have been described above; and also his efforts to further relations between the School and the young Rockefeller Foundation's newly established International Health Board since 1913. He had been personally rewarded with support for his research expeditions, and the School with the moral and financial support needed for its development into the LSHTM.[4]

Leiper also began applying for funds closer to home. Following the Great War, with its many problems including maintenance of healthy stock and crops to feed a nation at war, the Ministry of Agriculture agreed to fund a study of parasites of farm animals and plants. With a grant from the Development Commission's Fund, out of a special fund created by the Corn Reduction Repeal Act of 1921, Leiper was by 1924 in a position to establish a field station where he could pursue a second major strand of interests, in comparative parasitology. Describing him as 'one of the earliest of the comparative helminthologists', colleagues later recalled his three years as Director of Prosectorium of London's Zoological Gardens, and his lasting connection with the Zoo 'in a daily search for new and interesting parasites which could be used for teaching and research'.[5]

When Leiper, his grant assured, set about looking for suitable properties within a reasonable distance from London, and at an affordable price, he settled for Winches Farm at St.Albans in Hertfordshire. Bought from a Mr.John Lewis of the John Lewis store in Oxford Street, the existing farm buildings were derelict but cheap; that suited Leiper's limited budget as well as his taste for restoration and extension to suit his purpose. With its run-down buildings dating from the sixteenth and seventeenth centuries, Winches Farm was in need of sympathetic treatment.

Although the farm buildings could never compete, in terms of recorded history, with neighbouring St.Albans, its Abbey, and its remains of Roman Verulamium, the farm's name can be traced back as far as the fourteenth century, when one Alice ate Wynche (fl.1332) lived there, at Wynchepitt or Wynchewode (1312); by 1449 the name had become Wynchestrette. At the end of the sixteenth century (1591), Winchehill Farm on Winches Hill was farmed by John ate Wynche.[6] In its restored form the farmhouse, with its original fireplace stripped of unfortunate Victorian 'improvements', (Fig.00) housed the offices of the Professor; a near-by timbered barn – or stable – also thought to be 16th–17th century, emerged as a pleasant Common Room, still in use in 1990. The laboratories, designed by Leiper, remained unaltered for a long time. Blackie wrote at the beginning of the 1970s: 'The laboratories are rather makeshift buildings and we still await the promised day when the new labs are to be built.'[7] The day was not then far off. A year later the School's *Annual Report* noted:

> The long awaited rebuilding of laboratory accommodation commenced in April 1970. The new building will replace laboratories which were converted from farm buildings by the late Professor R.T.Leiper some 44 years ago ...

Also eventually overtaken by the march of time and progress were the animal quarters, which unlike the laboratories had been rebuilt and extended in the 1950s, and which at the beginning of the 1970s housed a representative variety of laboratory animals used in experimental pathology and parasitology: rats, mice, rabbits, guinea pigs, monkeys, baboons, and even 'Cherry, our chimpanzee'. Dogs, cats, and pigs enjoyed separate quarters, and pigeons and doves had their aviaries. The LSHTM Department of Helminthology maintained a large aquarium at its field station. Blackie added: '... to be a farm, we must have geese, ducks, sheep, calves, a cow and often other large animals'. Twenty years later, towards the end of Winches Farm's existence as the School's field station, all the large animals had gone. In an age of molecular biology, less controversial and more time-saving tissue culture techniques were, and are, rapidly obviating the need for increasingly problematic animal experimentation, although advances in parasitology will probably need some experiments involving live animals for longer than other areas of preventive and curative medicine concerned with transmissible diseases.

As soon as Leiper's Institute of Agricultural Parasitology was established at Winches Farm, staff already working on agriculturally related problems at the School in London began transferring to St.Albans. The *Annual Reports'* Appendix listing papers published by members of the department of Helminthology and the Institute of Agricultural Parasitology (from 1925–6 onwards) testify to the wide variety of subjects under scrutiny: from eelworm in potatoes, of importance through two World Wars, and nematode parasites in roots of barley and in pea-fowl gizzards, to rather more esoteric problems of ankylostomes in an African mongoose and helminths in wild birds in Aberystwyth.[8]

Throughout the inter-war years, and until Leiper's retirement from the School at the end of September, 1946, work at the Institute continued its comprehensive coverage of research into the four major groups of helminth diseases of economic importance, i.e. of: (a) farm stock; (b) poultry and game; (c) economic plants; and, (d) insect pests.[9]

The School Report which covered the end of the war in 1945 still referred to the 'Institute of Agricultural Parasitology' with Leiper as Director. A year later, Leiper had retired and the *Annual Report* now listed the 'Field Station (Winches Farm, St.Albans)'. It also announced wide-ranging changes in the future administration and concerns of the laboratories. Acknowledging Leiper's contribution – 'The important place the Institution had occupied in the field of Agricultural Parasitology had been due to him and it remains as a monument to his work'– the School decided to transfer all work on plant helminthology to Rothamsted Experimental Station. H.E.Shortt, who finally retired from the Indian Medical Service at the end of World War II to take up his appointment as Professor of Medical Protozoology and Director of the Department of Parasitology at the School in 1945, was 'Acting Director' during the transition period 1946–7 when the 'Institute' became the 'Field Station'; he subsequently used the Winches Farm facilities to continue a study begun in India with S.R.Christophers, on *Babesia canis*. But the move of the plant helminthologists to Rothamsted left only one senior member of the permanent staff at Winches Farm: John W.G.Leiper, MRCVS, Robert Leiper's son, who would act as administrator and as veterinary officer supervising animal health and husbandry at the farm. However, in December 1948 he resigned, moving to a new appointment elsewhere.[10]

With 'Winches Farm Field Station' finally part and parcel of the School after repayment of an agreed sum to compensate for the original Development Fund grant, the Winches Farm Committee unveiled ambitious plans for a development programme. Departments in Keppel Street interested in future use of laboratories at Winches Farm (Bacteriology, Parasitology, Entomology, Applied Physiology, Tropical Hygiene, and Biochemistry) were consulted, as was an architect. The development was planned to take place in three stages, the first stage being the erection of an animal breeding station.[11] In 1949, the School's *Annual Report* still sounded optimistic concerning the building plans; but the following year, the plans were adversely affected by 'national economic restrictions'. By 1951, at least the animal breeding station had been completed, providing mice, rabbits, and guinea pigs for the School, and:

> The monkey quarters house thirty baboons and here work on schistosomiasis is being carried out under the aegis of the Medical Research Council.

Apart from this morsel of good news, 'Treasury restrictions' prevented any further developments. No authority had been received to proceed

with Stage II, and 'the prospects of Stage III must be distinctly remote.'[12]
A year later, hope was finally abandoned:

> Little more can be added to last year's report on Winches Farm except to say that the prospects of any further building are now remote on account of financial stringency.[13]

Although total closure had been narrowly avoided at the beginning of the 1950s, for the remainder of the decade Winches Farm, if mentioned at all in the School's *Annual Reports*, was referred to only as 'Winches Farm Animal Breeding House'. What is not made clear in these official reports is how much of the actual research work of the Parasitology Department continued to be carried out there during the early years of Garnham's 'reign' as head of department, following Shortt's retirement and his own return to London after more than 20 years in the Colonial Medical Service in Kenya. He was fortunate indeed in the team assembled there, not all of whom bowed to the pressure to work on malaria parasites only.

Among the early recruits was W.E.Ormerod, who joined the department in 1953 as Garnham's 'No.2', in the belief that he would there be pursuing his interest in trypanosome studies; only to find that Garnham's own intense interest in malaria parasites outweighed other considerations: Ormerod, in spite of his appointment as Senior Lecturer, and his credentials which included a degree in chemistry in addition to his medical qualifications, was expected to act as research assistant to Garnham in his malaria work. He still remembers his initial difficulties in his ultimately successful fight to concentrate on studies of *Trypanosoma brucei*. Trypanosomes joined the list of subjects researched at Winches Farm. The range of fieldwork carried out there during the 1950s, as part and parcel of the *sum total* of the work in the Department of Parasitology, is reflected in the names of 'people at the Farm' referred to in the School Report for 1955–6:

> An Open Day was held at Winches Farm Field Station on 12th April, 1956, when demonstrations were shown illustrating the work of the people at the Farm, including Col.Shortt [who had by then been 'retired' for 3 years], Dr.Bird, Dr.Ormerod, Dr.Lainson, Mr.Mettrick, and the MRC Bilharzia Research Unit (Dr.Newsome).

Shortt was working on *Babesia;* R.G.('Dickie') Bird gave a demonstration of the morphology of *Entamoeba histolytica;* Ralph Lainson was working on toxoplasmosis; Mettrick on trematodes; and Ormerod, with C.B.Hill and R.Killick-Kendrick, on development of trypanosomes and effects of trypanocidal drugs.[14]

The range of problems associated with species of trypanosomes in Africa had, after a century, shifted considerably since the days of Bruce and Castellani. Developments in drug therapy, sanitary measures, and tsetse-fly control have over the years radically reduced the threat of sleeping sickness in man. Trypanosomiasis in cattle is, on the other hand, as much, and for various reasons perhaps more, of a threat to living standards in parts of Africa than when Bruce first began his study of *nagana* in the last decade of the nineteenth century.[15] In a developing world, the very results of well-meaning attempts to improve living standards in developing countries by organisations such as FAO/WHO and associated agencies and local governments, have paradoxically tended to aggravate rather than improve the outlook through ecological effects of overgrazing, competition for land use, and intensive disease control. For such reasons the study of animal trypanosomes and of the blood-sucking insects which transmit them, came to the fore during the years following the end of World War II. In 1947 P.A.Buxton, then in his last decade at the School, had suggested to the Colonial Medical Research Committee of the Colonial Office (which became the Commonwealth Office in August 1966) a programme of field and laboratory research into feeding habits and preferences of tsetse-flies and related species, with laboratory work done at the Lister Institute. The question of selective extermination of wild animals preferred by the tsetse was aired again for the first time since it had been rejected in May, 1914.[16]

Research on the trypanosomes, their hosts, their ecology, biology, metabolism, and other factors of importance for their control was carried out at the Field Station at Winches Farm in the 1950s and 1960s by Ormerod and a growing number of other medical protozoologists. J.R.Baker worked on vectors of bird trypanosomes; Ormerod, Bird, D.S.Ellis and D.A.Evans, and later W.H.R.Lumsden who succeeded Garnham in 1968, were primarily concerned with the *Trypanosoma brucei* group: *T.brucei gambiense* and *T.b.rhodiense,* and to some extent *T.cruzi* of Chagas' disease in South America. They were later joined by D.G.Godfrey's ODM/ODA trypanosomiasis research group which moved from the Lister Institute to the School in 1974, when the Lister's London Institute closed. The Lister had won the battle for the University Chair of Protozoology in the early days of the century, when Minchin chose to be based there; now the ODM Unit, facing exile because of the closure of its base at the Lister, found a new home at the LSHTM.[17]

Bird had begun his career as a student of Ormerod's, and had earned a Ph.D. with work on the morphology and pathology of amoebae. The *Annual Report* noted that he worked 'under conditions of some difficulty' because electron microscopy had to be carried out at the

Wright–Fleming Institute, ending with a plea for 'this essential instrument' to be available at the School. When this happened Bird, by then Reader in Cellular Fine Structure, became Director of the Electron Microscopy Laboratory, with D.S.Ellis as Assistant Electron Microscopist. From this position Ellis moved on to be Lecturer in Protozoology and electron microscopist in the department, before in the early 1980s he took over as Academic Head of the Electron Microscopy Laboratory. During the intervening years he formed a fruitful working relationship with D.A.Evans, his colleague in the department and a 'wizard at culturing'. In papers on the development of *Trypanosoma brucei* in the tsetse-fly Ellis and Evans provided the basis for establishing Ellis's thesis that 'there must be a sexual phase in trypanosomes as in other living things'; a view which was later confirmed by Swiss workers.[18]

In spite of the pioneering work of Bruce, Castellani, and others at the beginning of the century, and of all the resulting activity and intensity of study the complex problems surrounding the trypanosomes and the diseases they cause remained a subject of controversy for the better part of the twentieth century. Writing at the end of the 1970s, Ormerod summed up the reasons for lack of consensus among researchers over the years in terms which could apply to a number of other biological problems which have taken surprisingly long to resolve:

> ... on the one hand, valid observations have been made but misinterpreted and, on the other hand, adequate observations have been accepted because they happened to support a theory which was then in vogue.

By the mid-1980s Ormerod, with co-workers from Botswana, Kuwait, and Nigeria, had observed a crucial step in the development: the intracellular phase of *T.brucei* in ependymal brain cells, a discovery of importance for evaluation of different therapies used for sleeping sickness.[19]

During W.H.R.Lumsden's tenure of the Chair of Medical Protozoology, from 1968 to 1979, trypanosome research at the School continued its concern with the *Trypanosoma brucei* group causing African sleeping sickness in man, and with *T.cruzi*, which causes Chagas' disease in South America. J.R.Baker continued his work on trypanosomes in Cambridge, at the MRC Biochemical Parasitology Unit at the Molteno Institute, with studies of the subgenus *Schizotrypanum* in bats.[20] Of considerable help to trypanosome research generally has been the department's cryopreserved collection of parasitic protozoa. It consisted initially largely of trypanosome strains, but has since been one of the main suppliers of trypanosomes and leishmaniasis to researches both within the School and in a wider context, in its essential role as part of a WHO reference centre.

In the early 1960s, when expansion in the country's universities once again became possible, some reconstruction of long-neglected laboratories had coincided with the closing down of the animal breeding facilities, a corollary of a general improvement in commercially available experimental animals. Completion of work on the 'west block' also coincided with the appointment of George Nelson to the School's helminthology department in 1963. Fresh from years spent as medical officer and medical parasitologist in Uganda and Kenya, Nelson began to rebuild experimental helminthology at what from now on would be referred to as 'Winches Farm Field Station', and eventually 'Winches Farm Laboratories', or WFL.[21] With students from Egypt, Sudan, and Iran, as well as the UK, Nelson opened up a number of lines of research on schistosomes at Winches. One study concerned the effects of 'strain variation' in different geographical variants of schistosomes on their infectivity in snails and their behaviour in the mammalian host; another concern was the possibility of producing vaccines by exploitation of heterologous immunity – i.e., producing immunity to human schistosomes by exposure to cercariae of animal ones, a principle harking back to Jenner's use of cowpox to produce immunity to smallpox in man.

In 1967, Gerald Webbe came to the Department of Helminthology as Reader in Medical Parasitology. Webbe had spent the early part of his career in Tanzania, in the Colonial Medical Service, as medical entomologist and parasitologist to the Ministry of Health, and Assistant Director of the East African Institute for Medical Research. Subsequently he spent two years in Germany familiarising himself with pharmaceutical industry, conducting clinical trials of new compounds for the treatment of amoebiasis and Chagas' disease for Bayer's Clinical Tropical Trials Department, before joining the LSHTM. Within a year, he was appointed scientific director of Winches Farm Field Station, at a time of growth and revival of its activities and its laboratory accommodation, and when it once again, after more than ten years of anonymity, was given separate listing among the School's departments. At the same time, helminthology was not neglected in Keppel Street, where David Denham and his group have had a particular interest in the immunopathology of filarial infections (Chapter 10).[22]

In the new climate of improved facilities and consequent opportunity for broadly accelerating activity, Webbe and Nelson and their students began, with MRC support, an ambitious and many-faceted programme in schistosomiasis research. In Tanzania, Webbe had been involved in early experiments on *Schistosoma haematobium* in baboons for schistosomiasis research under the aegis of the MRC since 1950.[23] Thus the work of Nelson and of Webbe became an ever expanding and diversifying continuation of MRC sponsored work two decades earlier, when the young G.A.T.Targett had earned his Ph.D. there in 1961 in J.Newsome's Bilharzia Research Unit.[24]. This work was supported by several sponsors including, in addition to the MRC, the Wellcome Trust, the Edna McConnell Clark Foundation, and the Rockefeller Foundation.

Moving with the times, the increasing complexity of research took account of many new developments and techniques in studies in immunology, pathogenesis, vaccine production, and chemotherapy. Some of the first trials of praziquantel and metrifonate were carried out at Winches Farm; and considerable advances were made in the understanding of the immunology of all three schistosome species of man, as well as several of those parasitising livestock by an expanding group including also, in addition to Nelson and Webbe, Doenhoff, James, M.G.Taylor, and others. Winches Farm at this time housed the WHO Collaborating Centre for Research on Schistosomiasis, and there were strong links with field projects in Africa, Asia and the Caribbean[25].

Schistosomiasis was a key area of research pursued at WFL during the period between the changes of the 1960s and the field station's demise – or removal to Keppel Street – in 1992. On Garnham's retirement in 1968, it was found to be 'convenient to divide the department of parasitology into two new departments': medical helminthology under G.S.Nelson, and medical protozoology under W.H.R.Lumsden. Within this new arrangement, protozoology moved to Keppel Street, while helminthology resumed its old quarters at Winches Farm. Earlier the protozoologists had used the wild fauna of the buildings and surrounding land, with its pond, to maximum advantage, until the School Secretary, L.G.Ponsford, moved to Winches as his private residence and 'cleaned up' the site. Former members of the department still remember being awestruck by Garnham's unprecedented fury at the draining of the pond and consequent loss of a useful ecological site. Onchocerciasis – 'river blindness'– also rated high among research interests in the laboratories, ever since J.P.McMahon returned from eradication attempts in Kenya to explore local Hertfordshire rivers in a search for vector species suitable for laboratory research.[26] At the same time George Nelson, interested in *Onchocerca* parasites of local livestock, and their possible use as model systems in an exploration of host–parasite relationships and treatment of onchocerciasis, used such problems as research projects for his Ph.D. students. From these beginnings, aspects of onchocerciasis research were pursued by a growing group of enthusiastic workers at WFL. The technique of cryopreservation, initially studied at Winches by E.R.James for its potential value for storage of live attenuated organisms, necessary for development of a live attenuated vaccine against schistosomiasis, proved to be an important tool in studies of both *Onchocerca volvulus* and its blackfly vector. Such techniques were used in a number of studies, notably Wellcome Trust funded research on onchocerciasis carried out by A.E.Bianco and colleagues at Winches Farm between 1981 and 1986. This was a continuation of a WHO funded programme on onchocerciasis begun by George Nelson and Bianco in 1977.[27]

In the post-Leiper, post 1960s era of Winches Farm, subjects outside helminthology, but within tropical disease research, played considerable roles in the field station's programmes. The helminths include some of the largest parasites known to man; at the other end of the scale, viruses are among the smallest; the human arboviruses exhibit parasite-vector interactions as complex as many of the helminths. An Arbovirus Research Unit came to Winches Farm in the 1970s, as home support for the MRC Kisumu Project in Kenya under David Simpson. It closed in 1977, but was revived in 1979 as the School's Arbovirus Unit under the Professor of Medical Entomology, M.G.R.Varma. For a decade, during the deanship of C.E.Gordon Smith, himself an erstwhile virologist, enthusiastic staff at the Unit worked with new and developing techniques, producing monoclonal antibodies for diagnostic purposes, and also in the hope of using them to explore regions of viral proteins determining virulence and neutralisation. The ultimate aim was to further understanding of the role of virus sequence determinants for virulence and disease manifestations. Together with work on recombinant DNA technology, these studies as well as important fieldwork led by Colin Leake, had to be suspended when the Unit closed, and departments were reorganised in Keppel Street in 1989: Virology incorporated in the Department of Clinical Sciences, as its Viral Pathogenesis Unit; and Medical Entomology accommodated in the 'Vector Biology and Transmission Dynamics Unit' of the Department of Medical Parasitology, until more restructuring in the later 1990s.[28]

Another subject which enjoyed a short, late, span of research activity at WFL was malaria. Those involved ascribe this to the dominant part played by research in the Department of Parasitology of the School in Keppel Street, presided over by those towering figures in malaria research, H.E.Shortt (1887-1987) from 1945 to 1951, and P.C.C.Garnham (1901-94), from 1952 to 1968. The decade of malaria studies at Winches also coincided with the period of increasing emphasis on immune responses, and on their importance for the efficacy or otherwise of chemotherapy. When in 1970 G.A.T.Targett came to the School after the years with the MRC at Winches Farm, and subsequently at the NIMR and a spell at the University of St.Andrews, his research interests were beginning to move towards the problems of immunogenicity on which he focuses today. In the 1970s, back at WFL, he began studies of malaria as well as schistosomiasis. With M.J.Doenhoff and others, he explored the ways in which the effectiveness of chemotherapy may depend on the immunological status of the host. Former and current research interests were then combined in studies of interactions between schistosome infections and malaria in the mouse.[29]

Malaria research at WFL was also influenced by the appointment, from September, 1979, of Wallace Peters to the Chair of Medical Protozoology at the School, when W.H.R.Lumsden retired. Peters came to London from Liverpool, where he had been Dean of the School of Tropical Medicine since the departure of Brian Maegraith (1907–89) in 1975, after nearly thirty years not entirely free from controversy.[30] Like so many staff members at the two tropical schools, and his colleague at Winches Farm, Gerald Webbe, Wallace Peters had early experiences of practical tropical medicine in East and West Africa, before joining the WHO in Liberia and Nepal (1952–5), and spending five years directing the malariology section of the Health Department in Papua New Guinea. Also like Webbe, he spent five years in the pharmaceutical industry, in his case in the research department of CIBA in Basle. In 1966 he had moved to the Walter Myers Chair at the Liverpool School, serving as Dean after the departure of Maegraith, from 1975 to 1978. During those years there were attempts at a *rapprochement* between the two Schools, after long years of mutual isolation; but valiant efforts were unsuccessful. Even now, with both Schools nearing their centenaries, cooperation where it exists is on a personal rather than an official level. Very recently, though, the two Schools have at last joined forces to form the UK Malaria Consortium, to interact with the WHO, the World Bank, the CEC, and other agencies, to explore practical approaches to malaria control. Even then, financial constraints at Liverpool leave some doubts for the future of the Consortium.[31]

The removal of Wallace Peters to London, at a time when he was Chairman of the WHO Steering Committee on Malaria Chemotherapy, also meant the transfer of the WHO's collaborating Centre for the Evaluation of Antimalarial Drugs to the LSHTM. The Centre's *in vitro* research took place in London, directed by D.Warhurst, and *in vivo* studies at the WFL (Chapter 10).[32]

Leishmaniasis research at the School, at WFL, may on the face of it seem to have had only a short history in a unit set up in 1984 by Ralph Neal (1925–90). Neal came to Winches from the Wellcome Research Laboratories, where he had been Head of the Department of Parasitology. His experience of antiprotozoal chemotherapy shaped the unit's search for new drugs to be used against leishmaniasis and Chagas' disease. But long before the unit's arrival there had been a leishmaniasis research interest at Winches Farm. Ralph Lainson had come to the School as Garnham's first Ph.D. student the year he took over from Shortt, in 1952; three years later, he became lecturer in protozoology at the School before leaving, in 1959, to become Officer-in-Charge at the Dermal Leishmaniasis Unit in Baking-Pot, Belize. He chose to spend the rest of his working life in South America, but never cut his ties with Garnham and the School, even when he became Director of the Wellcome Parasitology Unit in the Evandro Chagas Institute in Belém, Brazil, in 1965. Today he still, although officially 'retired', and working with his colleague, J.J.Shaw, focuses on the leishmaniases, their sandfly vectors, and their epidemiology, work which earned him an FRS in 1982. At WFL, after Neal's death, the work on antileishmanial drugs continued under Simon Croft, who in 1991–2 transferred with the Unit to Keppel Street, where it is now the Parasite and Vector Biochemistry Unit, in the Department of Medical Parasitology. At the same time, W.Peters built on work begun in Liverpool on *Leishmania* surveys, identifying a number of new species, some not pathogenic for man, to be used in vaccination trials. After the changes in the early 1990s then, all the surviving activities from Winches Farm have transferred, in one form or another, to the various units concerned with parasites and vector biochemistry and biology, molecular biology, immunology and vaccine design, etc. All are incorporated in the new large Department of Medical Parasitology, headed by G.A.T.Targett, and Gerald Webbe, Sub-Dean at Winches, as Professor, now Emeritus Professor, of Applied Parasitology; Wallace Peters is also in the Department as Emeritus Professor of Medical Protozoology; and M.G.Taylor, who worked on schistosome vaccines at WFL throughout the 1970s and 1980s, is now Professor of Medical Helminthology in Keppel Street.[33]

With the latest moves and reorganisations between WFL and the School in Keppel Street, Leiper's creation has in a sense come full circle. Where he and his helminthologists had moved to the Institute of Agricultural Parasitology in 1924–5, his successors, almost seventy years later, have been transferred back to Keppel Street, to continue their research within the refurbished and reorganised School. The final closing down of Winches Farm also marked the end of the School's connection with other institutions established in Leiper's time, and developed under the auspices of Leiper's lively mind. From his earliest days in science, Leiper had been profoundly interested in the scientific literature. Introduced to Millport Marine Station by a cousin, James Gemmill, FRS (d.1926), he was appointed the Station's Hon.Librarian while still a student. Later, at Manson's School, he became 'acting' librarian to the School's developing library, a position he held, through his frequent absences abroad, until 1921, when Cyril Barnard took over as its first professional librarian. The LSTM librarianship has been seen as a natural link in Leiper's lifelong dedication to medical bibliography; but an extant letter in the School's archives suggests a possibly less disinterested motive: a letter from the Seamen's Hospital Society, which could not grant Leiper a £50 rise for 'existing duties', but offered an extra £50 if he would take on the School librarianship.[34] Nevertheless, the publication and dissemination of helminthological information was for Leiper a duty which never became a burden, but remained throughout his life a matter of keen interest.

There is no lack of evidence of his intense preoccupation with the literature of his subject, witnessed by his bibliographical contributions, and his countless and often inspired abstracts of papers for *Helminthological Abstracts* and for the *Tropical Diseases Bulletin*. His *Periodicals of Medicine and the Allied Sciences in British Libraries* of 1923, was a forerunner of the *World List of Periodicals;* the *bibliography of Helminthology* of 1930 and 1931 was incorporated in *Helminthological Abstracts* in 1932. Leiper's most important contribution to the publishing side of the helminthological literature was arguably the founding in 1923, the year before he arranged the purchase of Winches Farm, of the *Journal of Helminthology*. This he edited until 1947, the year of his retirement from the School; it still remains a valuable outlet for publication of the papers of helminthologists everywhere.

When Leiper, long retired from the School, finally left Winches Farm in the 1950s, it was in a move with the Bureau of Helminthology to nearby premises in St.Albans. The Bureau had come into existence not long after the Institute of Agricultural Parasitology. An Imperial Agricultural Research Conference held in 1927 recommended the establishment of an Imperial Bureau of Agricultural Parasitology, to serve as a source of information and advice available to all parts of the British Empire, and to interested foreign countries: agricultural parasitology's answer to the Bureau of Hygiene and Tropical Diseases. In 1932 the Bureau, influenced by Leiper's bibliographical efforts, began publishing *Helminthological Abstracts*. Until the outbreak of World War II, the *Abstracts* were 'issued by arrangement with the Imperial Bureau of Agricultural Parasitology'. Significantly, at the beginning of the post-war era, with the Empire crumbling, with Leiper retired from the School, and with Winches Farm entering a period of quiet stagnation, the Bureau was re-styled the 'Commonwealth Bureau of Agricultural Parasitology (Helminthology)'; and when Leiper finally left Winches Farm in 1953, the Bureau moved with him from 'Winches Farm Drive, Hatfield Road' to 'The White House, 103 St.Peter's Street, St.Albans.'[35]

Leiper did eventually retire from the Bureau also, but continued to be actively involved in its activities until a short time before his death in 1969. In 1982, the Bureau returned to a new building in the grounds of Winches Farm, as the Commonwealth Institute of Helminthology. Since the closure of the Winches Farm Laboratories in 1992, the Commonwealth Agricultural Bureaux have reorganised as the Centre for Agriculture and Biosciences International (CAB International, or CABI) with four constituent institutes offering scientific and information services:

> the International Institute of Parasitology has remained in Hatfield Road at St. Albans;
> the International Institute of Entomology in London, sharing some space with the Natural History Museum;
> the International Mycological Institute in Surrey;
> the International Institute of Biological Control at Silwood Park, Ascot, with field stations in Trinidad and Tobago, Switzerland, Pakistan, Malaysia, and Kenya.

Their information services include CABI's main databases, CAB ABSTRACTS, and the PHTM (Public Health and Tropical Medicine) database, produced by the Bureau of Hygiene and Tropical Diseases, incorporated in CABI in March, 1993.[36]

NOTES

[1] M.G.Taylor (ed), *A brief history of virology, protozoology and helminthology at Winches Farm Laboratories 1924-1992*, November 1992.

[2] Mary E.Gibson and Janet Foster, 'The development of Winches Farm Laboratories', in: *ibid.*, pp.1-4; also cf. chapter 1 and 2 above.

[3] P.C.C.Garnham, 'Robert Thomson Leiper 1881-1969', *Biogr.Mem.Fell.R.Soc.*, 1970, *16*:385-404;

Anne Hardy, 'Tuberculosis', in: *The epidemic streets,* Oxford, Clarendon Press, 1993;

R.T.Leiper, reply to tributes paid at his 80th birthday celebration, Suppl., *J.Helminthol.*, 1969, *43*, p.260.

[4] Sir Philip Manson-Bahr, *History of the School of Tropical Medicine in London 1899-1949,* London, H.K.Kewis & Co.Ltd., 1956, pp.227-9, and 'Research Expeditions', pp.304-5.

[5] Ian Clunies-Ross, T.W.M.Cameron, B.G.Peters, 'Professor Leiper's contribution to agricultural helminthology', Suppl., *J.Helminthol.*, 1961, pp.xvii-xx;

Corn Act (1921), 11 and 12, Geo 5, Chap.48.

[6] Eric J.Blackie, 'Winches Farm Field Station', MS for SSO News, c1970.

[7] *ibid.*, p.1.

[8] LSHTM *Annual Reports* 1925-6, pp.21-2, and 1944-5, p.27.

[9] LSHTM *Annual Reports* between 1925 and 1945.

[10] LSHTM *Annual Report* 1947-8, pp.108-9; Winches Farm Committee Minutes, 26.2.48.

[11] LSHTM *Annual Report* 1948-9, p.18; Winches Farm Committee Minutes 8.3.48;

C.M.Clark and J.M.Mackintosh, *The School and the Site,* London, H.K.Lewis & Co. Ltd., 1954, pp.83-6.

[12] LSHTM *Annual Reports* 1949-50, p.20; 1950-1, p.81.

[13] LSHTM *Annual Report* 1951-2, p.83.

[14] LSHTM *Annual Report* 1955-6, pp.79 and 118-20.

[15] H.Chick, M.Hume and M.MacFarlane, *War on Disease: a history of the Lister Institute,* [London], A.Deutsch, [1971], p.206; also Chapter 2.

[16] *War on Disease,* op.cit., p.207; also cf. Chapter 2.

[17] Chapter 1, pp.25-6;

LSHTM *Annual Report* 1974-5, pp.32-3. *A brief history*...... op.cit. note 1, p.39.

[18] D.A.Evans and D.S.Ellis, 'Penetration of mid-gut cells of *Glossina*

morsitans morsitans by *Trypanosoma brucei rhodesiense*' *Nature* 1975, *258*:231-3;
D.S.Ellis and D.A.Evans, 'Passage of *Trypanosoma brucei rhodesiense* through the peritrophic membrane of *Glossina morsitans morsitans*', *ibid.* 1977, *267*:834-5;
LSHTM *Annual Reports* 1972-3, 1973-4, 1974-5, and 1981-2.
[19] W.E.Ormerod, 'Development of *Trypanosoma brucei* in the mammalian host', in: *Biology of the Kinetoplastida,* W.H.R.Lumsden and D.A.Evans (eds), London etc., Academic Press, vol.2 1979, pp.339-94, p.340-1;
M.O.Abolarin, S.A.Stamford and W.R.Ormerod, 'Interaction between *Trypanosoma brucei* and the ependymal cell of the choroid plexus', *Trans.R.Soc.Trop.Med.Hyg.*, 1986, *80*:618-25;
W.E.Ormerod and M.S.-A.Hussein, 'The ventricular ependyma of mice infected with *Trypanosoma brucei*', *ibid.*, pp.626-33;
B.H.Raseroka and W.E.Ormerod, 'The trypanocidal effect of drugs in different parts of the brain', *ibid.* pp.634-41.
[20] D.A.Evans and S.L.Croft, 'Research on trypanosomiasis and leishmaniasis at Winches Farm Laboratories', in: *A brief history...,* op.cit. note 1, pp.39-42;
W.H.R.Lumsden and D.S.Ketteridge, 'Characterization, Nomenclature and Maintenance of Salivarian Trypanosomes' in: *Biology of the Kinetoplastida,* op.cit. note 19, pp.693-722;
J.R.Baker *et al.*, 'Biochemical characterization of some species of *Trypanosoma* (*Schizotrypanum*) from bats (Microchiroptera)', *Am.J.Trop.Med.Hyg.*, 1978, *27*:483-91.
[21] M.G.Taylor (ed), op.cit. note 1.
[22] LSHTM *Annual Report* 1969-70, p.139.
[23] LSHTM *Annual Report* 1950-1, p.81.
[24] MRC Reports 1957-8, p.105; 1960-1, p.134.
[25] M.G.Taylor and M.J.Doenhoff, 'Schistosomiasis research at Winches Farm Laboratories', in: *A brief history ...*, op.cit. note 1, pp.5-13, with list of key publications;
M.G.Taylor and G.Webbe, 'Prospects for the development of a vaccine for schistosomiasis', in: A.J.Zuckerman (ed), *Recent developments in prophylactic immunization,* Dordrecht, Kluwer, 1989, pp.289-312;
M.J.Doenhoff *et al.*, 'Evidence for an immune-dependent action of praziquantel on *Schistosoma mansoni* in mice', *Trans.R.Soc.Trop.Med.Hyg.*, 1987, *81*:947-51;
R.Sturrock, M.J.Doenhoff and G.Webbe, 'Schistosomiasis' in: O.Zak and M.A.Sande (eds), *Experimental models in antimicrobial chemotherapy,* vol.3, pp.241-79, London, Academic Press, 1986.
[26] LSHTM *Annual Report* 1968-9, p.15;

A.E.Bianco, 'Onchocerciasis research at Winches Farm Laboratories', in: *A brief history ...,* op.cit. note 1, pp.21-30;
R.Lainson and W.E.Ormerod, personal communications.
[27] G.S.Nelson, M.A.Amin, E.J.Blackie, and N.Robson, 'The maintenance of *Onchocerca gutturosa* microfilariae *in vitro* and *in vivo*' *Trans.R.Soc.Trop.Med.Hyg.*, 1966, *60:*17;
J.P.McMahon, 'Artificial feeding of *Simulium* vectors of human and bovine onchocerciasis', *Bull.WHO* 1968, *38:*957-66;
P.J.Ham and A.E.Bianco, 'Quantification of a cryopreservation technique for *Onchocerca* microfilariae in skin-snips', *J.Helminthol.,* 1981, *55:*59-61;
P.J.Ham, 'Cryopreservation of blackfly eggs (*Diptera- Simuliidae)*', *Cryobiology,* 1983, *20:*729;
A.E.Bianco, 'Onchocerciasis - River Blindness', in: C.N.L.Macpherson and P.S.Craig (eds), *Parasitic helminths, zoonoses, and human health in Africa,* London, Unwin Hyman Press, 1991, pp.138-203;
E.R.James, 'Cryopreservation research at Winches Farm Laboratories', in: *A brief history ...,* op.cit. note 1, pp.16-20.
[28] LSHTM *Annual Report* 1992-3, pp.39-40; *Research Report* 1990, pp.14-15 and 59-62;
M.G.R.Varma, Mary Pudney, C.J.Leake, 'Arthropod cell culture in medical virology', LSHTM *Annual Report* 1977-8, pp.61-7;
C.J.Leake, 'Arbovirology at Winches Farm Laboratories', in: *A brief history ...,* op.cit. note 1, pp.31-4;
D.I.H.Simpson, 'The Kisumu study', in: W.F.Stanley and M.P.Alpers (eds), *Manmade lakes and human health,* London, Academic Press, 1975, pp.193-208;
C.J.Leake, 'Arbovirus-mosquito interactions and vector specificity', *Parasitology Today,* 1992, *8:*123-8.
[29] LSHTM *Annual Report*s and *Research Report*s between 1989 and 1993;
G.A.T.Targett, 'Interactions between chemotherapy and immunity', in: W.Peters and W.H.G.Richards (eds), *Handbook of experimental pharmacology,* vol.68 (1), Berlin, Springer Verlag, 1984, pp.331-48.
[30] LSHTM *Annual Report*s 1978-9, p.33, and 1988-9, p.10.
[31] LSHTM *Annual Report* 1993-4, p.23, 'UK MALARIA CONSORTIUM';
Personal communications: D.Bradley; B.S.Drasar; R.Feachem; W.Peters; G.Webbe.
[32] G.A.T.Targett and W.Peters, 'Malaria research at Winches Farm Laboratories', in: *A brief history ...,* op.cit. note 1, pp.35-8;
W.Peters, *Chemotherapy and drug resistance in malaria,* 2nd ed., London, Academic Press, 1987.

[33] D.A.Evans and S.L.Croft, 'Research on trypanosomiasis and leishmaniasis at Winches Farm Laboratories', in: *A brief history ...*, op.cit. note 1, pp.39–40;
'Ralph Arthur Neal', obituary, LSHTM *Annual Report* 1989–90, p.24;
LSHTM *Research Report* 1992, pp.57–9;
R.A.Neal and A.Murphy, 'Tropical formulations for treatment of cutaneous leishmaniasis due to *Leishmania major*' in: P.A.Kager and A.M.Polderman (eds), *XII International Congress of Tropical Medicine and Malaria, Abstracts. Excerpta Medica Int.Cong.Series.810*, Amsterdam, Excerpta Medica, 1988, p.195;
R.Lainson, 'The middle years at the London School of Hygiene and Tropical Medicine', pp.129–30 of Garnham obituary, *Trans.Roy.Soc.Trop.Med.Hyg.*, 1995, 89:129–31;
R.Lainson and J.J.Shaw, 'The Role of Animals in the Epidemiology of South American Leishmaniasis', in: *Biology of the Kinetoplastida,* op.cit. note 19, vol.2, pp.2–116.

[34] LSHTM archives, MSS C1:S3, 7 July 1910.

[35] Title pages, *Helminthological Abstracts,* volumes 1 to 14, 1932–45; volumes 15–21, 1946–52; volume 22, 1953; for attitudes and implications, in a somewhat different vein, of the 'Imperial' prefix during this period, see David Cantor, 'Cortisone and the Politics of Empire: Imperialism and British Medicine 1918–55', *Bull.Hist.Med.,* 1993, 67:463–93.

[36] CAB International World Service to Agriculture Report: 1990 in Review, Wallingford, Oxon, CAB International, 1991; *Helminthological Abstracts* 1996, vol.65, information pages.

10

A MANY-FACETED SUBJECT:
TROPICAL MEDICINE IN A CHANGING WORLD 1919–89

For the first five years of its existence at the Albert Dock, Manson's School had based its teaching largely on clinical experience in the adjoining Seamen's Hospital, combined with lectures and laboratory analyses. In 1905, Leiper and Wenyon had been picked by Manson to establish helminthology and protozoology, respectively, as specialist subjects for teaching and research (Chapter 1). The pioneer specialists were followed into the School two years later by A.W.Alcock, appointed 'entomologist at £250 *per annum* with prospect of small increase for three years'. The salary for an entomologist was provided by a grant from the Colonial Office. The following year the salary for Robert McKay, who had joined the School at the age of 14 in 1899 as Manson's 'lab. boy', advancing to laboratory assistant before being killed in a road accident in 1928, was increased by 2s.6d. to a total of 17s.6d. a week.[1]

Two other specialist subjects had been taught at the School from its beginnings, but in a low-key, unemphasised way. Tanner Hewlett, described by Manson-Bahr as a 'mainstay of the Tropical School' in spite of his lack of tropical experience, lectured on bacteria of importance in the tropics, such as those of cholera, dysentery, and bubonic plague. Ritchie Simpson was a pioneer of tropical hygiene, serving on several government commissions on, e.g., enteric fever, plague in Hong Kong, sanitary conditions in Singapore; he also visited a number of African countries on similar missions. Both men held appointments at King's College London as well as at the School. When, at Simpson's suggestion, a course in Tropical Sanitation and Hygiene was established in 1913, only entomology, helminthology, and protozoology were to be taught exclusively by 'permanent staff'; bacteriology, chemistry, and hygiene depended for teaching to a considerable extent on 'visiting staff'.[2]

Between 1914 and 1918, the Great War inevitably affected the running of the School. Staff members were away on active service, or investigating disease in the theatres of war or in potential trouble spots. Student numbers dwindled: between October and December, 1917, only three students attended the 55th Session, and by the 56th Session, between January and April, 1918, there were only two. None of these students was able to complete a full course, and it was decided to suspend regular courses. Instead S.P.James (1870–1946), invalided from Mesopotamia at the end of 1916, and working in London on Malaria in returning troops, and on not infrequent local outbreaks at home, gave a series of lectures to officers of the Army Medical Corps. During May, June and July of 1918 a total of forty students attended, each for no more than ten days. Meanwhile the Hospital, with G.C.Low in charge, coped with a large influx of patients invalided from Egypt, Gallipoli, India, and Mesopotamia.[3]

The wartime experience reinforced a growing awareness of a need for changes in the circumstances of the School and the Hospital. At a Seamen's Hospital Society committee meeting attended by the School's Dean, Sir Havelock Charles, the possibility of obtaining a central London site was discussed. At the conclusion of war, plans for the implementation of such a scheme were accepted and, as described elsewhere above, were realised with help from the British Red Cross.[4]

The move to Endsleigh Gardens was completed during 1920; and with it began a new era for both research and postgraduate teaching of tropical medicine in London. It was reinforced by the changes in structure and administration during the 1920s, when Manson's Tropical School emerged in another incarnation as the LSHTM, under the leadership of Andrew Balfour. With the experience and expertise gained from his early exploits in the South African War, and later during World War I, and his long association with Henry Wellcome's developing scientific activities, he was well qualified for his new and growing responsibilities in the 1920s. For six years between 1924 and 1930, Balfour shaped the developing School, struggling to integrate new subjects and new 'Divisions', each with its own highly individualistic and committed department head, with the original Tropical Division and its equally strong characters leading the departments of entomology, helminthology, protozoology, and clinical tropical medicine. Amid the efforts to control work on the new building in Keppel Street, and the antics of the 'prima donnas' among the School's growing staff, he still managed to contribute a few published papers each year, although they were mostly papers on general topics. Certainly his novel-writing days were over; and it is doubtful if he ever found the time to set foot in the laboratory he had insisted on having installed across the corridor from his new office.[5]

At the same time, departments and divisions, old and new, were responding to developments: with increases in staff numbers and helped by financial support from the MRC, the Rockefeller Foundation, and even central government – in Leiper's case the Ministry of Agriculture – all were impressively productive, as evidenced by the School's annual reports. Until 1927 these covered, of necessity, only the work of the existing Tropical Division. It consisted then of the Department of Entomology, under P.A.Buxton (Alcock retired in 1925); the Department of Helminthology with its Institute of Agricultural Parasitology, under Leiper; and the Department of Protozoology, under J.G.Thomson. Each department contributed its own report and list of published papers. Separately listed were the papers of 'Clinical Tropical Medicine', from the Hospital for Tropical Diseases.[6]

With the move to Keppel Street in July, 1929, two main Divisions took over the teaching and research of the old tropical school: Medical Zoology, where Leiper presided over his own helminthology, J.G.Thomson's protozoology, and Buxton's entomology; and Tropical Medicine and Hygiene under Balfour until, in the following year, it emerged as the Division of Clinical Tropical Medicine under G.C.Low. Less than ten years later, the School's Board of Management decided to modify the system by replacing the existing 'divisions' with 'departments'. The only real effect of this largely semantic exercise seems to have been in 'Medical Zoology': 'Entomology' now became an independent department under Buxton, appointed Professor of Medical Entomology in 1933; and J.G.Thomson's Protozoology joined Leiper's Helminthology as sections in the larger Department of Parasitology.[7] This grouping was to continue until the major reorganisations during Gordon Smith's twenty years as Dean, in the 1970s and 1980s when, by degrees, the three subjects took up their independent positions as Medical Entomology, Medical Helminthology, and Medical Protozoology, each with its own complement of sub-specialists, under the umbrella of the new large Division of Communicable and Tropical Diseases. In these as in other disciplines, changing departmental structures reflected increasing complexity and sophistication of relevant subjects: in particular, immunology and molecular biology were leaving their respective marks on approaches to research, and to teaching, at the LSHTM as well as in other postgraduate schools at home and abroad.[8] In the following, the above disciplines will be considered separately in their LSHTM context. Work on malaria, a major contribution to tropical research at the LSHTM as elsewhere in the world in the twentieth century, requires and deserves a chapter of its own.

HELMINTHOLOGY

By the time the LSHTM, and his own department and Institute, had assumed their definitive shape, R.T.Leiper's major travels and expeditions were behind him. His activities in Keppel Street and at Winches Farm left limited time for travelling; but his students and younger associates were more than ready to follow in his footsteps. Even so, busy as he was during the 1920s, building up his department in the developing School, shaping the Institute of Agricultural Parasitology at Winches Farm, and editing the fledgling *Journal of Helminthology* and the *Tropical Diseases Bulletin*, Leiper himself never lost sight of his consuming interest in all aspects of helminthological research. In 1926, that led to a confrontation with his colleague L.W.Sambon, the colourful Italian of explosive temperament, who had been on the staff of the School and the Hospital since the very beginnings. His main interest lay in epidemiology; but even here, his arguments were rarely convincing, and the conclusions of his energetic research, and his theories, were too often proved subsequently to be inaccurate. Nevertheless, they always gave rise to fruitful scientific debate, and his hypothesis concerning the lateral-spined eggs of a new schistosome species, *Schistosoma mansoni*, had been proved correct by Leiper in 1915.[9]

Ten years later, a less fortunate excursion into the jungle of scientific ideas was made by Sambon in a different direction; and it was based on an even more unfortunate, though richly rewarded, association of ideas by one J.Fibiger. Johannes Fibiger (1867–1928), Professor of Pathological Anatomy at the University of Copenhagen, had claimed that the worm *Spirometry neoplastica (Gongylonema neoplasticum)* caused cancer of the stomach in rats, and that cockroaches might be involved as intermediate hosts, in man and in rats, in studies published between 1913 and 1920.[10]

Sambon in turn based his ideas on epidemiological observations in the Trentino region of Italy, which led him to form the concept of 'cancer houses': the uneven geographical distribution of cancer cases within certain areas, even among individual houses in a single street. Sambon found 'cancer houses' to be heavily infested with cockroaches, known vectors of *Gongylonema*. He followed Fibiger in postulating a causal relationship between presence of the worm and the formation of neoplasm in the inhabitants. It was left to Leiper to show the error of the ways of both Sambon and Fibiger; but not before Fibiger had been awarded the Nobel Prize in 1926 for 'his discovery of the *Spiroptera* carcinoma'.[11]

This was one of the more spectacular misjudgments of the Nobel committees, and one which cost cancer research dear. It was to be a full forty years before Stockholm had sufficiently recovered from the mistake to award another prize for cancer studies: the richly deserved, long overdue, Nobel prize to F.P.Rous (1879–1970), in 1966, for his work, in the century's first decade, on the transmissibility of spindle-celled sarcoma in Plymouth Rock hens.[12] Leiper could show that *Gongylonema neoplasticum* is not found in Italy, and that the species *G.pulchrum* which can, but rarely does, infect man, had never been found in the Trentino, the region studied by Sambon. The correspondence between Leiper and his, in the words of Garnham, 'exuberant Neapolitan colleague' was acrimonious; but Leiper was right, and in the final account, Fibiger's rat tumours were non-malignant.[13]

Meanwhile, a younger generation was coming to the fore in the School's helminthology department. T.M.W.Cameron (1894–1980) was Leiper's right-hand man in the running of the department, and the teaching, during the five years leading up to the School's move. His research contributions, some carried out at Winches Farm, included comparative studies of helminth parasites, especially lung worms, in man and in animals. During a tour of the West Indies in 1928, Cameron identified the wild monkeys of St.Kitts as natural reservoirs for frequent infection with intestinal schistosomiasis in the local population. In 1929 he left the School to take up appointments in parasitology at the University of Edinburgh and nearby Dick Veterinary College. His stay in Edinburgh was brief. Three years later he left for Canada and a distinguished career at McGill University, where his experience in Leiper's department was put to good use in his position as Professor of Parasitology, and founder and director of an Institute of Parasitology.[14]

Research students were soon filling the gap in the department. Some stayed at home: B.G. Peters, with a Grocers' Company Research Scholarship, pursued the relatively prosaic, though not unimportant, subject of the helminth fauna of sewage; and Joyce Leishman, Milner Research Student, worked in Keppel Street on a 'miscellaneous collection of worms' kindly brought back from West Africa by V.B.Wigglesworth (1899–1994) in Entomology, just returned from his first expedition to Nigeria, Ghana and Sierra Leone.[15]

Other research students went further afield; for these were also the years when the young J.J.C.Buckley, who twenty years later would succeed Leiper in the Courtauld Chair of Helminthology, began his travels and his heroic exercises in self-experimentation. His early notebooks, recently 'saved from the incinerator' by David Denham, bear witness to his selfless disregard for the risks he took, and continued to take, in the name of investigative science, and which would eventually leave him with a seriously compromised immune system.

An Irishman among the high proportion of Scots at the London School, even long after it had ceased to be 'Manson's School', John Joseph Cronin Buckley (1904-72) was educated in his native Dublin, at the Catholic University School and University College Dublin. In 1927 he left the National University of Ireland for London, and Leiper's department, the holder of a prestigious Travelling Studentship in Zoology. For the next few years he worked, while completing his doctoral thesis on the liver fluke of sheep, *Fasciola hepatica,* on such varied subjects as fungal invasion of helminth eggs, and lungworm infestation in Kinkajous. Working under Leiper, his subjects in those years were inevitably in the field of comparative parasitology, much of it forming part of the department's collaboration with the London Zoo. Then, in 1931, in keeping with the School's Manson tradition of encouraging promising young researchers to work in the field abroad, he was awarded a Wandsworth Scholarship to investigate the unsolved problem of the transmission of *Mansonella ozzardi*, a filarial parasite infecting millions of inhabitants of the West Indies and South America, although with no serious effects. John Buckley sailed for St.Vincent, and within a few months he had identified the midge *Culicoides furens* as the vector of *Mansonella ozzardi*; he also observed and described the development of the parasite in the vector.[16]

For Buckley, the successful demonstration of the course of the lifecycle of *Mansonella ozzardi* was only the beginning of a long line of observations and experiments including, when necessary, self-inoculation, which he pursued over a period of more than thirty years, through World War II, and from 1946 as Leiper's successor in the William Julien Courtauld Chair of Helminthology at the LSHTM. As a consequence of his heroic experimentation he was, for the last fifteen years of his life until his death at the relatively early age of sixty-seven, partially paralysed and in constant pain. He bore his sufferings stoically, and continued to teach, ably supported by the department's technicians, W.Cooper and F.N.N.Pester.[17]

Historians of the School and of tropical medicine research at this time are indeed fortunate in Dr.Denham's rescue of the Buckley papers during recent alterations and building work in Keppel Street. The notebooks cover the long period of J.J.C.Buckley's most active research, from 1931 and throughout the war years, and are revealing of his working methods. For although in published papers he did not specify self-inoculation, but rather referred to the use of 'a human volunteer' (or 'volunteers' when some of his associates were involved in later years), the notebooks freely record details, and contain sketches such as the one of his own arm with inoculation sites and results, shown in Fig.00.[18]

Historically, self-inoculation was of course nothing new. John Hunter's rather more public and spectacular self-inoculations and observations before he published *A treatise of the Venereal Disease* in 1786 are well known; so is the episode of Max Pettenkofer imbibing a virulent culture of *Vibrio cholerae* in a misguided effort to disprove the germ theory. At the turn of the century, the United States Army Board, with Walter Reed in charge, took risks studying mosquitoes infected with yellow fever in Cuba; they achieved results, but at a cost, when one worker died after being bitten accidentally.[19] In the 1920s, a number of workers put to the test a long held belief that human *Ascaris* and pig *Ascaris* were specific species and not interchangeable with regard to their respective hosts. Shimesu Koino (1897–1971) in Japan, and Payne, Ackert and Hartman in the United States, swallowed eggs of *Ascaris suum* without causing infestation, although there were symptoms of respiratory disturbances. In August, 1922, Koino also bravely ingested no less than 2,000 eggs of *A.lumbricoides,* the human roundworm, and made a full recovery. Leiper, and Buckley himself, elaborated such experiments with pig roundworms by swallowing migrating larvae (on an open sandwich) in 1931.[20]

In the West Indies in the early 1930s Buckley, having completed his Mansonella studies, turned to the American pig hookworm *Necator suillus,* beginning his self-inoculations. Here he was able to show that the pig hookworm, although a species distinct from the *Nector americanus* of man, could be infectious for humans and hence could cause diagnostic confusion. After eighteen months in the West Indies Buckley travelled via Venezuela to India where, in Assam, he began work on a fluke first described in 1876, and renamed *Gastrodiscoides hominis* by Leiper in 1913. Common in parts of northeastern India, where the incidence in local populations may be as high as 40 per cent, this trematode is thought to have a complex life-cycle which even now has not been definitively determined. Pigs and various species of monkey have been found to serve as reservoir hosts; a snail, *Helicorbis coenosus,* has been infected experimentally; humans can suffer massive infestation.[21]

In Assam in 1934–5, Buckley had worked hard in an attempt to determine possible snail vectors for *Gastrodiscoides*. There was no lack of local patients to produce specimens; fortunately mere soap and water enemas serve as successful therapy in a majority of cases. By such means

PREVENTION AND CURE

Buckley could treat his patients and at the same time gain ample material for further research: from one individual no less than 999 worms were recovered. His long lists of patients, his drawings of cercariae (larval stages of the trematodes), and of several local snails under suspicion as intermediate hosts testify to his dogged perseverance, which in the end left only inconclusive results.[22]

John Buckley's next port of call was Malaya. The problem there was again one of transmission of a parasite, in this case a parasite of cattle. Well schooled in the study of animal parasites in Leiper's department and at Winches Farm, Buckley was quite ready to begin investigating bovine onchocerciasis. 'Worm nodules' of cattle had been under scrutiny since the beginning of the century, notably in Australia, where *Onchocerca gibsoni* was widely distributed and caused great losses to the beef industry; Leiper had studied aspects of the parasite as early as 1911. In spite of much valuable experimental work carried out in a number of places, determination of the mode of spread of the disease, and its potential control, let alone its eradication, had so far eluded the investigators. On the other hand, as so often happens, even the largely negative results of the studies carried out over a period of thirty years had provided useful information, defining possible further lines of research and excluding others.

By the time Buckley set to work in Malaya, other investigators had been able to eliminate considerable numbers of species from the multitude of cattle-biting insects under suspicion as vectors for *Onchocerca gibsoni*. Rodolfo Robles (1878–1939) in Guatemala City had suggested, on circumstantial evidence, that *Simulium* species might be involved as vectors in the transmission of human onchocerciasis in Central America in 1917. Nearly ten years later D.B.Blacklock, Director of the Liverpool School's Research Laboratory at Freetown, Sierra Leone, was able to demonstrate that the black-fly *Simulium damnosum* was the vector responsible for the transmission of *Onchocerca volvulus* in man. This discovery led him to suggest that *Simulium* species might also be involved in the transmission of *Onchocerca gibsoni* in Australia, a conclusion disputed by others.[23]

Then, in 1935 the veterinarian John S.Steward incriminated midges of the genus *Culicoides* as vectors for *Onchocerca cervicalis* in the horse; and Buckley decided to test this genus, so far largely overlooked in the search for the vector of the bovine disease in Malaya: *O. gibsoni* had originally been introduced into northern Australia from this source. Dissecting and examining large numbers of cattle-biting insects in Kuala Lumpur, Buckley could conclude that midges of the genus *Culicoides* were responsible for transmission of bovine onchocerciasis; statistical evidence showed *C.pungens* to be the main species involved.[24]

It was an important observation for veterinary medicine, and for the economics of cattle breeding. It was also a portent for the future research of Buckley himself, and for that of the department to which he belonged. Human onchocerciasis was to play a very important role in the research carried out at Winches Farm, where *Onchocerca* species and their *Simulium* vectors, especially those of river blindness, would figure prominently in the 1970s and 1980s. The human onchocerciasis programme at the LSHTM originated with Buckley's work during World War II, when the Governor of Kenya requested help with the problem of river blindness in Nyanza Province. During the pre-war period, a number of new foci of this debilitating disease had been found on the African continent. Many areas recorded blindness rates of more than 10 per cent.; one such area was Kenya's 'Valley of the Blind'. The Governor's appeal to the Colonial Office went to the LSHTM and Buckley, fresh from his study of onchocerciasis in cattle left for Kenya in 1941. In the Valley of the Blind he was able to observe the development of *Onchocerca volvulus* in the black-fly *Simulium neavei* (rather than *S.damnosum* as in the hill country of Sierra Leone, demonstrated by Blacklock in 1926). At the same time, he could assist the local authorities by recommending a method for epidemiological control which proved effective: preventing the vector from breeding by clearing shade trees from the edge of rivers in the affected area. Like Carpenter's attempt to control sleeping sickness in Uganda during the years before the Great War, Buckley was using interruption of the transmission cycle to prevent spread of the disease; only where Carpenter had tried to remove the hosts from the vector by moving whole populations, Buckley was obtaining results by preventing the vector from breeding. With the advent of DDT shortly afterwards, the outlook for control was radically changed. By 1947, Garnham and McMahon had succeeded in eradicating *S.naevei* from one area in Kenya by application of an oil/water emulsion of DDT to the limited breeding areas in local rivers, where early stages of the *Simulium* larvae were carried on freshwater crabs.[25]

At the end of the war, Buckley was appointed to the Courtauld Chair of Helminthology in succession to Leiper. He could now have settled down to his teaching – his students held him in great esteem as well as affection – and research at home. He chose instead to travel once more to Malaya, there to wrestle with problems which Leiper had pursued in British Guiana more than twenty years before: taxonomic identity, life-cycle, and pathogenicity of the parasites causing elephantiasis in man. But where Leiper and his associates had relied on observation, of clinical aspects, pathology and histopathology, combined with evaluation of early chemotherapy and vaccine therapy (i.e. detoxicated staphylococcal and streptococcal vaccines to combat secondary infections in filarial abscesses which ended in septicaemia), Buckley went further. He began experiments involving self-inoculation.

It was of course not the first time he had resorted to self-experimentation; but the roundworm and hookworm infestations referred to above were far more easily controlled with known antihelminthics than the tropical pulmonary eosinophilia resulting from infection with filarial parasites of animal origin. It was in Malaya that Buckley produced the evidence which allowed him to finally separate the helminths causing elephantiasis in man into two distinct genera, *Wuchereria* and *Brugia*, the latter a new genus erected by Buckley; it was also in Malaya that Buckley and Edeson began their self-experimentation with animal parasites, of cats, dogs, and monkeys. Both Edeson and others collaborating with Buckley, R.H.Wharton and A.B.G.Laing, practised self-inoculation; but Buckley seems to have suffered more lasting effects than his younger associates. After his death, it has been suggested that an accidentally acquired schistosome infection may have contributed to his medical problems.[26]

After a final visit in 1955 Buckley himself returned to London, leaving his fieldwork to his younger associates. Edeson, Wharton, and Laing continued to keep in close touch, by airmail letters and 'VIA IMPERIAL' cablegrams, from their bases at Kuantan and Kuala Lumpur. Laing and Wharton wrote respectfully to 'Dear Professor Buckley' throughout the correspondence; Edeson, Buckley's pupil and friend, endearingly addressed him as 'Dear Himself'. During 1958–9, Edeson was at the Institute for Medical Research in Kuala Lumpur, and the branch laboratories at Kuantan Pahang, collaborating with Laing and Wharton, who were there on a more permanent basis. The ensuing correspondence with Buckley at home in Keppel Street vividly depicts the excitement and the pitfalls and the inevitable occasional disappointments of tropical research and long-distance collaboration. As Manson-Bahr had recalled, it was to the Kuala Lumpur Institute for Medical Research that C.W.Daniels had gone as Director, as a first step in Manson's unfulfilled dream of a permanent exchange scheme between the Institute and the old tropical school: 'Manson's underlying idea ... that the Malayan Institute and the LSTM should grow up together ... and should interchange personnel and material ...'.[27] It never became a permanent arrangement; but the Buckley papers testify to lasting links, however informal, which have also been reinforced by large numbers of Malaysian alumni enjoyed by the School over the years. Gordon Smith was head of virology at the Kuala Lumpur Institute (IMR) from 1952 before joining the London School in 1957.

The men on the spot in Malaya worked on both *Wuchereria* and *Brugia* infections in a variety of species, ranging from cats and monkeys to more exotic species and 'human volunteers'. Reading of the letters leaves no doubt as to the identities of those volunteers. In October, 1958, Edeson wrote to 'Himself': 'Total and differential W.B.C. counts are being done on the human volunteers. Since last writing I have developed a swelling over the lower end of the ulna and I can now feel the epitrochlear gland. The axillary lump is going down but Barry's [Laing] "untut" has been more serious and it has interfered with his golf.' He added a PS: 'My skin test was violently positive and the area of erythema (ignored as per instructions) covered about half of my arm. Eosinophils now 15 per cent and I have a slight cough.' And Buckley wrote back by return of post: 'The news of your eosinophils and cough is very satisfactory. ... If the cough gets really bad there will be no point in withholding Banocide treatment in the hopes of finding microfilariae in the blood. You might have to wait too long for your own convenience and comfort.'[28]

The letters from Malaya in 1958–9 also reflect a continuing desire on the part of Edeson and the others for a visit by Buckley to his old hunting grounds in Malaya. But it was not to be; increasing disability was affecting their mentor. At the end of April, 1959, he dashed their hopes finally: 'I never "promised" to visit Malaya this year: it was just a pious hope, and not even a hope just now.' Running like a red thread through this correspondence in the late 1950s is the question of *Wuchereria* taxonomy and whether it would be justifiable to establish a new genus of *Brugia* (after S.L.Brug, 1927), with *Brugia malayi* a species separate from *Wuchereria bancrofti*. After all the self-inoculations and animal experiments, Buckley finally suggested this innovation in print in 1960, a move which was opposed by a number of other specialists. It was eventually accepted when other species of *Brugia* were identified in Malaya as well as in East Africa and the United States. Since then, *Brugia* species have played a major role in research carried out in the department by David Denham and his group, including Patrick McGreavy. Together with work on other filariae, their studies then had roots in both Manson's early work and in the much more recent achievements of Buckley and his associates. Over the years *Brugia pahangi* in particular featured prominently in investigations of the immunology of lymphatic filariasis and as a vehicle for testing and evaluating growing numbers of new anthelmintics. Less exotic investigations have involved the group in public health aspects closer to home, such as a delicate matter of tapeworm infections in a girls' public school.[29]

In 1967, George Nelson (b.1923) succeeded Buckley, who as Professor Emeritus continued to edit the *Journal of Helminthology* until his death in 1972. Nelson had first joined the School in 1963; he had come to helminthology by a path very different from that of Buckley. Graduating in medicine at St.Andrews in 1948, he had spent a year at Dundee Royal Infirmary before returning to St.Andrews to lecture on pathology. After another year there he left for Africa, joining the Uganda Medical Service as Medical Officer for the West Nile District, in over-all charge of health services for a population of not much less than half a million. During six years there, he still found time for research on prevailing problems of leprosy, onchocerciasis, and schistosomiasis, before he transferred to Kenya, and the Division of Vector Borne Disease. This was the well-known centre of parasitological research where P.C.C.Garnham had spent more than twenty years before his return to London as Leiper's successor as Director of the School's Department of Parasitology after World War II.[30]

In Kenya Nelson turned his pathologist's mind to public health problems presented by zoonoses, in Africa and elsewhere, e.g. trichinosis, which Nelson described for the first time in Sub-Saharan Africa.[31] On leave from Kenya in 1959, Nelson allowed himself the time to gain the DAP&E (Diploma in Applied Parasitology and Entomology), having taken the DTM&H at Liverpool in 1952. In 1963 he returned to the London School as Reader in Medical Parasitology, when Garnham was Director of the department, and Buckley still occupied the Courtauld Chair which Nelson would inherit three years later, fulfilling an ambition concerning which he had needed, in the meantime, much reassurance from colleagues. His work at Winches Farm has been described in the chapter on the field station. In 1980 Nelson left London for the Liverpool School and its Walter Myers Chair of Parasitology.[32]

During the 1980s, the work of the department which now became designated 'Medical Helminthology' continued to be closely linked to developments at Winches Farm until, in the early 1990s, with the closure of the field station, all helminthological activities returned once again to Keppel Street, albeit in a very different form from that of its early days in the hands of Manson and of Leiper. Today, most of the School's helminthologists are located in the Immunology Unit of the Department of Infectious and Tropical Diseases, working on the immunology, molecular biology and biochemistry of the schistosomes and of several nematode parasites. Elsewhere in the School, other staff are concerned with the epidemiology and control of helminth infections. For example, in the Disease Control and Vector Biology Unit, Sandy Cairncross, collaborating with colleagues in Nigeria and Ghana, and supported by UNICEF/WHO, is heavily involved in an ambitious Guinea worm eradication programme in West Africa. Towards the end of the century which began with Leiper's definitive description of the life-cycle of the Guinea worm *(Dracunculus medinensis)* (Chapter 3), global eradication of dracunculiasis seems at last to be within reach. The disease was in fact targeted for worldwide eradication in 1995 by the UNICEF/WHO Interagency Team for Dracunculiasis Eradication. With logistic difficulties in endemic countries both in Africa and on the Indian subcontinent – in particular difficulties in identifying endemic villages – the deadline has passed with only a 90 per cent reduction in cases achieved, but hopes of an early positive outcome remain high. Although there is not effective chemotherapy, implementation of strategies developed during the International Water Decade (1981–90) promises eventual success: involvement of local populations in control by employing volunteer village health workers in both surveillance activities and health education. Such networks of local volunteers may then become a permanent fixture. With an initial goal of dracunculiasis eradication the village health workers should, once that goal is achieved, play a more general role in health promotion in their respective villages.[33]

PROTOZOOLOGY

Charles Morley Wenyon (1878–1948) and protozoology arrived at the Albert Dock at the same time as Leiper and helminthology. Manson-Bahr described protozoology as a then 'new' science; and although some protozoa had been described during the nineteenth century, they had certainly received less attention than the worms of helminthology, until the acceleration in observations heralded by the studies of plasmodia by Ross and by Grassi, and of trypanosomes by Bruce, Dutton and Todd, and others, around the turn of the century. Also at this time, the rise of protozoology in Britain was fostered by the work of E.A.Minchin (1866–1915), first holder of the London University Chair in Protozoology, at the Lister Institute, where he worked with H.M.Woodcock and Muriel Robertson. In 1905, the year before his appointment to the Chair, Minchin had been a member of the Royal

Society Commission on Sleeping Sickness; and trypanosomes, of man and of animals, their transmission by and development in tsetse-flies (*Glossina* species) became a focal point for research in his department, where after his death Woodcock and Robertson continued studies of trypanosomes in a wide range of animal species.[34]

Three years older than Leiper, Wenyon had counted zoology and physiology among his main interests before coming to the School; after Manchester and Leeds he came to University College London, graduating B.Sc. with first-class honours in his favourite subjects, having been taught zoology by Minchin and physiology by E.H.Starling. His examination results earned him a scholarship enabling him to complete his medical training at Guy's Hospital Medical School. His student notebooks from his years in the Zoology Department at UCL have been preserved, and testify to his early interest in the minute creatures which became the cornerstone of his life's work. The collection also contains the young C.M.Wenyon's 'Zoology notes of lectures by Professor E.A.Minchin, U.C.L. 1900-1', with 'Protozoa' figuring prominently.[35]

Having qualified in medicine, Wenyon had none of Leiper's hang-ups about the practice of clinical medicine, and had immediately bought a general practice in Camberwell for the magnificent sum of £15; but an offer to head protozoology at Manson's School proved irresistible, and Wenyon, like Leiper, was launched on a career in research. Like Leiper, Wenyon spent extended periods abroad, at first educating himself for his new task, at the Pasteur Institute with Mesnil, and in Munich with Oscar Hertwig (1849-1922); later he worked with Andrew Balfour in the Sudan, aboard a 'floating laboratory', donated to the Sudan government by Henry Wellcome, on the upper reaches of the Nile. The last years before the outbreak of war in 1914 found Wenyon in Baghdad, Aleppo, and Malta, studying oriental sore and increasingly becoming convinced that the leishmaniae were transmitted by sandflies, although proof evaded him: final, crucial, evidence definitively incriminating *Phlebotomus argentipes* as vector of oriental sore and kala-azar came only in 1940, after many years of determined efforts by Sir Rickard Christophers and Colonel H.E.Shortt, and their Indian collaborators including C.S.Swaminath, and not forgetting the inspired intervention of R.O.Smith in 1939.[36]

In 1914, after less than ten years, Wenyon left the School (having been solely responsible for writing and editing the *Kala Azar Bulletin 1911-12*), to join Balfour at the Wellcome Bureau of Scientific Research as Director of Research in the Tropics. He was succeeded at the School by John Gordon Thomson (1878-1937). An Edinburgh educated Scot, he came to London after three years in Liverpool, at the Royal Southern

Hospital and the School of Tropical Medicine. After a brush with helminthology early in the Great War, accompanying Leiper on the Bilharzia Mission in Egypt in 1915 as Captain in the RAMC, Thomson was free to concentrate on protozoology; in 1918 he returned to London in charge of the malaria research laboratory at the War Office. His wartime experiences stood him in good stead back at the School at the end of the war: with his gift for teaching, he was instrumental in rebuilding the course in protozoology which, like other courses, had suffered through enforced neglect during the war.[37]

In the post-war years, Thomson's interests centred particularly on malaria and blackwater fever. In the early 1920s he went twice to Southern Rhodesia with Willie Cooper, his technical assistant, to study blackwater fever; in 1936 he lectured in Singapore for the League of Nations' special course on malaria.[38]

Thomson's death in office in 1937 marked the end of protozoology as a separate department in the London School. The Board of Management grasped the opportunity to 'unite the departments of helminthology and protozoology in a single Department of Parasitology under Professor Leiper ...'; at the same time, the Board secured, from the University of London, a Readership in Medical Parasitology in the new, larger, department. The new post was earmarked for H.E.Shortt (1887–1987), who was about to retire from the IMS. He was duly appointed, only to return to India, by request, on the outbreak of World War II in 1939. He was to take up the appointment in earnest after the war, when he was joined in Medical Parasitology by P.C.C.Garnham (1901–94) in 1947. The reorganisation of the department then signalled a new era for protozoology in the School; one in which malaria became a subject of increasing concern in a number of departments, in parasitology, entomology, epidemiology, and the recently incorporated Ross Institute.[39]

When Shortt, his war duties over, finally took up his appointment at the LSHTM, Leiper was retiring in September, 1946; Shortt stepped in as Professor of Medical Protozoology and Director of the department. Born in India, he had been brought up in Inverness by a Scottish grandmother; in 1910 he graduated in medicine at the University of Aberdeen and went straight into the IMS embarking for India in 1911. Apart from short periods of home leave, he spent the next thirty years on the Indian subcontinent. Details of the career of Shortt, who survived official 'retirement' from the LSHTM for more than thirty-five years and lived to the age of a hundred, serve to emphasise the remarkable resistance and longevity enjoyed by a surprising number of twentieth-century pioneers in tropical medicine, who built up the discipline initially unprotected by the preventive measures they worked so hard to develop. In Shortt's case, his service in Mesopotamia was forcibly interrupted by sick leave in 1916, when he was suffering from dysentery, ankylostomiasis, and malaria; he promptly fell ill with a, fortunately mild, attack of bubonic plague; shooting wild buffalo in Assam in 1924 he narrowly escaped being gored by the herd. Throughout the years of arduous clinical service and tireless research, he never lost an air of thoroughly enjoying himself, like his similarly long lived friend and colleague, Sir Rickard Christophers (1873–1978), and the younger member of this remarkable trio of heroes of twentieth century service in India and Africa, and of malaria research, P.C.C.Garnham.[40]

Both born well before the turn of the century and the opening of the two schools of tropical medicine, Christophers and Shortt cut their tropical teeth in the Indian Medical Service, and later joined the select band of 42 Fellows of the Royal Society produced by the IMS between its inception in 1680 and the end of the British rule in 1947. Outside of their contributions, singly and jointly, to malariology, perhaps the second most fruitful collaboration of Christophers and Shortt in research in protozoology was their work on the vexed question of control of the leishmaniases, both the cutaneous form and the visceral disease, kala-azar. Transmission of those diseases had long presented a major problem to the IMS. Leonard Rogers had worked long and hard on kala-azar in Assam, discovering the flagellate stage of the parasite, and pioneering the therapeutic use of intravenous doses of tartar emetic; and Christophers had been introduced to the problem in his earliest days in the IMS. Shortly after qualifying, he had served with J.W.W.Stephens (1865–1946), later of the Liverpool School, on the Malaria Commission of the Royal Society and the Colonial Office between 1898 in 1902, in Africa and India. Then, passing into the IMS he had, with S.P.James, directed anti-malarial operations at Mian Mir, only to move on to clinical investigations of patients infected with *Leishmania donovani,* newly described, newly named, cause of kala-azar.[41]

Twenty years later began Christopher's collaboration with Shortt, when the Kala-azar Commission was established in 1924–5. This work culminated in the identification of the sandfly *Phlebotomus argentipes* as vector of kala-azar, although final evidence for transmission to man was, for technical reasons – the long period necessary for the development of infective forms of the parasite, and the need for raisin feeds to prolong the life of the sandflies – not obtained until 1942.[42]

The experiments necessary to draw valid conclusions concerning the life-cycle and transmission of the parasite of kala-azar had involved the use of both animals and human volunteers. Shortt's experimental work with animals, for the benefit of animals, were first inspired by the death in India, soon after his arrival there, of his own dog: he found the piroplasm *Babesia canis* in its tissues. Newly arrived in India, Shortt had not known of the necessity of deticking dogs, a procedure routinely performed by European dog owners in India and Africa. Transmission of *Babesia* species was in fact a subject preoccupying medical and veterinary protozoologists in the early years of the century, ever since Smith and Kilborne's classic reports on the transmission by ticks of *Babesia* species causing Texas fever in cattle in the Southern United States.[43] Encouraged by Christophers, who had studied the disease in India since 1907, and compared the *Babesia* life-cycle to that of the malaria parasite, Shortt later studied the piroplasm in dogs (and in one leopard in India); in much later years he continued *Babesia* studies in a number of small mammals at Winches Farm after its revival, and his own formal retirement, in the 1960s and 1970s. By then administrative changes were once again affecting the department. The School's infrastructure was about to undergo the first of its readjustments of the 1970s and 1980s, coinciding with a change of Dean – Gordon Smith was beginning his two decades at the head of the School – and four new heads of departments were taking office between October, 1968, and October 1970 (J.N.Morris in Public Health; W.H.R.Lumsden in Medical Protozoology; L.J.Bruce-Chwatt in Tropical Hygiene at the Ross Institute; and J.C.Waterlow in Human Nutrition). At the same time, throughout the School, diplomas and diploma courses were being replaced by one-year M.Sc. courses, except for the even more revolutionary two-year course for the M.Sc. in Social Medicine (Chapter 6). The large Department of Parasitology was divided into its original components: Medical Helminthology under George Nelson; and Medical Protozoology under W.H.R.Lumsden.

In this post-Garnham era, protozoology research – on trypanosomones and on malaria – shared the Winches Farm Laboratories at St.Albans, with students commuting on a regular basis, an arrangement involving even more practical difficulties than the position of the Hospital for Tropical Diseases at St.Pancras. Trypanosome research often involved collaboration between the School's departments of Protozoology and of Clinical Tropical Medicine, sometimes also with the Ross Institute, and various overseas centres. In 1969 the Wellcome Trust initiated an ambitious international scheme with a grant of a million pounds, to be spent on research in tropical diseases. It was to be a collaboration between the Harvard School of Public Health, the LSHTM, and units attached to institutes in the tropics such as those under Lainson in Brazil, and R.S.Bray in Ethiopia. Between 1975 and 1984 the project yielded nearly forty papers on aspects of diseases caused by schistosomes, trypanosomes, leishmanias, and filariae, in collaborative studies involving the two Schools and South American bases at the Federal University of Bahia and the Oswaldo Cruz Institute; although the funding body was thought at the time to consider the LSHTM input into the scheme to be rather less than expected. The work of Lainson and of Shaw on leishmaniasis epidemiology in South America has been referred to above (Chapter 9). At the same time, M.A.Miles and associates at the School were working on unresolved problems of the epidemiology and immunopathology of Chagas' disease, the South American trypanosomiasis caused by *Trypanosoma cruzi*. In the 1980s, the work of Miles's group benefited from the introduction of techniques using monoclonal antibodies, supported by Wellcome Trust facilities for the development of monoclonal antibodies against protozoal infections.[44] Into the 1990s, the long battle to control the protozoa continues. In Miles's laboratories, the molecular work first begun under the auspices of the Wolfson Molecular Parasitology Unit, now focuses on applications of genetic transformation and similar techniques; in Paul Kaye's group the emphasis is on the host immune response to *Leishmania*, and in Martin Taylor's group on immune response to schistosomes; while in Alan Fairlamb's laboratory the focus is on chemotherapy and development of drug resistance in the same diseases.

ENTOMOLOGY

Entomology – more specifically, medical entomology – can be seen as a subsidiary discipline supporting the mainline subjects making up the vast canvas of medical parasitology. But it can also be perceived as a central plank, a core subject, without which none of the other constituents of parasitology can be fully realised, let alone be able to reach definitive conclusions in overall medical terms – be it in therapy or prevention. As it evolved at the London School, it had its roots in zoology and natural sciences. Alcock had joined Manson's School after twenty years in the IMS, an accomplished surgeon and naturalist intent on studies in marine zoology and teaching in the Medical College of Bengal. His legacy of acquired excellence in a naturalist's imaginatively constructive approach to medical entomology was continued by his successor, when in 1925 Patrick Buxton (1892–1955) took over as director of the Department of

Entomology. Brought up in a family where a classical education was considered the norm – his father's family had strong Quaker leanings, his mother was one of the spirited Jex-Blake sisters – he only found his academic feet and true vocation at Cambridge, under the tutelage of Walter Fletcher; with a Natural Sciences Tripos and an MB under his belt, he was elected to a Trinity Fellowship in 1916, and qualified in medicine at St.George's Hospital in 1917. Taking up a commission in the Royal Army Medical Corps, he was posted to Mesopotamia and North West Persia, where he seems to have spent most of his time collecting insects and bird skins and preparing a survey of the fauna of Iraq – a relatively peaceful pastime, which left him with fewer scars from the Great War than a number of his future colleagues at the LSHTM.[45]

At the end of 1919, Buxton returned to England, to work on itch mites in G.H.F.Nuttall's laboratory at Cambridge. He also attended the tropical medicine course at the School where, according to Wigglesworth, he 'was chiefly noted for his habit of arriving late and reading the newspaper during lectures – characteristics which in later times he found impossible to tolerate in his students'.[46] After a spell as entomologist in the Medical Department in Palestine, his chance to experience life as a 'real tropical entomologist' came in 1923, when the School's Milner Research Fund enabled Buxton, assisted by G.H.E.Hopkins, to spend two years in Samoa, studying filariasis in the Manson-Leiper tradition: charting the breeding biology of the *Aedes* vector with a view to control; collecting Samoan insects; and surveying human diseases and welfare in an area of the Pacific defined by the islands of Ellice, Tokelau, Samoa, and the New Hebrides.

The insect collection brought back from this expedition by Buxton and Hopkins formed the nucleus of the Insect Collection of the School's Department of Entomology. With later additions – Leeson and Gillett's African collections from the 1930s, and Wigglesworth's mosquitoes and tsetse flies from Nigeria in 1928 among them – it has been preserved as an invaluable specialist reference collection.[47]

Buxton returned to London in January, 1926; Alcock had retired and Buxton had been appointed his successor. By the time of his retirement Alcock, who had built up the subject of medical entomology at the School from modest beginnings to a new and flourishing science, was according to Wigglesworth's tactful assessment, 'sadly aged'. The department was ripe for the sweeping of new brooms, with the helpful injection of part of the Rockefeller cash available to revitalise the School. Buxton himself defined his plans for the future in a letter to *Nature*, in which he wrote that 'real progress will not be made in applied entomology until ... we devote time and labour to the study of the fundamentals of insect physiology'; at the same time persuading the Board of Management that 'contribution of the School to medical entomology should be to go deep and to produce a science of insect physiology'.[48]

These were prophetic words for the shaping of the department and the choice of an assistant: Buxton specified the need for someone with experience in biochemistry or physiology. He was supported by his old tutor Walter Fletcher, by now Secretary of the MRC and an active member of the School's Board of Management. Fletcher also supported Buxton in the eventual choice of V.B.Wigglesworth (1899–1994) to fill the post. At this time Wigglesworth was twenty-six and, although with a double First in the Cambridge Tripos was only just about to qualify in medicine. He himself disarmingly quoted, in his obituary of Buxton, the less than enthusiastic comments made by the appointing committee: that he 'had had a good academic career, had written half a dozen papers, some jointly with J.B.S.Haldane, was about to qualify in medicine – and was very silent and unimpressive at interview. Against him were middle-aged people, with lots of experience in anti-malarial work etc.' Balfour himself did not spare the successful candidate, confronting him with the opinion that the appointment was 'a very queer one'.

If it were perceived as 'queer' by the School authorities at the time, it should be remembered that this was the period of transition, when Manson's tropical school was preparing for its amalgamation with a new school of public health, with all that implied. In the new LSHTM, physiology was to play a rapidly increasing part in more than one discipline, as in all biological disciplines everywhere during the inter-war period. The study of insect physiology in particular would become of paramount importance with the advent of DDT during World War II; but long before that, Buxton and his staff had been actively involved in a search for 'lasting' chemical insecticides suitable for impregnating clothes, and hence for replacing the inadequate, short-term, de-lousing methods developed during the Great War. In fact, from the very early days of amalgamation, tropical and temperate public health at the School came together in medical entomology as much as in epidemiology.

Newly appointed, Wigglesworth within a year set off for Nigeria, Ghana, and Sierra Leone, earning his tropical spurs: travelling by poling canoe down the Benue River system in Nigeria with crew and equipment, he encountered most of the destructive diseases haunting the African continent, including malaria, sleeping sickness, yellow fever, and cases of plague. In northern Nigeria, he worked in the Tsetse Research Camp studying the recondite physiology of digestion and nutrition of the tsetse.

He eventually arrived in Accra, on that Bight of Benin of ill repute in the nineteenth century jingle:

> Beware and betide of the Bight of Benin
> For few come out, though many go in

Accra and Lagos on that coast were also the sites of Yellow Fever Stations, where Adrian Stokes and Hideo Noguchi had died of the disease they were researching, shortly before Wigglesworth's arrival in 1927. In a decade of no yellow fever vaccine and, then as now, no cure for yellow fever or indeed for most other virus diseases, Wigglesworth returned home hale and hearty, with a couple of new mosquito species named after him: *Aedes (Aedimorphus) wigglesworthi,* and *Culex (Eumelanomyia) wigglesworthi.*[49]

Once back in Keppel Street, Wigglesworth re-entered life in the department with enthusiasm, both in teaching and research. J.D.Gillett, who attended his lectures in the early 1930s, remembered them as 'models of good planning and clarity ... If he perhaps lacked some of the entertaining sparkle of Buxton, he more than made up for this in clear and ordered exposition ... he was the antithesis of Buxton in almost every facet of his behaviour and philosophy.' According to Gillett, their so different personalities were reflected in their respective attitudes to work and time spent in the laboratories. Wigglesworth always arrived punctually by train from his home in Beaconsfield at 9.20 am, and left as punctually at precisely 17.10; Buxton kept far less regimented hours, and his working methods were far more casual. John Updike, who did not know Wigglesworth, but had talked to colleagues of his during a visit to Cambridge shortly after the appointment of V.B.Wigglesworth (VBW) to the Quick Chair of Biology in 1952, almost miraculously caught the flavour of his working life in the thumbnail sketch of a poem reprinted here. Wigglesworth himself was less than pleased by this piece of publicity, but before his death agreed, generously if somewhat reluctantly, to its re-publication. Others find it an irresistible and witty example of a layman's view of goings-on in a biological laboratory.[50]

V.B.NIMBLE, V.B. QUICK

V.B. Wigglesworth wakes at noon,
Washes, shaves and very soon
Is at the lab; he reads his mail,

PREVENTION AND CURE

Swings a tadpole by the tail,
Undoes his coat, removes his hat,
Dips a spider in a vat
Of alkaline, phones the press,
Tells them he is FRS,
subdivides six protocells,
Kills a rat by ringing bells,
writes a treatise, edits two
Symposia on 'Will Man Do?',
Gives a lecture, audits three,
Has the Sperm Club in for tea,
Pensions off an ageing spore,
Cracks a test-tube, take some pure
Science and applies it, finds
His hat, adjusts it, pulls the blinds,
instructs the jellyfish to spawn,
And, by one o'clock, is gone.
John Updike

Professor J.D.Gillett, who supplied much of the above personal and professional information on Buxton and Wigglesworth before his death in October, 1995 had arrived in the department in September, 1930, at the age of just 17, and with the distinction of having failed in nine O-level (School Certificate) subjects. His consuming interests lay in natural history and music; it was his lively participation in the activities of the London Natural History Society which led to an introduction to Buxton, and a job in a 'very junior capacity' in the department. His initial task was the feeding and general upkeep of the department's colonies of living insects; the School would, Buxton assured him, 'be willing to pay 75 pence per week' for his services. He never looked back, and over the next six years in the department learned so well that he published seven papers, four of them jointly with Wigglesworth. In 1936, he went with H.S.Leeson to East Africa to further educate himself in the study of mosquitoes – the scheduled flying time from London to Entebbe was then 5½ days. For the next twenty-six years Gillett stayed on in Uganda's Medical Department with few interruptions, except for visits home to obtain the degrees he had so misguidedly avoided before. There was also an interlude during the last war when, with his recent bride, he spent a year on an island in Lake Victoria, in an attempt to control sleeping sickness there by reducing the number of tsetse in the infected area in order to 'break contact between man and fly'. In the short term, the measures taken were successful; in the longer term, the tsetse and the disease returned and, as had happened in the time of Bruce and of Carpenter in Uganda more than thirty years before, it became necessary eventually to evacuate the island's entire population. In 1962, Gillett returned to Britain and the Chair of Applied Biology at Brunel University. Since retiring from there at the age of sixty-five in 1978, he was until his death a Senior Research Fellow, initially with MRC support, in the department he joined by great good chance nearly half a century earlier.[51]

In spite of their so different styles, the work of Buxton and of Wigglesworth in the 1930s combined to shape the fortunes of the department, and of developing insect physiology, in a way which raised the subject to unprecedented levels of excellence and importance in tropical disease research. By 1935, Wigglesworth was travelling again, this time to the Indian subcontinent and as far afield as Burma and Indonesia. In Ceylon (now Sri Lanka) he was present during the devastating malaria epidemic of 1934–5, and has left two graphic accounts of his harrowing experience, when at the peak of the epidemic malaria accounted for a death toll of 80,000 per week.[52]

In the meantime Buxton, at home and abroad during a brief visit to Palestine, and a more extended expedition, with D.J.Lewis, to Northern Nigeria, pursued the study of relations between insect physiology and ecology, particularly in that border line area where interactions between the study of physiology in the laboratory, and of microclimatic conditions in an actual environment, meet and serve to define the limitations of existence of a given insect in a given field.[53] Another recruit to work in this field was Kenneth Mellanby (1908–93), who like Gillett, but five years older and with a more conventional academic background, also arrived in 1930, with MRC support, to assist in Buxton's research on the physiological response of insects to heat and desiccation. Paradoxically, from this more academic background, Mellanby ultimately achieved less academic distinction, but became eventually 'outstandingly valuable' in what one anonymous obituarist has called 'the half-world of scientific administration'. But his achievements here, both at home and abroad, should not be dismissed so easily. He played a central role in establishing, and developing as its first Principal, the University College at Ibadan in Nigeria (1947–53); and later on home ground as first Director of Monks Wood Experimental Station (1961–74).[54] In his scientific endeavours, outside his brief periods at the LSHTM, he was known more for their controversial nature than their actual results.

During World War II, as Director of the Sorby Research Institute at Sheffield, it was his work with a group of conscientious objectors which propelled Mellanby into the forefront of a debate on the legitimacy of human experimentation. To quote his obituarist again, many colleagues 'felt strongly that "live" experiments should stop with the chimpanzee', even though the conscientious objectors themselves were eager enough to prove their courage in general by taking part. In any case, the stakes were less than high, if uncomfortable: the human 'guinea pigs' were being asked to wear dirty underwear discarded by scabies patients and to test the effects of different levels of calcium and vitamin C in their diets. More potentially hazardous were attempts to determine levels of fluid intake needed for human survival. Matters came to a head when Mellanby went, as observer for the *British Medical Journal*, to the Nüremberg trials, and argued for the release of results obtained by Nazi doctors in 'scientific experiments' in concentration camps, in order to have them evaluated by *bona fide* investigators. His later career was spent as Director of the Nature Conservancy's Monks Wood Experimental Station, and as consultant for environmental pressure groups.

In the late 1930s, Buxton was, in addition to other duties, working on a projected textbook of medical entomology; only one chapter, on the louse, was finished when war broke out in 1939. The lessons of the role of lice in the transmission of typhus in the earlier war were not forgotten. Now the results of applied entomology obtained in the intervening years were there to suggest ways of controlling such potential secondary disasters in wartime. The results of de-lousing procedures were woefully inadequate in the longer term, and only insecticides for treatment of clothing held out any hope of success. Yet, for all the advances made in development of insecticides in the course of twenty years, none had so far proved satisfactory: skin irritation was a factor militating against general use of all agents then developed. As in Mellanby's scabies experiments, so in experiments with lice which played such a prominent role in the activities of the department before and during World War II: dirty underwear and human volunteers were a *sine qua non*. But Buxton did not need conscientious objectors. His volunteers included, for the breeding of lice, students, staff, and family as well as himself; and for the provision of dirty and infected underwear, tramps ('verminous vagrants') who were handsomely remunerated, at 5 shillings per visit, plus insecticide-sprayed underwear.[55]

Friends and colleagues have described the discomforts of all involved. Wigglesworth wrote in 1956: '... everyone possible, including most of Buxton's family, were pressed into the service of rearing lice in small containers under their socks or vest to provide the material for controlled experiments in the laboratory'; and 'Buxton's methods of conducting this investigation were energetic, unconventional and Buxtonian. They were not very popular with the authorities of the London School of Hygiene'. Sidney Chave, writing twenty years later, recalled 'Buxton who clawed his legs red and raw to relieve the irritation caused by the lice he carried inside his socks to maintain his cultures – as we were to do later for Professor Busvine.'[56]

For all the hard, and sometimes slightly questionable, experiments the results, although useful, were far short of reaching the standards required for general use. By 1942, even Buxton was discouraged; and approached by Dr. G.A.Campbell of the Manchester branch of the Swiss Company Geigy, Buxton and Wigglesworth were sceptical. The Swiss parent company had produced a new synthetic insecticide, which they called 'Gessarol'; it was claimed to be highly toxic to insects, non-volatile and long-lasting, but also non-irritating and harmless to man. In fact it was everything Buxton had hoped for through the long years of louse research, and it seemed just too good to be true. Nevertheless, tests in the department, and simultaneously in the United States, proved the new insecticide to be at least as promising as Geigy's specifications had claimed. Chemically, 'Gessarol' was dichloro-diphenyl-trichloro-ethane: Ian Heilbron (1886–1959), chairman of the Insecticides Research and Development Committee coined the name DDT, and the compound was launched on its meteoric rise to fame, and the inevitable later disappointments, as the physiology of individual insect species began to adjust and develop defences against the threat to their survival. DDT was first used against a large-scale epidemic of typhus in Naples in 1944, with dramatic results: the epidemic was under control within three weeks. P.H.Müller (1899–1965) received a Nobel Prize in 1948 for his painstaking testing of countless contact poisons for insects, which led to the choice of DDT.[57]

Buxton's war was the department's war; and the louse problem, and the resulting textbook, was only one among many contributions. The department had close relations with the medical departments of the War Office, the Admiralty, and the Air Ministry; Buxton became chairman of an MRC Entomological Sub-Committee, later replaced by the Pyrethrum Development Panel, with responsibility for that useful natural insecticide; this in turn became the Insecticides Research and Development Committee referred to above. Other projects undertaken included work on mosquito repellents, fly sprays, control of bed bugs in air raid shelters, control of head lice in children evacuated from large towns and in girls in the Women's Services. The end of the war came almost as an anti-climax, although for the next ten years Buxton was kept more than busy on MRC committees concerned with typhus, malaria, and Colonial Medical Research, and the Colonial Office's Tsetse-Fly and Trypanosomiasis Committee, in the dying days of the Empire and the Colonial Office. At the same time, he never forsook his travels: studying tsetse flies in Southern Sudan, blackfly and mosquito induced problems in the far north of Canada, jungle yellow fever epidemics in Central America, etc. Wigglesworth's move to Cambridge in 1945 put an end to their close working relationship; the Research Unit of Insect Physiology, established in the School with Wigglesworth as Director, on the recommendation of the SRC Committee on Insecticides, went with him to Cambridge. When Buxton died at the too early age of 63 in 1955, it was the end of an era for applied insect physiology in the School.[58]

Buxton's death left the Department of Entomology as one of the smallest in the School, with the academic staff consisting of his two Readers, D.S.Bertram (1913–88), and J.R.Busvine (b.1912). Bertram succeeded Buxton as Professor and Director of the Department; in 1964, the University conferred on Busvine the title of Professor of Entomology as applied to Hygiene. Busvine had completed his Ph.D. thesis while working for ICI in 1938, at a time when insecticides were high on the agenda both in the School's entomology department and in the research laboratories of chemical and pharmaceutical industries everywhere; during World War II he was entomological adviser to the Ministry of Health. By the time he joined the School at the end of the war, his insecticide credentials were impeccable, and throughout his career – both he and Bertram retired in 1976 – he divided his time between research and teaching, and service on WHO and FAO Expert Panels on Insecticides and Pest Resistance. Through this work the department's involvement with insecticide development was continued, forming an uninterrupted pattern from Buxton's pre-war search for louse control measures to the post-war hopes and disappointments of the era of DDT.[59]

Buxton and Wigglesworth had both qualified in medicine before focusing on insect physiology and applied entomology at the LSHTM, at a time when medical degrees were required for teachers in a postgraduate medical school. Bertram and Busvine were both trained as entomologists, at Glasgow and Imperial College London, respectively, with no medical qualifications. When they both retired in 1976, the incoming professor and Director of the Department, William Weir Macdonald (b.1927) was also a graduate of Glasgow University in entomology. Macdonald did not stay long, certainly not long enough to make an impact in the department; after three years in Keppel Street he left for the Chair of Medical Entomology at the Liverpool School. His departure marked something of a change in direction for the department, a change which would soon become part of a wider redefinition of concerns, and gradual integration between departments and new units of rapidly developing subjects, old and new: epidemiology, immunology, molecular biology, vaccine design, medical entomology and applied parasitology, etc.[60]

In this changing world, within and without the School, a major reorganisation of departments was on the way: the creation for the 1980s of the three main Divisions, each with a full complement of departments. Between Macdonald's departure in 1980 and the introduction two years later of the divisional structure, G.Davidson, Reader in Entomology in the Ross Institute, moved to the Department of Entomology as 'caretaker' Director and Professor of Entomology as applied to Malaria until he retired as Emeritus Professor at the end of December, 1982. By the time of his move to Entomology, he had spent more than thirty years as the Ross Institute's chief entomologist since he had joined as 'entomological research assistant' after World War II; like Busvine, Bertram and W.W.Macdonald he had a B.Sc. in entomology rather than any medical qualifications. Eventually he became 'Reader in Entomology as Applied to Malaria' in the Ross Institute; and his final move to the Department of Entomology coincided with the transfer of the Ross anopheles collection, in what may be seen as a 're-uniting of the anophelines' of the two departments. Davidson's particular interests and achievements lay in anopheline genetics, with special reference to the genetics of insecticide resistance, and the possibilities of alternative genetic control measures involving introduction of sterile males into mosquito populations, which became of increasing interest in the later 1960s when the enthusiasm for the use of insecticides faltered in the face of irreversible setbacks. The genetic nature of anopheline resistance had first been demonstrated in the Ross Institute by Davidson and Draper as early as 1956. Later, as increasing numbers of mosquito and other insect species developed resistance to increasing numbers of synthetic insecticides – at the end of the 1970s no less than 44 anopheline species had been reported to show resistance, variously, to different insecticides: to DDT, to dieldrin and other organochlorines, to organophosphates, carbamates and even new synthetic pyrethroids. In the 1970s the work of Davidson, of C.F.Curtis, and others in the Ross Institute, focused especially on *Anopheles* species. Within the *Anopheles gambiae* complex matters are complicated by the presence of some genes with recessive resistance (e.g. to DDT), and others with dominant resistance (eg to dieldrin).[61] From then on, until the next major and radical reshaping of the structure of the School's departments as it entered its final decade before its centenary, and the millennium, Entomology began a period of close links with the Arbovirus Unit, with a joint Head, M.G.R. Varma, and with research collaborations with the Department of Medical Microbiology, and the Department of Tropical Hygiene, as well as the Arbovirus Unit. There was also an innovation. The 1986-7 *Annual Report* noted: 'The Department of Entomology has been strengthened, as has its links with other Schools of the University. An academic initiative post, provided by the University, has enabled us to recruit a specialist in insect behaviour who holds a joint appointment with Imperial College. She not only provides a new dimension to research on preventing disease vectors from biting man, but also links it with research on tsetse-flies at Imperial College and with the complementary expertise of the insect physiology group at Birkbeck College. Collaboration in seminars and research with Birkbeck College is developing and cooperation in teaching is being explored.'[62]

Barely ten years later, the LSHTM entered the 1990s with a new Dean, and a complete restructuring with four large main departments. Until 1996-7, the Department of Medical Parasitology included, among staff in its five Units, entomologists and medical entomologists in 'Vector Biology and Epidemiology'; and biochemists – 'insect biochemists'– investigating insecticide resistance, an area of growing concern, in 'Parasite and Vector Biochemistry'. The very titles of the units, and of their respective staff members, illustrate vividly both the growth in knowledge and understanding, and the increasing complexities of research in entomology, in an age when molecular biochemistry plays an decisive role in all the biological sciences, including tropical parasitology. As a result of the latest review of the School's departmental structure, completed in September, 1996, it consists as of August 1997 of three large departments: the Department of Epidemiology and Population Health; the Department of Infectious and Tropical Diseases; and the Department of Public Health and Policy; Medical Parasitology is now part of the Department of Infectious and Tropical Diseases.[63]

CLINICAL TROPICAL MEDICINE

When Manson's Tropical School opened its doors at the Albert Dock in October, 1899, the School and the Branch Hospital of the Seamen's Hospital Society formed an inseparable whole. The School was unthinkable without the Hospital, and the clinical experience it offered for students and staff alike; the School's research in turn opened up new avenues of prevention and therapy. When the School and Hospital moved together to the Endsleigh Gardens site in 1920, the close-working relationship looked set to continue unabated, the teaching presented with an added advantage in the shape of the collections of the neighbouring Wellcome Tropical Museum. But only a year later the Athlone Committee published its recommendations; Leiper began negotiating with the Rockefeller Foundation; and by 1924, firm plans for the new LSHTM were evolving, and the Seamen's Hospital Society abdicated responsibility for the Tropical School it had nurtured for a quarter of a century.

Sir Philip Manson-Bahr, who as Manson's son-in-law, one-time Director of the LSHTM's Department of Clinical Tropical Medicine, and senior physician, later consultant (he also had a lucrative Harley Street practice) to the Hospital, felt himself to be very much the custodian of the values and traditions of School and Hospital, commented bitterly on the events that led to their relative separation:

> The Hospital became the whipping boy of medical politics. The pendulum swayed from one side to another and for this indecision the Hospital and the teaching of tropical medicine had to suffer. It had to suffer because of the puzzling attitude of many members of the Board of the Seamen's Hospital Society. There was always a representative body of admirals whose interest lay in the sailor, but not in tropical medicine which they thought lay outside the scope of their charter. ...

One could of course argue that the admirals' primary concern for their sailors did them credit, and that Manson-Bahr's remarks came perilously close to an arrogant medical conceit which perceived the patient as an instrument to be used in the teaching of tropical medicine. On the other hand, the dilemma was a real one. G.C.Cook, Consultant at the HTD who retired as Clinical Senior Lecturer in the School in 1997, quoted part of this outburst from Manson–Bahr in 1989, more in sorrow than in anger. He also emphasised the 'valuable and productive' effects of the former cohabitation of School and Hospital, which came to an end when the School moved to its new premises in Keppel Street in 1929. He characterised the resulting geographical division – by however short a walking distance – as 'the greatest disaster which was to befall [the discipline of clinical tropical medicine]'.[64]

Until the opening of the Keppel Street building in 1929, 'Clinical Papers', the vast majority written by Manson–Bahr and George Carmichael Low, were included in the lists of published papers in appendices to the School's annual reports. Most of these papers described case histories and observations in the Hospital: the therapeutic value of anti-malaria compounds; the effects of blood transfusion on pernicious anaemia in sprue patients; observations on human filariidae; blood transfusion in blackwater fever; and so on. Even Low, who had made such fundamental contributions to the early discoveries, was now approaching retiring age, and was preoccupied with his patients, his interest in ornithology, and his presidency of the Royal Society of Tropical Medicine and Hygiene of which he had been such an influential founder member back in 1907. Manson-Bahr also devoted most of his time to his patients and to teaching, and to the successive editions of that enduring text, *Manson's Tropical Diseases*.[65]

Into this atmosphere of quiet solid clinical work there arrived, in 1929, a younger Australian, Neil Hamilton Fairley, known to Manson-Bahr from work on schistosomiasis in Egypt during the Great War, when Manson-Bahr was serving in the RAMC and Hamilton Fairley with the Australian Imperial Forces. Fairley, ten years younger than Manson-Bahr, had enlisted in 1916, after graduation from the University of Melbourne, where he had been taught according to the methods developed by Charles Martin during his years in Australia. By the time Fairley arrived at university, Martin was back in London, Director of the Lister Institute, but the spirit of his teaching survived in Melbourne. He himself had said of his Australian medical students that 'They all meant business and the experimental method of approach came naturally to them and intellectual adventure was congenial.' That certainly applied to Hamilton Fairley, and some months spent at the Lister in London with Martin and Muriel Robertson in 1919, reinforced his belief in the importance of correlation between clinical and laboratory observations, which characterised his life's work. It also convinced him of a need for team work; he became an early exponent of this form of collaborative effort which was to develop so rapidly and with such outstanding successes throughout a second European war and its aftermath.[66]

Hamilton Fairley had not been long at the School and the Hospital when he wrote, in the *Annual Report* a note on 'Research Work at the Hospital for Tropical Diseases'. Here he emphasised his certain belief in the importance of biochemical studies, both in blackwater fever, and in tropical sprue, that puzzling condition under scrutiny since the time of Manson. Fairley himself had suffered from sprue in India before coming to London; at the Haffkine Institute he had worked on the disease, and introduced a high protein diet to help recovery from the malabsorption caused. After three years in India, the diet he had developed helped his own recovery from a severe attack. In 1931 he wrote: 'Our recent work at the Hospital for Tropical Diseases has shown that there is a definite biochemical background to sprue'; and of blackwater fever: '... biochemical data are being used with increasing degrees of success in indicating the need for special lines of treatment'.[67] Thus Hamilton Fairley's arrival in the Department of Clinical Tropical Medicine marked the introduction of a more biochemical approach to clinical problems; and also a growing interest in the development of serological tests for early diagnosis in a number of diseases.

Throughout the 1930s Hamilton Fairley continued to shape tropical clinical research at the School, where work on blackwater fever led him to distinguish between the different haemoglobin derivatives found during the acute haemolytic crisis in cases of the disease. In the course of these studies Fairley visited, on a number of occasions, the League of Nations' Malaria Research Laboratory at Salonika. It was an experience which would stand him in good stead during World War II in a famous incident when he and a colleague – Sir John Boyd – in the Medical Directorate had a fierce argument with General Wavell in order to convince the General of the dangers of malaria, and the policy for avoidance, during the planning of Allied intervention in Greece in 1941.[68]

In 1942, Fairley went with the Australian Forces first to Java, and afterwards to the South Pacific theatre of war, where malaria was a major threat to troops fighting in the jungles. Realising the critical importance of convincing both the authorities, and serving personnel, of the necessity of using preventive medication, he was able to establish two research groups at Cairns, and eventually to prove the benefits of regular daily doses of atebrin.[69]

Released from his army appointments in 1946, Fairley returned to London, to succeed Manson-Bahr as Director of the Department of Clinical Tropical Medicine, and to take up a newly created Chair in an expanding subject; for the first time, there was a Deputy Director, Frederick Murgatroyd (1902–50), and a full-time Lecturer, A.W.Woodruff (1916–92). At the LSHTM, Fairley soon found kindred souls, whose work complemented his own wartime activities in Cairns: he was able to give essential advice to Garnham and Shortt in their pioneering work on the exoerythrocytic cycle of *Plasmodium* species. Unfortunately, serious illness, from which he never completely recovered, forced Fairley to resign his newly acquired Chair in 1948, and Murgatroyd succeeded him, the appointment to date from October 1st, 1950; alas, it was not to be. Murgatroyd died, suddenly and unexpectedly, in December, 1951; and the Chair of Clinical Tropical Medicine was again vacant, though not for long: A.W.Woodruff

(1916–93), Senior Lecturer, not yet thirty-five, inherited the Chair, where he was to stay for nearly thirty years, until he retired at the age limit in 1981.[70]

In his first report, Woodruff made clear his intentions to divide the department's research activities into two distinct, but interdependent, parts: clinical problems being studied in the Hospital's Medical Unit; basic research, including animal experiments, being undertaken in the Keppel Street laboratories, with their advantage of an animal house on the premises. Fat absorption was studied in both places, at the Hospital in its dependence on emulsifying substances in the treatment of sprue, in Keppel Street in relation to vitamin deficiencies. Other subjects for research included chemotherapy in onchocerciasis, and terramycin treatment of amoebic dysentery. Clinical trials were carried out with therapy for leprosy and malaria, in collaboration with Sir Neil Hamilton Fairley and Sir George Reid McRobert (1895–1976), another survivor of the IMS, who after the 1939–45 war and final retirement from India was senior consulting physician to the Hospital for Tropical Diseases. With Sir Philip Manson-Bahr, Fairley and McRobert formed a formidable trio, which in the 1950s was referred to by students and younger staff, affectionately albeit somewhat irreverently, as 'The Galloping Knights of Tropical Medicine'. To the students, Hamilton Fairley's superiority in academic terms was unquestionable; and his early retirement from teaching, due to ill health, was a setback for the department, aggravated by the almost immediate death of his successor, Murgatroyd. It was left to Woodruff to revive a temporarily demoralised department. To his credit, he succeeded at a time which was difficult for other reasons.[71]

During World War II, precautionary measures involving evacuation of patients from the Hospital on the corner of Gordon Street and Endsleigh Gardens had been followed by major bomb damage. The Seamen's Hospital Society had been able to arrange for temporary, though far from satisfactory, premises in Devonshire Street.[72] In the early post-war years negotiations began with University College Hospital (UCH). As a result, a new clinical unit of 68 beds was opened by the Duchess of Kent in May, 1951, in St.Pancras way. It was not ideal accommodation, but the arrangements did at least improve facilities for clinical teaching and ward demonstrations. Cynics might question the disinterestedness of UCH's generosity: the building allocated to the Hospital for Tropical Diseases had initially been planned as an obstetric unit. According to one observer, the gynaecologists and obstetricians had unanimously rejected the idea of such unsuitable, even potentially insanitary, accommodation for their purposes. The closeness of the site to the St.Pancras railway stables was regarded as a major potential source of pollution and invading flies.[73]

At St.Pancras, the improved accommodation also improved the outlook for teaching. It became possible to enlarge the groups of students taught at anyone time, and hence to increase their period of attendance from one month to six weeks. The Medical Unit also increased its numbers of both in-patients and of out-patients seen at its thrice weekly clinics. In a recent volume, G.C.Cook has recorded the fate and the struggle of the Department and the Hospital before and during those years in meticulous detail.[74]

A.W.Woodruff served the Department of Tropical Medicine and the Hospital for Tropical Diseases for more than thirty years, from his arrival at the School as Senior Lecturer in 1948, until he retired from the Wellcome Chair in 1981. His preoccupations during those years reflected the changing concerns of clinical tropical medicine in London and elsewhere, from the erstwhile approaches of the 'Colonial Medicine' of the days of Manson and of Low, to the very different attitudes following World War II and the independence of, first, India, and by degrees other parts of what was once the British Empire, as well as the possessions of other colonial powers. There was also a change from the never quite realised good intentions of the League of Nations between the wars, to the far more comprehensive measures pioneered on a global scale by the United Nations and the World Health Organization. Woodruff pursued a number of interests in parasitic diseases at home and abroad, from the problems presented by transmission of the roundworm *Toxocara canis* through dog faeces as a threat to children frequenting parks in Britain, to sickle-cell anaemia, sprue, and malaria. The involvement of Woodruff, and of his department, in the changing priorities of the developing world, was reflected in his long-term memberships of WHO Expert Advisory Committees on onchocerciasis, and on resistance of malaria parasites to chemotherapy; of the Medical Committee of Overseas Development Administration; and of MRC Committees on Haemoglobin Variants and on Travellers' Diarrhoea. His life-long determination to improve education in tropical medicine where it mattered abroad is evidenced by his many periods spent in visiting professorships at countless universities in Africa and the Middle East. Former colleagues remember Woodruff's impressive frame, and the whiff of a colonial Medical Officer of a bygone age which characterised his appearance. In Woodruff's case, this aspect of his demeanour was accepted, even admired, in parts of the former empire not otherwise markedly tolerant of British influence in the post-colonial age. When he retired from the School in 1981, he left immediately, with a small team, for Juba in the Sudan, there to assist in the development of a new medical school. He stayed on, as Professor of Medicine in the University of Juba until, no less active at the age of 76, he died suddenly in Khartoum, in October, 1992.[75]

Following Woodruff's retirement and departure for Juba, the Department of Clinical Medicine had one of its Senior Lecturers, H.A.K.Rowland, as 'acting Head' until Keith P.W.J.McAdam returned to Britain to the Wellcome Chair after seven years in Boston, Mass. at Tufts University School of Medicine. His arrival coincided with preparations for another period of change in administration and structure of the School's departments. The divisions structure of the 1980s was heading for the mega department structure of the 1990s, with its proliferation of units each with its own sub-specialty, with increasing emphasis on molecular, biochemical studies. McAdam's new Department of Clinical Sciences had four research units which supported and complemented the Hospital for Tropical Diseases, the whole designed to 'span the interface between clinical investigation and biomedical science'. On arrival from Tufts he brought with him a group of laboratory scientists; and supported by the Wellcome Trust and other foundations, he introduced laboratory-based clinical research in infectious diseases. It was a major change from the Woodruff era, placing the School's clinical tropical medicine on a level with contemporary clinical science, and with a strong scientific base in programmes on tuberculosis and sexually transmitted diseases (STDs). Additional skills in studies of chlamydial infections and STDs came with the appointment of David Mabey from the MRC Unit in The Gambia. The TB programmes also benefited when J.D.H.Porter was recruited from the Centre for Disease Control (CDC) at Atlanta, Georgia. The programmes centred around an overseas unit in Lusaka, Zambia, where Peter Godfrey-Fausset and Alison Elliott developed a number of collaborative studies. In 1995, on the eve of the most recent restructuring of the School McAdam, on secondment, took over as Director of the MRC Laboratories in the Gambia from Brian Greenwood, who then came to the School as Professor of Communicable Diseases.[76]

REFUGEE HEALTH CARE

In 1978, the Ross Institute under David Bradley was planning to establish a new research unit to be called the Evaluation and Planning Centre for Health Care (cf. Chapter 11), supported by funds from the ODA Health and Population Division. Staffed by an interdisciplinary group under Patrick Vaughan and including Dr.Bruce Dick and Stephanie Simmonds, it became an important factor in planning and developing emergency international health care in a number of long-term refugee situations throughout the 1980s; since 1981 as a separate **Refugee Health Group (RHG)** within the department, individually funded by the New York Office of the Edna McConnell Clark Foundation. Over the years the group was involved in the increasingly critical, global, problems of health in refugee camps and refugee populations: nutrition and supplementary and therapeutic feeding programmes, general health surveillance, provision of drugs in emergency situations, etc. More recently, within the Health Policy Unit, attention has been focused on policies adopted by host nations towards incoming refugees.[77]

A DEVELOPING LIBRARY IN AN EXPANDING SCHOOL

Development and extension of the School's existing library, to serve the twin objectives of Tropical Medicine and Public Health, and their post-war offspring, Tropical Public Health, was long overdue when it was finally realised. The growing scope in teaching and research, and hence in sheer numbers of students and staff since World War II, inevitably brought pressure on accommodation and facilities throughout the School, not least on library services, for long in need of updating and reorganisation. In the early 1960s, substantial benefactions from a number of sources made it possible to begin an ambitious programme of restructuring, to take place in three stages. Stage I, generously supported by donations from the Wolfson Trust and Marks and Spencer, yielded 1,200 square feet of additional space for teaching and research, space to be put to good use by allowing acceptance of more students for the Diploma in Tropical Public Health, as well as accommodating a number of new lecturers funded by the Ministry of Overseas Development.

    A new large refectory and kitchens were completed by January 1965 in the basement, freeing space elsewhere for teaching and research. The structural work was undertaken by the architectural firm of Verner Rees, who had so successfully carried out the original building of the School in Keppel Street in the 1920s. Stages II and III involved conversion of the 2nd and 3rd floors, and the construction of a 4th floor above them; at all stages substantial help was also received in the form of grants from the University of London. In step with these structural improvements, the library also had a face-lift, funded by the Wellcome

PREVENTION AND CURE

Trust. 'Open' book stacks were added, and research facilities substantially improved;[78] but ten years later it became obvious that more improvements were necessary. Problems increasingly affecting professional libraries everywhere in the country were making themselves felt. The School Report for 1974–5 explained the dilemma in euphemistic terms:

> ... outhousing of less-used material should be kept abreast of accessions. Over the years, there has been growing non-observance of library rules and an increasing part of the current literature has been disappearing without trace for short or longer periods. The new plans, of which only the first phase can be afforded at present, take account of both factors. ...[79]

At the same time, inflation and the growing volume and costs of current periodicals made cuts necessary, and consequently 'Co-operation with the Bureau of Hygiene and Tropical Diseases, with the Interim Library Resources Coordinating Committee of the University and with the British Library, is increasingly important in the provision of an adequate service .' Since then, the outlook for Library Services has improved radically, thanks largely to the growing volume of information technology becoming available (cf. Chapter 6, p.150).

NOTES

[1] Sir Philip Manson-Bahr, *History of the School of Tropical Medicine in London, 1899-1949,* London, H.K.Lewis, 1956, 'Diary', 1907 and 1908, p.273.
[2] *ibid.*, 'Diary' 1913, p.276.
[3] *ibid.*, p.59.
LSTM Student Register, vol.6, 55th (October-December, 1917) and 56th (January-April, 1918) Sessions;
S.R.Christophers, 'Sydney Price James 1870-1946', *Biogr.Mem.Fell.R.Soc.* 1945-8, 5:507-23, p.514.
[4] Chap.3, p.6 above.
SHSMB, *15,* 12 July, 1918; *ibid., 16,* 9 January, 26 June, and 12 February, 1920.
[5] Sidney Chave, 'The School through fifty years', LSHTM MSS Collection, acc.No.83461, 1976, pp.13-14;
LSHTM *Annual Reports* 1924-5, p.14; 1926-7, p.18; 1927-8, p.27; 1928-9, p.30; 1929-30, p.30;
E.M.Tansey and R.C.E.Milligan, 'The early history of the Wellcome Research Laboratories, 1894-1914', *in:* J.Liebenau *et al., Pill peddlers: essays on the history of the pharmaceutical industry,* Madison, WI, American Institute for the History of Pharmacy, 1990, pp.91-106.
[6] LSHTM *Annual Reports* as above.
[7] LSHTM *Annual Report* 1937-8, pp.12-13.
[8] LSHTM *Annual Report* 1970-1, p.24.
[9] Chapter 2, p.10 and note 22.
[10] 'Johannes Fibiger (1867-1928), *in:* T.L.Sourkes, ed., *Nobel Prize Winners in Medicine and Physiology 1901-65,* London etc., 1967, pp.123-7;
J.Fibiger, 'Ueber eine durch nematoden (*Spiroptera sp.*) hervorgerufene papillomatöse und carcinomatöse Geschwulstbildung in Magen der Ratte', *Berl.klin,Wschr.,* 1913, *i*:289-98;
idem, 'Sur la transmission au rats de la *Spiroptera neoplastica) Gongylonema neoplasticum).* Méthode pour la production expérimentale du cancer', *C.r.hebd.Séanc.Mém.Soc.Biol.,* 1920, *83:*321-4.
[11] The Nobel Foundation (ed), *Nobel The man and his prizes*, New York etc., 3rd ed. 1972, pp.188-9.
[12] F.P.Rous. 'Transmission of a malignant new growth by means of a cellfree filtrate', *J.Am.med.Ass.,* 1911, *56:*198.
[13] L.W.Sambon, 'Observations and researches on epidemiology of cancer made in Holland and Italy (May-September, 1925)', *J.Trop.Med.Hyg.,*

1926, *29*:233-87;
H.A.Bayliss, '*Gongylonema* and cancer', *Br.med.J.*, 1926, *ii*:503-4;
R.T.Leiper, '*Gongylonema* and cancer', *ibid.*, p.504;
L.W.Sambon, 'Refutation of statements made by Professor R.T.Leiper, MD, D.Sc., FRS, concerning African schistosomes, "American" gongylonemes, zoo vermin and Italian cancer houses', *J.Trop.Med.Hyg.*, 1926, *29*:314-22;
Anon, 'Fibiger's tumour of the rat's stomach', *Lancet* 1938, *i*:735-6.
[14] T.W.M.Cameron, 'A new definitive host for *Schistosoma mansoni*', *J.Helminth.*, 1928, *6*:219-22;
idem, 'Helminth parasites of man and monkeys', *Proc.Roy.Soc.Med. (Sect.Trop.Dis.Parasit).*, 1929, *22*, April.
LSHTM *Annual Report* 1928-9.
[15] LSHTM *Annual Report* 1928-9, p.14.
[16] J.J.C.Buckley, 'On the development of *Culicoides furens* Poey of *Filaria (Mansonella) ozzardi* Manson, 1897', *J.Helminth.*, 1934, *12*:99-118.
[17] [George Nelson], Buckley obituaries in *Nature, Lancet*, 1972, *i*:968; *Br.med.J.*, 1972, *i*:355;
for Cooper and Pester see Chapter 11, p.23 and note 44, p.45.
[18] 'Exercise Book' marked 'keep', with, largely, hookworm experiments dated 1932-3; Buckley Collection in authors' possession.
[19] William B.Dean, 'Walter Reed and the ordeal of yellow fever experiments', *Bull.Hist.Med.*, 1977, *51*:75-92.
[20] D.I.Grove, *A history of human helminthology*, Oxon, CAB International, 1990, pp.477-8;
J.J.C.Buckley, 'An observation on human resistance to infection with ascaris from the pig', *J.Helminth.*, 1931, *9*:45-6.
[21] Grove, op.cit. above, p.302.
[22] Buckley, 'Bull-Dog' Exercise Book No.6, labelled *Gastrodiscoides hominis* in Buckley's handwriting;
J.J.C.Buckley, 'Observations on *Gastrodiscoides hominis* and *Fasciolopsis buski* in Assam', *J.Helminth.*, 1939, *17*:1-12.
[23] D.B.Blacklock, 'The development of *Onchocerca volvulus* in *Simulium damnosum*', *Ann.Trop.Med.Parasit.*, 1926, *20*:1-40.
[24] J.J.C.Buckley, 'On *Culicoides* as a vector of *Onchocerca gibsoni* (Cleland and Johnston 1910)', *J.Helminth.*, 1938, *16*:121-58.
[25] J.J.C.Buckley, 'Studies on human onchocerciasis and *Simulium* in Nyanza Province, Kenya. I. Distribution and incidence of *O.volvulus*', *J.Helminth.*, 1949, *23*:1-24;
idem., 'II. The disappearance of *S.naevei* from a bush-cleared focus', *J.Helminth.*, 1951, *25*:213-22;

P.C.C.Garnham and J.P.McMahon, 'The eradication of *Simulium naevei* Roubaud, from an onchocerciasis area in Kenya Colony', *Bull.Entomol.Res.*, 1947, *37:*619–28;
idem, 'Final results of an experiment on the control of onchocerciasis by eradication of the vector', *ibid.*, 1954, *45:*175–6;
V.D.van Someren and J.P.McMahon, 'Phoretic association between *Afronurus* and *Simulium* species, and the discovery of the early stages of *Simulium naevei* on crabs', *Nature,* 1950, *166:*350–2.

[26] Several former friends and associates have speculated on likely causes, but there is no hard evidence.

[27] P.Manson-Bahr op.cit. note 1, p.164.

[28] Edeson to Buckley, dated Kuala Lumpur, 27 October, 1958; Buckley to Edeson, dated Keppel Street, 6 November, 1958.

[29] J.J.C.Buckley, 'On *Brugia* gen.nov. for *Wuchereria* ssp. of the "malayi" group i.e. *W.malayi* Brug, 1927, *W.pahangi* Buckley and Edeson, 1956, and *W.patei* Buckley, Nelson and Heisch, 1958', *Ann.Trop.Med.Parasit.,* 1960, *54:*75–7;
Grove, op.cit. note 20, pp.604–5;
D.A.Denham *et al.,* 'The effect of metrifonate on *Brugia pahangi* infections in domestic cats', *Bull.Wld.Hlth.Org.*, 1971, *45:*423–9;
D.A.Denham, 'The diagnosis of filariasis', *Ann.Soc.Belg.Med.Trop.*, 1975, *55:*517–24;
D.A.Denham, R.R.Suswillo, *et al.,* 'Studies on *Brugia pahangi* 13. The anthelmintic effect of compounds F151(Friedheim), HOE 33258(Hoechst) and their reaction product', *J.Helminth.,* 1976, *50:*243–50;
D.A.Denham *et al.,* 'Studies with *Brugia pahangi* 20. An investigation of 23 anthelmintics using different screening techniques', *Trans.R.Soc.Trop.Med.Hyg.,* 1978, *72:*615–8;
D.A.Denham, E.Brandt and D.A.Liron, 'Anthelmintic effects of oxibendazole on *Brugia pahangi*', *J.Parasit.,* 1981, *67:*123.

[30] George Kinoti, 'Professor George S.Nelson An appreciation', *in:* C.N.L.Macpherson and P.S.Craig (eds), *Parasitic helminths and zoonoses in Africa,* London, Unwin Hyman, 1991, pp.ix–xiii.

[31] W.C.Campbell, 'Trichinella in Africa and the *nelsoni* affair', *in: ibid.,* pp.83–100.

[32] LSHTM *Annual Report* 1979–80.
LSHTM Report of the Working Group on Departmental Structure, October 1996.

[33] LSHTM *Research Report* 1992, pp.53–6;
Ahmed Tayeh and Sandy Cairncross, 'Dracunculiasis eradication by 1995. Will endemic countries meet target?', *Health Policy and Planning,* 1993,

*8(3):*191-207;
Sandy Cairncross, E.I.Braide and Sam Z.Bugri, 'Community participation in the eradication of Guinea worm disease', *Acta tropica,* 1996, *61: 121-36;*
Sandy Cairncross, personal communication.
[34] Harriette Chick, Margaret Hume and Marjorie MacFarlane, *War on disease: a history of the Lister Institute,* [London], A.Deutsch. [1971].
[35] CMAC, G.C./57, 1-6.
[36] Cecil A Hoare, 'Charles Morley Wenyon 1878-1948', *Obit.Not.Fell.R.Soc.,* 1948-9, *6:*627-42;
Robert S.Desowitz, *The Malaria Capers,* New York and London, W.W.Norton & Co., 1991, p.57.
[37] 'John Gordon Thomson', *Lancet,* 1937, *ii:*473;
LSHTM *Annual Report* 1936-7, p.1;
LSTM Research Memoir, vol.III, 'Reports on the results of the Bilharzia Mission in Egypt, 1915', *JRAMC,* 1915, *25:*1-55; 147-92; 253-67;
'Egyptian mollusca. Based largely upon a typical set partly collected and arranged by J.Gordon Thomson', *ibid.,* 1916, *27:*171-90.
[38] P.Manson-Bahr, op.cit. note 1, p.219;
Ibid., p.305: J.G.Thomson (Milner Research Fund), 'Researches on blackwater fever in Southern Rhodesia, J.Gordon Thomson accompanied by W.Cooper, technical assistant. A very complete study of blackwater fever with special reference to association with the subtertian malaria parasite *(Plasmodium falciparum).* Volume VI, Research Memoirs, LSTM;
LSHTM *Annual Report* 1935-6.
[39] P.C.C.Garnham, 'Henry Edward Shortt 15 April 1887-9 November 1987', *Biogr.Mem.Fell.R.Soc.,* 1988, *34:*715-51.
[40] Shortt and Garnham co-wrote the Royal Society obituary of Christophers; Garnham alone that of Shortt.
[41] Garnham, op.cit. note 39, p.715;
H.E.Shortt and P.C.C.Garnham, 'Samuel Rickards Christophers 27 November 1873 - 19 February 1978 Elected FRS 1926', *Biogr.Mem.Fell.Roy.Soc.,* 1979, *25:*179-207, pp.180-1.
[42] *ibid.,* pp.732-5;
R.S.Desowitz, op.cit. note 36.
[43] L.Wilkinson, *Animals and Disease,* Cambridge University Press, 1992, pp.209-10.
[44] LSHTM *Annual Report* 1968-9;
Report to the Board of Management on the School Council's views concerning the future policy of the School. January 1970, pp.10-12;

LSHTM *Annual Report* 1968-9, p.24;
List of publications in the Ross Institute and D.Bradley, personal communication;
M.A.Miles, 'Transmission cycles and the heterogeneity of *Trypanosoma cruzi*, in: W.H.R.Lumsden and D.A.Evans (eds), *Biology of the Kinetoplastida,* vol.2, London etc., 1979, pp.117-95;
LSHTM *Annual Report* 1980-1, pp.42-3.
[45] V.B.Wigglesworth, 'Patrick Alfred Buxton 1892-1955', *Biogr.Mem.Fell.R.Soc.,* 1956, 2:69-84.
[46] *ibid.,* p.71.
[47] P.A.Buxton and G.H.E.Hopkins, *Researches in Polynesia and Melanesia: medical entomology,* London School of Hygiene and Tropical Medicine, Memoir No,1, 1927; and
Researches in Polynesia and Melanesia: human diseases and welfare, LSHTM Memoir No.2.;
John Lane, 'The insect collection of the Department of Entomology, LSHTM: 1885-1985', *Trop.Dis.Bull.,* 1985, 82 (3):R1-R2.
[48] P.A.Buxton, 'Applied entomology', *Nature,* 1926, *117*:623-4. Wigglesworth, op.cit. note 45, p.73.
[49] J.D.Gillett, 'Professor Sir Vincent B.Wigglesworth, CBE, MA, MD, FRS', an 85th birthday address for Sir Vincent, 1985;
'Professor Sir Vincent Wigglesworth', *The Times* obituary, 15 February, 1994.
Michael Locke, 'Sir Vincent Brian Wigglesworth, CBE 17 April 1899-12 February 1994' *Biog.Mem.Fell.Roy.Soc.* 1996, *42*:541-53.
[50] The poem was first published in the New Yorker, and in slightly altered form in John Updike, *Hoping for a Hoopoe: Poems,* London, 1959, Gollancz. Apparently Updike's imagination was also caught by 'a talk listed in the BBC *Radio Times*: Science, Pure and Applied, by V.B.Wigglesworth, FRS, Quick Professor of Biology in the University of Cambridge'; it also appears with an author's disclaimer: 'The V.B.Wigglesworth in the poem *V.B.Nimble, V.B.Quick* (page 17) bears no resemblance whatever to the real V.B.Wigglesworth.'
[51] 'Biography of John David Gillett, OBE, D.Sc.', *Mosquito Systematics,* 1984, *16*:317-28.
[52] J.D.Gillett, op.cit. note 49;
Col.C.A.Gill, IMS etc., 'Report on the Malaria Epidemic in Ceylon in 1934-5', Sessional Paper XXIII, Colombo, Ceylon Government Press, 1935;
R.Briercliffe, W.Dalrymple-Champneys, V.B.Wigglesworth and others, 'Discussion on the malaria epidemic in Ceylon 1934-5',

Proc.R.Soc.Med., 1936, *29*:537–62.

[53] P.A.Buxton and D.J.Lewis, 'Climate and tsetse flies, laboratory studies upon *Glossina submorsitans* and *tachinoides*', *Phil.Trans.Roy.Soc.B*, 1934, *224*:175–240.

[54] 'Kenneth Mellanby', *The Times* obituary, 24 December, 1993.

[55] Wigglesworth, op.cit. note 45, p.75.
J.R.Busvine, *Disease transmission by insects,* Berlin etc., Springer-Verlag, 1993, p.212.

[56] Sidney Chave, op.cit. note 5, p.13.

[57] Wigglesworth, as note 55;
Wigglesworth, op.cit. note 45, pp.75-6.

[58] *ibid.*, p.77;
LSHTM *Annual Report* 1955–6, pp.14–15.

[59] Busvine, op.cit. note 55;
'Emeritus Professor Douglas Somerville Bertram', LSHTM *Annual Report* 1988–9, pp.9–10.

[60] LSHTM *Annual Report* 1979–80, p.26.

[61] G.Davidson and C.F.Curtis, 'Insecticide resistance and the upsurge of malaria problems and alternative solutions', LSHTM *Annual Report* 1978–9, pp.78–82;
G.Davidson, 'Prospects of genetic control for medically important insects;, in: *Proceedings of the Medical entomology centenary symposium*, London, *Roy.Soc.Trop.Med.Hyg.*, 1978, pp.111–19.
C.F.Curtis, 'Hybrid sterility in the *Anopheles gambiae* complex: mechanism and possible means of using it for genetic control; in *ibid.*, pp.133;
James R.Busvine, *Disease transmission by insects,* Berlin etc., Springer Verlag, 1993, pp.305–25.

[62] LSHTM *Annual Report* 1986–7, pp.23–4;
C.J.Leake, 'Arbovirology at Winches Farm Laboratories', *in:* M.G.Taylor (ed), *A brief history of virology protozoology and helminthology at Winches Farm 1924-92,* LSHTM, 1992, p.31.

[63] LSHTM *Research Report,* 1992, pp.47–63.

[64] P.Manson-Bahr, op.cit. note 1, p.67;
G.C.Cook, 'Early history of clinical tropical medicine in London', *J.Roy.Soc.Med.*, 1990, *83*:38–41.

[65] LSHTM *Annual Report*s between 1924–5 and 1929–30.

[66] John Boyd, 'Neil Hamilton Fairley 1891–1966', *Biogr.Mem.Fell.Roy.Soc.*, 1926, *12*:123–41;
'Fairley, Sir Neil Hamilton (15 July 1891–19 April 1966), *Roll of the RACP,* pp.86–9.

[67] 'Note by Dr.Hamilton Fairley on research work at the Hospital for Tropical Diseases', LSHTM *Annual Report* 1930-1, Appendix No.2.
[68] Boyd, op.cit. note 65, pp.133-4.
[69] *ibid.,* pp.135-8.
[70] LSHTM *Annual Reports* between 1949-50 and 1980-1;
Murgatroyd obituaries, *Lancet,* 1951, *ii:*1229; *Br.med.J.,* 1951, *ii:*1586-7.
[71] LSHTM *Annual Report* 1951-2, pp.26-7;
vivid sketches of life in the department and the hospital are given in letters to the authors from Professor P.D.Marsden, who was in the department between 1958 and 1976, and who is now at the University of Brazil (died October 1997).
[72] LSHTM *Annual Report* 1949-50, p.33.
[73] LSHTM *Annual Reports* 1950-1, 1951-2, and 1952-3, p.32;
G.C.Cook, *From the Greenwich Hulks to Old St Pancras,* London, Athlone Press, 1992, pp.287-99.
[74] *ibid.*
[75] 'Professor Alan Woodruff', *The Times* obituary, 20 October, 1992; W.E.Ormerod, personal communication.
[76] LSHTM *Research Report,* 1992, p.4;
On the eve of yet another round of changes in administration and organisation of the School's infrastructure, first announced in August, 1994, the 'likely secondment' of Keith McAdam to be Director of the MRC Laboratories in The Gambia is mentioned among the circumstances justifying thoughts of restructuring.
Professor E.H.O.Parry, Senior Research Fellow at the School, personal communication.
[77] Papers on the work of the Refugee Health Group of the Evaluation and Planning Centre for Health Care, LSHTM archives;
LSHTM *Research Report* 1990, p.65.
[78] LSHTM *Annual Reports* 1962-3, 1963-4, p.15, and 1964-5 p.94.
[79] LSHTM *Annual Report* 1974-5, p.36.

11

MALARIA: A CENTURY OF ADVANCES AND REVERSALS IN THE FIGHT AGAINST AN INTRACTABLE THREAT

As noted in other chapters above malaria, known and feared long before the Christian era, and not only in the tropics, was a focus of interest and activity for tropical medicine from its beginnings as an academic discipline, and the inauguration of the two tropical schools. Two of the Nobel Prizes in Physiology or Medicine during the first ten years of the award's existence were given for discoveries concerning malaria: to Ronald Ross in 1902 for 'his work on malaria, by which he has shown how it enters the organism and thereby has laid the foundation for successful research on this disease and methods of combating it'; and to Alphonse Laveran in 1907 'in recognition of his work regarding the role played by protozoa in causing diseases'. To many observers, the two prizes came in the wrong order; but the early statutes, insisting on no delay in the awards, had had to be circumvented in order to allow consideration of Laveran's discovery of twenty years before. Nor did Ross's receipt of the prize take account of the contributions of Manson, who had guided him all the way, or of the simultaneous, independent, work of Grassi and his associates. It has been suggested that Robert Koch, out of personal spite (he and Grassi had been involved in acrimonious arguments) prevented the Nobel committee from awarding a shared prize to Ross and Grassi.[1]

    Ross of course accepted the Prize as his due; and spent the rest of his life and career seeking further recognition and financial rewards, comparable to the parliamentary grants received by Jenner for cow pox vaccination in the early nineteenth century. He also made very real contributions to developing epidemiology, with his algebraic expression for endemic malaria, his 'theory of happenings', and his studies in the context of the Liverpool School's early expeditions. The outbreak of the Great War in 1914 concentrated the minds of medical authorities and of staff members at both schools on diseases presenting major threats to troops in the theatres of war. Alongside studies of transmission of typhus and of schistosomiasis, malaria, malaria therapy and possible malaria prevention assumed an overall importance in the eyes of the military medical services, from southern Europe – Italy in particular – to far-flung areas in Africa, India and even Australia.

    In London, the Hospital for Tropical Diseases played a major role in treating incoming cases, and dealing with minor outbreaks at home, at a time when the incidence of indigenous malaria, drastically reduced during the nineteenth century, was reduced to low levels of endemicity, with only mild symptoms, in the marshes of northern Kent. Philip Manson-Bahr, still in the early stages of his career in tropical medicine (after marrying Manson's daughter), served in the Middle East and later in Egypt with the RAMC. His greatest contribution to malaria control during the Great War was the establishment, on his insistence, of six Malaria Diagnosis Stations in forward areas, prior to the final Palestine Campaign. It proved to be a practical and invaluable control measure, which prevented undue rises in malaria morbidity and mortality statistics in troops passing through heavily infected areas on their way to Galilee and Damascus.[2] During the same period, the first scientific malaria surveys of the war were carried out by two stalwarts of malaria research, who only much later would take their places at the London School, there to continue to make outstanding contributions to malaria research in the post-war years. For the young H.E.Shortt, and his mentor S.R.Christophers, it was a chance to apply in a different environment lessons already learnt in malaria surveys in India, where Christophers had been put in charge of the recently formed Central Malaria Bureau in the grounds of the Central Research Institute of Kasauli.[3]

The first decades of the twentieth century had been dominated by practical applications of what Bradley has called the 'rapid translation of parasitological research to preventive action'. Ross's emphasis on the importance of control of the mosquito vector and of its breeding potential in the field led to early successes in Panama and in Malaysia; and in some areas, this epidemiological approach could be combined with an alternative approach, using quinine prophylaxis in groups considered to be particularly at risk.[4] In the late 1920s, the search for new synthetic quinine substitutes accelerated within the two tropical schools, under the umbrella of the MRC, and in collaboration with certain commercially funded research laboratories.

Developments in the late 1920s coincided with the years of expansion of the London School, when the old tropical school was emerging as the LSHTM. The period was also marked by a series of other events, which combined to influence approaches to malaria research both within tropical schools, and in other centres and laboratories working to defeat the old enemy. Ross, who by now had dissociated himself from either school, and whose eccentricities it was becoming increasingly difficult to ignore, had few real friends left; but two colleagues who had remained faithful from the early days, combined forces to head an appeal for a Ross 'Clinic'. The idea was first ventilated by Aldo Castellani in

1917; it was enthusiastically supported by W.J.Ritchie Simpson, who became Sir William Simpson in the same year the appeal was finally launched, in 1923.[5] A few years later, the MRC, in collaboration with the Department of Scientific and Industrial Research, began work to encourage and evaluate the development of new synthetic substances to be used in chemotherapy, for malaria and a number of other diseases. Finally, in the 1930s, P.H.Müller (1899–1965), an industrial chemist working for the Geigy pharmaceuticals firm in Basle, was studying insecticides of potential importance for agriculture. Searching for a chemically stable 'contact' poison among the numerous synthetic substances prepared in the Geigy laboratories Müller, on the eve of World War II, found dichloro-diphenyl-trichloro-ethane – DDT. In different ways, all three events were major influences on malaria research generally, and on work in a number of new departments and divisions in the LSHTM between the wars, and after.[6]

THE ROSS INSTITUTE

The two prime movers in the original appeal for, and the eventual establishment of, the Ross Institute, Simpson and Castellani, were very different characters. Simpson was Ross's exact contemporary; the two of them were born, and died, within a year of each other. A pioneer of tropical hygiene, teacher and organiser of tropical hygiene courses at the LSHTM, he was an admirer and staunch friend of Ross. His experiences, particularly in South Africa and India, with plague control, had made him a convinced camp follower of Ross's environmental, epidemiological approach.[7] Castellani on the other hand, bacteriologist, hot-tempered Italian, self-styled trypanosome discoverer, eventually ennobled by Mussolini, probably had more complex motives, as his later career at the Ross Institute would suggest. He was also an admirer of Ross's epidemiological methods and early discoveries; but he came to consider the Ross Institute as a convenient base and suitable outlet for his own ambitions. When the letter to the *The Times* appeared, at his and Simpson's instigation, on June 22nd, 1923, it had many distinguished signatories, headed by H.H.Asquith. Despite this, and its stirring title: 'Tropical diseases. The debt to Sir Ronald Ross. Proposed Institute as a monument', there were still obstacles to a successful outcome. By November, 1923, Simpson wrote to Ross, who was being kept fully informed about the fate of the appeal:

My dear Ross,

Sir Dorabji Tata had a conversation with me today on the telephone. ... He said it was quite useless his circularising the Princes of India. He had done so many times [sic] for different objects scientific and otherwise but all without success. They were indifferent to any appeal that did not come from a member of Council of India or the Viceroy, that they had no sense of philanthropy ... or a good cause. ... honours ... was the only moving impulse. ... I wonder how we can get hold of Lord Reading. If we could add his name to those of Lord Lansdowne and Lord Hardinge as a Vice President it might be good. ...[8]

Other old friends had signed, or reacted to the subsequent appeal; some regretting that in their relatively impecunious dotage they could afford 'Only a humble little guinea dear Sir Ronald', others professing themselves unsure whether they had signed or not, pleading 'faulty memory' since being gassed in the last years of the war.[9]

After three years of intensive fund raising by Simpson and Castellani, the 'Ross Institute and Hospital for Tropical Diseases' was opened by the Prince of Wales 'on a healthy site facing Putney Heath'. Ross himself was Director-in-Chief, with Castellani Director of tropical medicine and dermatology, and Simpson, by now retired from his other appointments, Director of tropical hygiene. It was a cause of satisfaction, at last, for Ross, and some compensation for the long years of struggle for added recognition; but from his point of view, it was too little, too late. His health was failing, and a serious stroke the following year left him with impaired mobility, and unable to influence developments at the Institute to any great extent.[10]

To describe the three years between 1923 and 1926 in such simple terms as 'fund raising' is a gross understatement. The reality was far more complex. We owe knowledge of the true situation to the man who eventually, successfully, organised the appeal work after Simpson and Castellani's initial attempt had miserably failed: Major H.Lockwood Stevens (d.1964). In an extraordinary letter, which has miraculously survived in Professor Bradley's Ross Institute files, he described, thirty years later, the creation and the development of the Ross Institute, from the shaky start of the appeal in 1923, through the years of consolidation of the Institute and its incorporation in the LSHTM, and the war years and their aftermath. The letter was a personal one, written solely for the benefit of Lockwood Stevens's trusted secretary, Miss E.Roberts, who joined him at the Ross Institute in 1926 and transferred with him and it to the School in 1934, staying for more than thirty years until she retired at the end of 1965. Between them Lockwood Stevens and Miss Roberts guided, administratively, the Institute – and during the war the School – through critical times, and a number of 'incidents'.[11]

Stevens began by pointing out that the original appeal was titled *The War Against Malaria*, albeit the 'memorial' was meant to be a 'Ross Clinic', somewhat a contradiction in terms, inasmuch as Ross's primary concern had always been preventive work in the field, rather than clinical research. For this and other reasons, the original appeal was a resounding failure. The loyal Simpson, in desperation, approached an old friend from his ten years in Calcutta in the 1880s and 1890s, Sir Charles McLeod (1858–1936), pleading with him to act as Chairman for a renewed appeal for a memorial to Ross. McLeod, involved with another charity, in which he was helped by Lockwood Stevens, was not enthusiastic. Asking Stevens to investigate 'the so-called Ross Memorial Committee', he declared himself interested only in prevention of malaria within tropical industries; if Stevens considered the appeal worthwhile, he would become chairman only with Stevens's support.

Stevens wrote of his meetings with the Ross Memorial Committee that he had never attended meetings like it – 'Gilbert and Sullivan could have doubled their fortunes could they have dramatised those meetings.' He was not impressed, and was inclined to advise McLeod to have nothing to do with the project, until he came to know Simpson better and realised his absolute commitment to tropical hygiene and preventive medicine research. With McLeod's help the 'clinic' idea was dropped, and a new appeal launched for the 'Ross Institute and Hospital for Tropical Diseases'. Lockwood Stevens became 'part-time Organising Secretary' and began 'gaily raising money for malaria control in the tropics'. By 1925, enough funds had been collected to acquire Bath House in Putney, and to equip its two wards and its research laboratories.[12]

A month before the official opening of the Institute in 1926, the organising committee found to their dismay that the Institute's acting secretary – a friend of Castellani's – had made no attempt to make arrangements, issue invitations, or indeed carry out any work at all. Lockwood Stevens was called in to replace him, and with the assistance of Miss Roberts the arrangements were completed in the nick of time. For the next twenty-five years, Stevens and Miss Roberts effectively ran the Institute's administration and accounting between them. They did not have long to wait before they had to deal with serious 'crises' and 'incidents'. For although Simpson did his level best to shape research work in laboratories, it soon transpired that the bulk of money raised for malaria prevention work was being 'frittered away on a small hospital which was virtually a private nursing home for patients of one of the Directors'. It is not difficult to guess at the identity of that Director. Ross was too ill to work in the hospital; Simpson was primarily interested in preventive tropical hygiene; but Castellani was known for his predilection for fashionable, even royal, patients.[13]

By the autumn of 1927, Stevens was insisting on a different orientation in the work of the Institute: he would continue his efforts to raise money for malaria control only if Sir Malcolm Watson (1873-1955), about to retire from his eminently successful pioneering work on malaria control in Malaya, could be persuaded to join the Institute to head its appeal and conduct its malaria control policy. Watson was duly appointed, and he and Lockwood Stevens travelled in India, Burma, Malaya and Ceylon adding fund-raising activities to their malaria control services; but it was not the end of the fledgling Institute's troubles. During their absence, Castellani made the Committee appoint an 'ex-officer patient who was hard up' as Stevens's deputy. The man proceeded to embezzle a considerable sum from the Institute's funds, and was dismissed. From problem to problem the Institute just managed to survive until the death of Ross in September, 1932, when a need for radical assessment of its future had become only too obvious.

It was a sad, but inescapable, fact that London had never needed a Ross Institute and Hospital in addition to the Seamen's Hospital and Manson's existing Tropical School. The Institute had been founded by the faithful Simpson as a final gesture to soothe Ross's insatiable ambition and perennially wounded pride; and by Castellani for his own purposes. When Ross and Simpson died within a year of each other, negotiations regarding amalgamation with the London School of Hygiene & Tropical Medicine were soon under way. From January 1st, 1934, the Ross Institute of Tropical Hygiene became an integral part of the School. Its hospital was translated into 'The Ross Ward' of the Hospital for Tropical Diseases, a manoeuvre facilitated by 'a substantial grant from the Ross Institute to the Seamen's Hospital Society'. The incorporation of the Institute into the School was on the face of it an amiable affair, with full cooperation on both sides; the only voice of dissent was that of Castellani, who 'did everything in his power to prevent the amalgamation', but nevertheless accepted a position as 'Director of Studies on Tropical Mycoses' until he returned to Italy, there to participate in the Ethiopian campaign. For his troubles he was created Count of Chisimaio by his friend Mussolini; he eventually accompanied the Italian Royal family into exile in Portugal, where he ended his days at the age of 94 in 1971.[14]

From its first full year as an integral part of the LSHTM, the work of the Ross Institute under Sir Malcolm Watson added new dimensions to the School's existing departments, although relations later deteriorated under the strain of personal rivalries. The Institute brought with it wide-ranging interests in overseas industries, from Indian tea plantations to Anglo-Iranian oil companies, many of which contributed substantial sums to the running of the Institute, which in turn ran a much used advisory service supported by other departments in the School. Tropical Hygiene, in abeyance in the School since the death of Andrew Balfour, now flourished under Malcolm Watson.

The choice of Watson as the man to put the Ross Institute on its feet in the late 1920s had been an inspired one. Having qualified at Glasgow in 1895, he immediately set out to satisfy his taste for travel, serving as ships's surgeon, to destinations in South Africa, Australia, Singapore, and the Philippines. After a short spell at home at the Glasgow Royal Infirmary, and having obtained the Cambridge DPH, he joined the Malayan Medical Service at the turn of the century, at the age of 27. Malaya and its public health problems were then a formidable challenge to a young physician and would-be epidemiologist. It was an outpost of Empire where a newly begun and rapidly expanding rubber industry promised potentially unlimited prosperity – if a solution could be found to the problem of frequent, devastating, malaria epidemics. Ross had only recently convincingly demonstrated the cycle of transmission in malaria, and was making extravagant claims for consequent possibilities of eradication of the disease; but his principles had yet to be applied to practical control. In Malaya, Watson became one of the early pioneers as were, at the same time, Le Prince and Gorgas in Havana and Panama.[15]

Ross himself was impressed by the initial results, and later called Watson's Malayan campaign 'the greatest sanitary achievement ever accomplished in the British Empire'.[16] When the call came to the Ross Institute, Watson was about to retire from his years in the tropics. Ross's assessment of the Malayan campaign had not been empty praise. Malaya at the beginning of the century was a society under threat: the life and welfare of the whole community, the developing rubber industry, the whole economic fabric of the Straits Settlement and the Federated Malay States, were in danger of collapse under the impact of the frequent severe epidemics of malaria. It was Watson's flair for combining knowledge of the new discoveries with application of epidemiological principles, and his adaptability, intellectual honesty and readiness to embrace new techniques of civil engineering which combined to enable him to design effective control measures. Within a few years, the overwhelming threat to the country and its rubber industry had receded. Advocates of the 'medicine as a tool of Empire building' perception may prefer to ignore such developments, or regard them as just another example of high-handed colonialists' interference in local affairs, in the name of medical advance. In the case of malaria in Malaya, Watson's pioneering control campaign led the way for many later successful control programmes elsewhere, and at the same time benefited not just the rubber industry, but also the economic and social fabric of local populations.

Watson's work in Malaya, beginning in the first decade of the twentieth century, as the Far-East answer to Gorgas's Panama campaign, demonstrated the principles and possibilities of a rational approach to what became known as 'species sanitation': the logical exploitation of the relation between malaria and local ecosystems, which had been suspected since the time of Hippocrates and which now became possible in the wake of the discoveries of Laveran, of the malaria parasites, and of Ross, of the role of the anopheline mosquito vectors. Watson was working in Malaya, where British interests were paramount; in Dutch Indonesia, Nicolaas Hendrik Swellengrebel (1885–1970) matched Watson's achievements in the field.[17] With a common purpose, and both relying on field studies, the two men were different in background and approach. Watson, medically qualified and with much practical common sense, was dogmatic in his unquestioning adherence and dogged determination to follow closely the principles to be derived from Ross's discovery. Swellengrebel, trained as a zoologist in Amsterdam had, as Bradley has pointed out with an apt metaphor,

> an ability to conceptualize processes, to explain a wood where Watson would simply describe trees

Between them, Watson and Swellengrebel established the principle of 'species sanitation', the corollary of a growing understanding of the relations between malaria and ecosystems, and of individual species of *Anopheles* mosquitoes – or even, as found later in Rockefeller sponsored research in Europe from 1930 onwards, different races of one species (*A.maculipennis*) with different breeding places and different biting habits.[18] Watson had begun using the method in Malaya early in the century; Swellengrebel turned to malaria research in 1911 at the same age of 27, only ten years later, at which Watson had begun his studies in Malaya. Helped by his wife, he adopted and developed Watson's method in Indonesia in the following decade, introducing the term 'species sanitation'. Swellengrebel later acknowledged that ' ... Watson ... [invented] the method of malaria control to which he afterwards allowed me to give the name of "species sanitation"'.[19]

In January 1950 Swellengrebel lectured at the LSHTM on the creation of the Malaria Service in Indonesia, in the context of the discoveries and the growth of understanding of the disease and its pathogenesis over the fifty years between 1898 and 1948.[20] It is a story which reflects parallels between the situation in Dutch Indonesia, and the later internecine relations between the main departments concerned with malaria studies at the LSHTM: Epidemiology, Tropical Hygiene, Entomology and Parasitology; and also the underlying mistrust between medically trained malariologists and the zoologists who had arrived at malaria research via entomology.

But Swellengrebel did not stop at entomological aspects of species sanitation. With his wide-ranging experience and taste for conceptualisation he, and Watson too, became influential members of the Malaria Committee of the League of Nations between the wars; and in the early 1930s Swellengrebel the zoologist, with no formal medical training, made a brave initial foray along the rocky path of clinical trials.

Having been involved in studies of naturally acquired malaria infections in Holland, Swellengrebel with de Buck decided to test the prophylactic powers of the promising new drugs plasmoquine and atebrin, with or without quinine, in 15 healthy volunteers. Contrary to expectations, all volunteers became infected, and even showed patterns of recurrence almost identical to those suffered by naturally infected patients. Swellengrebel commented:

> What we had actually done was this: we had started an experimental epidemic of benign tertian malaria, the disadvantage of small numbers being compensated to some extent by the circumstances that all our subjects were infected on known dates and by one and the same parasite, conditions warranting a uniformity of results hardly to be obtained under field conditions.[21]

Having inadvertently started an epidemic among their volunteers, the authors were forced to test the curative powers of the drugs used; again, the results were discouraging, although S.P.James at Horton reported more favourable outcomes at the same time. Discussing the discrepancies Swellengrebel speculated, without touching on any ethical aspects of the original experimentation, that the negative result could possibly be explained by the particularly resistant strain of *P.vivax* used, and the 'unusually large number of infecting mosquito bites'. He concluded that the system of combined prophylaxis and treatment ' ... which has definitely proved its great practical value, may occasionally break down under the stress of unusual conditions'.[22]

Once the Ross Institute was part of the School, Watson's personal and professional qualities as a pioneer in malaria control added new dimensions to the work of the entomologists and parasitologists already researching and teaching other aspects of the problems of malaria. At the same time, the Ross Institute Industrial Advisory Committee was strengthened by new members representing a wide spectrum of commercial interests in the tropics. Its meetings provided a forum for informal discussions on potential practical applications of the School's work in an industrial context, as its members linked their industrial interests to the work in tropical hygiene taking place in the Institute. Mines in the Rhodesian 'Copper Belt' had been included in these industrial interests since Watson's first visit there in 1930; his book *African Highway*, published three years before his death, is dedicated to 'the venturers of the Copper Belt', and has as a frontispiece a portrait photograph of Sir Chester Beatty (1875–1968). In turn, financial support was received from a number of sources, reflected also in the occupations and destinations of the students attending the 'Malaria Control Course for Laymen'. Both the School itself and the Institute had begun such courses in the late 1920s; now run by the Institute within the School, the students attending the course included tea planters, sugar planters, sisal planters and even 'Tea Company Directors', in addition to missionaries, Imperial Airway Cadets, engineers and oil industry employees.[23]

By 1939 the Associations, Banks, Chemical Companies (including ICI), Colonial Governments, Merchants, Mining Companies, Oil, Railway and Rubber Companies etc., contributing donations ranging from a few pounds annually to, in rare cases (ICI, Banks, certain Colonial Governments and Mining Companies), hundreds of pounds, covered an average of 15 pages of small print in the School's annual reports. The Institute had no difficulty in maintaining its role as a centre to which overseas industrial concerns came as a matter of course, when advice was needed concerning public health and disease prevention for staff members and labour forces in the tropics and sub-tropics.[24] In the year before the outbreak of World War II, the total number of students attending the Malaria Control Course for Laymen reached an all-time high of 222. This was felt to represent the maximum number of students which the department could possibly handle efficiently during one course. The possibility of holding two annual courses would have to be considered.

In the event, the outbreak of war altered the outlook for courses of any kind in the School.[25]

As the role and responsibilities of the Ross Institute and its teaching programmes within the School grew, Malcolm Watson felt the need for younger expert assistance. His choice for a new post of Assistant Director of the Institute was George Macdonald (1903-67), who in the thirty years he was associated with the School shaped the department's approach to quantitative epidemiology of tropical diseases through mathematical modelling of the dynamics of disease transmission, with particular reference to malaria and later also schistosomiasis.[26]

Son of the physiologist John Smyth Macdonald, FRS (1867-1941), George Macdonald graduated MB, Ch.B. at the University of Liverpool at the age of 21, taking the Diploma in Tropical Medicine in the same year. Committed to research from his early years, he was research assistant at the Liverpool School's laboratories in Freetown, Sierra Leone, until 1929, when he joined the Malaria Survey of India. In 1931 he returned to England, to take the MD at Liverpool and the Diploma of Public Health in London. It was his subsequent work in India as Principal Medical Officer to the tea estates of the Mariani Medical Association in Assam which brought him to the attention of Malcolm Watson and led to his appointment at the Ross Institute and the London School in 1937. War duties apart – commanding Field Malaria Laboratories in the Middle East and eventually, as Consultant Malariologist, advising Montgomery as the allied armies struggled from North Africa through Sicily to the Italian mainland – Macdonald spent the next thirty years at the London School until his untimely illness and death in 1967.[27]

Of all the work and the many papers published by George Macdonald, three stand out as representative of his approach to tropical epidemiology. One, written two years before his death, states his passionate belief in the importance of maintaining a 'proper balance between the prevention of [infectious diseases] and the development of sociological and educational activities within general health services, always with proper attention to the demographic consequences of improved health'.[28] The present incumbent of the Chair of Tropical Hygiene, which was created for Macdonald at the end of the war, and who had been influenced in his choice of career by an earlier paper of Macdonald's, calls it 'the best paper ever written on tropical hygiene'; Macdonald here addresses the problems of prevention strategy, dynamics of infection, and the use of mathematical modelling, all topics central to his life's work in theory and practice.[29]

In two other papers, one read to a meeting of the Royal Society of

Medicine in November 1967, a month before his death, the other published two years earlier, he discussed in more detail the use of modelling in the case of schistosomiasis, even more complex in its path of transmission because of the bisexual nature of the infecting helminths, and its effect on the dynamics of the infection.[30] But it was a paper published in 1951, discussing the basis of group immunity, and the balance between concern for the individual and for the community in attitudes to immunity to malaria, which was most controversial in particular in its harsh criticism of papers by Garnham, Swellengrebel, and Wilson that caused a lasting rift within the School between the departments of Tropical Hygiene (the Ross Institute) and of Parasitology – on a personal level between Macdonald and P.C.C.Garnham, who are said to have been 'not on speakers' ever since.

Parallel situations had existed before, and were to exist again decades later. The contrast between a clinical approach concerned with diseases of the individual, and an epidemiological approach emphasising concern with protection of whole communities had first become evident in the schism between the work of Manson in the old London School and its Hospital, and that of Ross working in the field abroad, although those differences have sometimes been exaggerated. Elsewhere within the School, there were to be long-standing difficulties between the departments of epidemiology and of bacteriology, as discussed elsewhere.[31]

The polarisation of views causing such difficulties between two departments within the School followed the conclusion of World War II in 1945, when the parasitology department was reorganised. Robert Leiper, at the age of 65, 'retired' to Winches Farm; H.E.Shortt, back from additional special duties in Assam and Burma between 1941 and 1945, took over as Director of the Department of Parasitology, and Professor of Medical Protozoology, until 1951, when he also reached retirement age. Garnham, until then Reader in Parasitology, succeeded him, and relations with Macdonald's department deteriorated.[32]

THE MRC MALARIA UNIT AT THE LSHTM

It was an unfortunate end to hitherto amiable relations between several departments concerned with different aspects of malaria research and control within the School, which had existed since the Ross Institute had first been incorporated as a Department of Tropical Hygiene. At about the same time as its amalgamation with the LSHTM, the MRC had received a Leverhulme grant to aid the Council in establishing a Malaria Unit at the School. The Unit was to operate under the direction of Sir Rickard Christophers, also appointed Professor of Malaria Studies in the University of London, on his return from his years as Director of the Malaria Survey of India at the age of 60, marking the end of his inspired fieldwork and malaria surveys.[33]

For all the depth and variety of Christophers' activities during an exceptionally long working life, referred to elsewhere, it is above all for his achievements in malaria research that he will be remembered. His life's work ranged from the early series of Reports to the Malaria Committee of the Royal Society, written with J.W.W.Stephens, later of the Liverpool School, between 1900 and 1903 (Chapter 2), via the pioneering work of the malaria surveys, including predictions of epidemic years, to entomological studies of anophelines and other arthropods, which included the application of the Barcroft respirometric technique to isolated malaria parasites; and finally to the work carried out by the MRC Unit at the School in the 1930s: evaluations of synthetic antimalarials, and of mosquito repellents.[34]

Between 1933 and the outbreak of war in 1939, relations between the Ross Institute under Malcolm Watson, and the MRC Unit under Christophers, and related interests in the departments of entomology and protozoology, were, according to the School's annual reports, marked by 'friendly cooperation'.[35] Christophers' charm and outgoing personality smoothed over any rough passages which might have risen where so many strong and disparate personalities were pursuing different aspects of malaria research. The Ross Institute, and its teaching, remained largely preoccupied with matters of hygiene and sanitation as factors in disease control, especially in areas served by its overseas branches: in Watson's old stamping ground of Malaya, in India, in Ceylon (now Sri Lanka) and in East and West Africa. About the Institute's work in Northern Rhodesia the 1937–8 School Report had this to say:

> Steady progress is being made on the Copper mines; and the standard of health, in spite of a great influx of new labour, is being well maintained. The great improvement in the health of the African after working a year on a mine, during which he is freed from many of his diseases and well fed, suggests how greatly the African is handicapped in ordinary life. It explains the lack of energy in the African and his inability to work efficiently, so often attributed to a national inertia. It is interesting to see how care for the African leads to an improvement similar to that with which we

are familiar in Indian, Chinese, Malay and other labourers.[36]

A would-be engaging picture of colonial paternalism presenting work in the Copper Mines as therapy.

After five years of war, after inevitable changes in staff and heads of departments which were being reorganised, tensions so far suppressed in the service of a common cause, surfaced between Macdonald, now Professor of Tropical Hygiene, and Garnham, Head of an enlarged Department of Parasitology from 1951. The reverberations also reached the Department of Entomology: Buxton was prevented from studying anophelines, and had to turn instead to lice and tsetse-flies, writing outstanding monographs on both subjects, which were in any case his main interests. It should also be noted that former colleagues find it 'difficult to believe that Buxton was ever prevented from doing anything that he wanted to do'.[37]

THE LSHTM AND MALARIA RESEARCH AFTER 1950

Once it had settled down after the war, there was a new look to the School and many of its departments. The 'Old Guard', who had seen the LSHTM through its teething troubles since 1927 had retired or moved on. In the Ross Institute, now the 'School Department of Tropical Hygiene', the emphasis was on mathematical modelling with Macdonald in charge; in Parasitology, with first Shortt and then Garnham as Director of the Department, the emphasis was on malaria, and above all on the stages in the development of its *Plasmodium* parasites in the mosquito vector, and in man. There was little common ground for malaria research in the two departments, and relations were uneasy as already indicated, involving also the entomology department: the rightful place for malaria research should be in the Department of Parasitology, under the watchful eye of its Professor of Medical Protozoology. It was an unfortunate and, seen from the outside unnecessary, rift between departments with interests which should have been common, but which were instead pursued in an atmosphere of sharp divisions and unremitting isolation. There was no attempt to marry the approaches of biological epidemiology concerned with the complex cycle of development of the parasite in vector and host, and the mathematical epidemiology initiated by Ross and subsequently studied by Macdonald and others in Germany, the United States, and the USSR.[38]

Ten years before he died, Macdonald set out to explain his

mathematical approach to the epidemiology of malaria, and its interactions with other factors to be taken into consideration, including the biological one. He wrote:

> The aim of mathematical epidemiology is to integrate biological and circumstantial data into one coherent whole; with the other two branches it completes the science of epidemiology. Emphatically it gives a sense of proportion, relating the various factors of the transmission cycle to each other and to relevant biological characteristics of the mosquito. It can show the scale of changes in infection rates to be expected following changes in one of the transmission factors, and why this scale should differ greatly under different conditions. It can supply the principle which connects happenings in two countries and explain the detail of happenings in any individual country. It does not attempt to usurp the place of either of the other branches, being dependent on both, but to round them off as a complete whole, giving a rational understanding of disease.[39]

It is a statement which does little to explain the lack of understanding between Macdonald and Garnham; but their radically different approaches can be illustrated by comparing Macdonald's above statement with Garnham's introduction to his volume on the haemosporidia:

> This is a book about malaria parasites and not malaria; it is concerned with protozoology and only deals with the clinical aspects, epidemiology, or eradication of infections, when these subjects have a direct bearing on the parasite ...

Nevertheless, what Macdonald called the 'various factors of the transmission cycle' and the 'relevant biological characteristics of the mosquito' were of course precisely the subjects which preoccupied the parasitology department at this time. H.E.Shortt, with K.P.Menon and P.V.S.Iyer, had made certain observations on so-called pre-erythrocytic schizogony in the jungle fowl in India during World War II. Back in London after the war, he set out to explore those still unknown stages in the development of the malaria parasite in man in association with P.C.C.Garnham (1901-94), who joined the department as Reader in Medical Parasitology in 1947, after more than 20 years in the Colonial Medical Service.[40] It became a famous partnership when together they unravelled the full cycle of development of malaria parasites, with its pre-erythrocytic and exo-erythrocytic stages, in monkeys and in man during the late 1940s and early 1950s, before Shortt's retirement from the School in 1952.[41]

The malaria parasite used by Shortt, Menon, and Iyer in the 1940 experiments had been found in domestic fowls in Ceylon in 1935, and had been studied in Cambridge, at the Molteno Institute, by S.P.James, who with P.Tate went on to observe the striking exo-erythrocytic development of the parasite (*Plasmodium gallinaceum*) in the brain capillaries of inoculated birds.[42]

Bird malaria had of course served Ross well enough in his early experiments; as a model for studies of other aspects of malaria it is less well suited, and developments in brain capillaries of birds did not solve the problem of suspected liver involvement in parasite development in man. It was to this problem that Shortt and Garnham turned in 1947 when they were both back in London from India and Africa, respectively. They were both long past their first youth, but still working with undiminished enthusiasm. Shortt had been introduced to the problems of malaria while serving in the IMS before the Great War; he had suffered from the disease himself – and there were indeed those of the Old School at that time who firmly believed that you could not work on the pathology of any disease unless you had suffered from it yourself. With Christophers he had carried out the malaria surveys in Mesopotamia between 1916 and 1918. Now it was with Garnham that he began to clear up the uncertainties still surrounding the stages of development, and especially what became known as the pre-erythrocytic and exo-erythrocytic stages, in human malaria: what happened between the injection of sporozoites by the biting mosquito, and the appearance of the parasites in the circulating blood of the patient? And how to account scientifically for the frequent relapses suffered by malaria patients, at varying intervals after apparently successful treatment with quinine and a number of synthetic anti-malarials on a rapidly increasing list?

In the immediate post-war period, Shortt and Garnham began to seek answers to the questions with a series of experiments involving rhesus monkeys, two 'outside' volunteers, and themselves and their co-workers. It is worth recording here that this was the period when, on a wave of euphoria following the discovery of DDT, it was hoped and believed that eradication of malaria was in sight. Desowitz has recorded how, having completed his studies at the LSHTM under 'the Colonel', i.e. Shortt, he entered the Colonial Medical Research Service and arrived in Nigeria only to be told, by another eminent malariologist, to work on trypanosomes, because 'malaria is about to be eradicated, and you will never make a career, let alone a living, from it'.[43]

Shortt and Garnham began their experiments with monkeys, supplied by Frank Hawking at the National Institute of Medical Research. After two years of painstaking work they could publish their first findings of pre-erythrocytic forms of the monkey parasite *Plasmodium cynomolgi* in the liver of the monkeys; after another six months they had linked what they called 'a persisting exo-erythrocytic cycle' to the occurrence of relapses.[44] It was time to turn to the study of the cycle in man.

For this last stage of completion of their study of the cycle of development of malaria parasites in mammals, including man, Shortt and Garnham were helped by access to patients being treated for General Paralysis of the Insane (GPI), that euphemism for chronic syphilitic meningoencephalitis, the late stage of untreated syphilis, by malaria therapy. This was a possibly unique instance of therapeutic procedures in one serious disease being legitimately used to elucidate the pathology of another. By this time, malaria therapy for GPI had quite a long history behind it, even in its more rational aspects. The effects of quartan fever on certain other diseases had been observed from the time of Hippocrates and of Galen, and on general paralysis and psychoses throughout the nineteenth century in Europe and America. Wagner-Jauregg (1857–1940) in Vienna had first begun speculating on the possibility of using induced fevers to arrest the path of destruction of brain cells in patients in the later stages of neurosyphilis soon after the turn of the century. Since 1917 he had been putting his theory to the test in clinical experiments on patients who had little to lose, and a number of whom had benefited to a considerable extent.[45]

After the Great War, Warrington Yorke (1883–1943) had pioneered the use of malaria therapy by mosquito inoculation for GPI at Liverpool since 1922; in the same year, S.P.James attempted malaria therapy at Epsom where, in the words of one observer, he had 'crossed the boundary fence between the Manor War Hospital and the adjoining Horton Hospital'.[46] As knowledge of the treatment spread, more mental hospitals adopted it, and research was undertaken also in malaria centres in other countries, notably in Rumania and in the United States. By 1925, the Ministry of Health acted, by arrangement with the Board of Control and the London County Council, to establish a central hospital for malaria therapy, with its own laboratory specialising in malaria studies: the Horton Malaria Laboratory came into existence. For nearly fifty years until 1973, it served as the country's Malaria Reference Laboratory; eventually, after World War II, it became the WHO Regional Malaria Centre for Europe. When its resident self-made (with the help of Ronald

Ross, S.P.James, and later Directors) 'international expert' P.G.Shute (1894–1977) retired in 1973 at the age of 78, it transferred to the LSHTM, joining the School's other WHO Reference centres: the Anopheles Centre in the Ross Institute; the Mycological Reference Laboratory and the WHO/FAO International Reference Laboratory for Leptospirosis in the Department of Microbiology; and the WHO International Reference Centre for Filarial Nematodes in the Department of Medical Helminthology. The work of the Malaria Reference Laboratory within the School was shared between the Department of Medical Protozoology (diagnostics), and the Ross Institute, where Brian Southgate was responsible for the epidemiological side. Long before this move, in the time of its early Directors S.P.James and J.A.Sinton (1884–1956), the institution had played a major role in crucial experiments begun at the School, where Shortt and Garnham and their associates carried out their heroic (on the part of the volunteers) malaria experiments.[47]

Liver involvement in the pathogenesis of the disease had long been suspected, but evidence was lacking, although experiments with birds and monkeys supported the hypothesis. At the end of 1947 an anonymous patient, about to receive malaria therapy with the parasite of benign tertian malaria agreed – this being a mental patient, permission was also sought, and granted, by his wife – to have a small piece of liver removed for biopsy during the incubation period of the infection. The resulting material, when examined in sections, showed the presence of bodies very similar to those found a few months before in rhesus monkeys, and already suggested as being pre-erythrocytic forms of the parasite. A major step had been taken towards confirming hypotheses of developments between the act of injection of the parasite by mosquito bite, and its appearance in the blood of the patient. The experiments had established the close resemblance between the parasite of monkey malaria and that of human tertian malaria, and also between the pre-erythrocytic stages of the disease in the livers of both hosts. Moreover, the existence of a persisting exo-erythrocytic cycle would account for the relapses in patients with this type of malaria.[48]

The more severe falciparum malaria (aestivo-autumnal fever, malignant tertian malaria, cerebral malaria) presented different problems. There was no suitable monkey parasite for comparison, and so no alternative to human experimentation. But the luck of the investigators held. A healthy volunteer offered himself – cheerfully and on his own initiative – to serve as the essential human guinea pig: C.H.Howard, a civil servant from the Ministry of Aviation. There were of course still serious ethical problems, no matter how positive and committed the volunteer; and there was some delay before experiments could begin: approval was sought, and eventually granted, by Wilson Jameson, former Dean of the LSHTM and now Chief Medical Officer at the Ministry of Health, and by the School's then Dean, James Mackintosh. The 'very willing' volunteer was inoculated through the bites of 770 mosquitoes – there is no information as to how they were counted, and by whom – infected by feeding on a patient at Horton Hospital who was receiving malaria therapy. The results were published in November 1949: liver biopsy samples revealed the progressive stages of maturing schizonts. After successful completion of the experiment Mr.Howard made a complete recovery, and was appointed MBE in recognition of his service to medical science.[49]

Five years later Garnham – Shortt had meanwhile 'retired' – began with five staff members of the Department of Parasitology at the LSHTM, a last definitive series of experiments. His staff included his invaluable chief 'technical assistant', one Willie Cooper, who, like others at the School, had begun life there before technicians became professionalised union members, when departments trained their own, who in turn became dedicated members of the departmental community (although Cooper's relations with the students are said to have left something to be desired). He had begun his career straight from school in 1916 when, with a War Office grant, he came to work on malaria with David and John Gordon Thomson, under the general direction of Ronald Ross, in the laboratories of the 4th London General Hospital. In 1919 he worked at Shoreham Malaria Concentration Camp as technician with special knowledge of malaria; and later in the same year he came to the School at the Albert Dock as assistant in Gordon Thomson's protozoology department. Cooper was one of six such outstanding 'home-grown' technicians who served the School in its early years: Robert McKay (1886–1928), Manson's first 'lab.boy' at the Albert Dock; W.A.McDonald (1895–1941), originally employed by Alcock as laboratory assistant but soon 'poached' by Leiper for the Helminthology Department; R.J.Bromfield, who was the demonstrator originally infected in the yellow fever tragedy at the Hospital for Tropical Diseases in July 1930 (Chapter 3); F.N.N.Pester, Cooper's colleague and contemporary in Parasitology as chief technician in helminthology to Cooper's protozoology, and with rather more flair than Cooper for dealing with students in laboratory exercises; and the, in his time indispensable, Museum technician, W.T.Bush.

The experiments in 1954 using staff volunteers involved

plasmodium ovale, yet another malaria parasite, relatively common only in the Lagos and Accra areas of West Africa. Again, there was no simian equivalent, and so once again the use of human volunteers was essential. Garnham's team of six, including himself, all took part, thus minimalising ethical problems, and patients at Horton served only marginally as sources of infection – the paper noted that the 'practical difficulty today is the scarcity of cases of general paralysis available for experiments'. The list of Garnham's students and colleagues who infected themselves over the years is impressive: F.Awad, malaria (once); R.S.Bray, malaria (4x), leishmaniasis (once); R.Killick-Kendrick, leishmaniasis (once); R.Lainson, malaria (2x), leishmaniasis (2x); J.Shaw, leishmaniasis (once); and J.Williamson, malaria (once). The clinical course of resulting disease was mapped, and the blood cycle studied. In the last part of the experiment Willie Cooper was infected in December 1953; after 9 days a portion of his liver, 'about 10g in weight', was excised 'from the lower margin of the left lobe' for biopsy at the Hospital for Tropical Diseases. Cooper himself sectioned, stained, and photographed his own liver samples (Fig. 00). An asthma sufferer and heavy smoker never in robust health, he recovered from what should have been a routine operation only with difficulty. The experience left him, as other self inoculation experiments had left Buckley, with long-term problems; he later worked only part-time, and died in 1964. Although many questions regarding the life-cycles of malaria parasites were answered by these experiments of Shortt and Garnham and their associates, uncertainties remained concerning different species of *Plasmodium*, and above all about the nature of relapses. Garnham himself was increasingly uneasy about the hypothesis he and Shortt had developed in the 1940s and 1950s. In 'retirement' at Imperial College's Field Station at Silwood Park he joined enthusiastically in team work with W.A.Krotoski, who eventually discovered the hypnozoite, the resting stage in the liver, of *Plasmodium vivax*. Even so, the mechanism of delayed clinical relapse in *P.malariae* infections remains so far unknown.[50]

The case of Cooper, as that of J.C.C.Buckley, serves to emphasise such ethical questions as might be raised concerning the use of human volunteers, however willing, however dedicated to their cause. Years later, Garnham himself touched more explicitly on the problem, when he referred to 'certain ethical and personal problems' confronting parasitologists and other research workers. Garnham wrote, in 1971:

> The experimentalist is often faced with the problem of volunteers, and in spite of the rules for ethics of their use issued by the

Medical Research Council (1967), the ardent research worker may have to find a way around them, just as he has to overcome any other obstacle, and it is classical for him to use himself...[51]

He went on to acknowledge the advice of Hamilton Fairley on an occasion when he, Garnham, had planned to use volunteer medical students in a comparative study of two pathogenic amoebae: never use human volunteers when there is no certain cure for the potential disease involved. He concluded:

> Apart from human experimentation, the exposure of one's staff to dangerous work has always been a problem, which sometimes is not recognised. It is doubtful if anyone can go through the parasitic life without incurring some penalty in the next world or some parasites in this...[52]

Clothed in a lightness of style masking the serious message underneath, Garnham in these passages summed up his philosophy of experimentation in parasitology, with no apology for the right of the individual to use his own body when necessary to achieve the result craved by his enthusiasm for the subject. They also reflect his lasting irritation with the WHO's opposition to the use of human subjects in experimental parasitology, 'spelling as it did an end to his use of volunteers in his malaria programme'. It was a polished piece of writing, very different from his first paper, written at the age of seventeen, and rejected for publication by *St.Bart's Journal* in 1918. Titled 'On a very definite something which pervades the human body', it deals with the possibilities of photographing the 'human aura', phenomena of spiritism, and occult phenomena ('Alternative title: "The Astral Body"') – all subjects discussed in certain circles at the time. The handwritten paper is a youthful effort, a long way from sophisticated studies of malaria cycles, but which nevertheless documents the precocious thoughts of the young Garnham, able and willing to take philosophical flight on a subject 'either much scoffed at or totally disregarded by the conventional medical world...'.[53]

It was in any case an isolated episode, although in his final 'retirement' since 1980, Garnham returned to his 'life-long fascination with mysticism' by writing a work on Edgar Allen Poe, barely completed at the time of his death. From the time P.C.C.Garnham first joined the Colonial Medical Service in Africa and went on his first expedition to Kisumu in Kenya in 1925, having qualified at Bart's in 1923 and then obtained the DPH, malaria remained the theme of his research: malaria controls and malaria parasites, of man and of other mammals, birds, and even lizards.[54] Throughout his working life and long into 'retirement', malaria was always the focus of his interests. Into his nineties, he remained an occasional stimulating influence around the School and in the Royal Society of Tropical Medicine and Hygiene until his death on Christmas day 1994.

The personal and professional distancing between MacDonald and Garnham, driving a wedge through the research interests in their two departments, fortunately did not affect their respective teaching programmes. The Department of Parasitology in Garnham's time ran two courses for the DTM&H, in addition to six sessions for the general DPH course, and a full complement of Ph.D. and other advanced students. In October 1955, teaching began for a new Diploma in Applied Parasitology and Entomology (DAP&E), open to medical, veterinary and zoology graduates. The different professional training of students entering the latter course led to a need for careful adjustments to be made to its syllabus in the early years. The Diploma in Tropical Public Health (DTPH) was introduced by Macdonald in October, 1963, and needed changes when Bradley took over in 1974; all other courses continued unchanged until the further overall adjustments following the gradual conversions of diploma courses to M.Sc. syllabus status in the 1970s.[55]

MALARIA AND TROPICAL HYGIENE IN THE 1970S AND 1980S

George Macdonald died in December, 1967; Garnham retired at the end of the same academic year, in 1968. The resulting changes in the two departments became in the event part of a general restructuring within the School, in two phases, during the period when C.E.Gordon Smith was Dean, from 1971 to 1989. As noted elsewhere, the awarding of diplomas was gradually discontinued, beginning with the DPH in 1968, and replaced by full M.Sc. courses in the subjects offered by the School. The M.Sc. courses were in line with developments in other Schools of the University of London. The restructuring of departments was another matter. According to observers within the School, who are in a position to review developments during the 1970s and 1980s, it was less than successful; some use even stronger terms and regard it as unmitigated disaster. As far as malaria and epidemiology were concerned, those who had hoped for better relations between established departments of Tropical Hygiene, Parasitology, Epidemiology, and what became Medical Microbiology, were to be disappointed. The feud between Macdonald and Garnham had left a legacy of awkwardness which was not overcome until many years later, under a new Dean, and with further restructuring. In the event, the damage done had more complex reasons than a mere feud between Macdonald and Garnham; it was greatly assisted by an outright structural blunder in the School's building programme. The unhappy effects on the departments concerned has been wryly summed up by a current member of staff of one of them: 'Co-operation – that was never a problem – none of the professors were ever on speakers'.

Macdonald was succeeded by Leonard Bruce-Chwatt (1907–89), who then had only five years left before retirement. The appointment gave great offence to B.B.Waddy, reader in the department, who had threatened to resign, and now duly did, if he himself were not appointed. Born in Poland, Chwatt (as he then was) had qualified at the University of Warsaw before completing his studies in Paris. At the outbreak of World War II he joined the British Army in France, serving with the Polish Army Medical Corps and the RAMC; having survived internment and escape to Britain, where he obtained the DTM&H at the School, he later served with No.7 Malaria Field Laboratory. His post-war career included more than ten years with the Colonial Medical Service in Nigeria, where he worked on both yellow fever and malaria. His years of practical experience as Senior Malariologist in Nigeria gave him incomparable insight into the malaria situation in tropical Africa; experience which served him well when ten years later he was appointed to head the Research and Technical Intelligence department of the Malaria Division of the WHO. In that position, and from 1968 at the LSHTM, he was regarded, with hindsight, as the man who 'probably did more than any other individual to steer the world's malaria experts back from the failure of eradication to a more reasonable and rational programme to contain malaria'.[56] Former colleagues, speaking without rancour but with a certain amount of healthy realism, suggest this may be to some extent the hyperbole often associated with obituaries; and that one might add that he had helped to steer the experts towards failure in the first place, before reversing the process. The failure of eradication was to cast a shadow over Bruce-Chwatt's later years with the WHO and the School, which coincided with the great disappointment of the resurgence of malaria, just when consolidation of eradication seemed possible; but when instead it gradually became only too evident that mosquitoes were outwitting DDT by developing resistance, and that *Plasmodium* species were likewise beginning to resist the onslaught of many of the synthetic antimalarials, in step with their development. Other factors contributing to failure included organisational difficulties and the erroneous perception of malaria as a single global disease. Bradley has recently put it bluntly: 'Nobody can look at the list of available antimalarials today with any complacency: the safe drugs are rapidly becoming ineffective, and the more effective drugs are either new or relatively toxic or both, and are expensive.'[57]

In 1974 Bruce-Chwatt retired, to concentrate in retirement on his contributions to the study of medical history, and David Bradley was appointed to the Chair of Tropical Hygiene and the Directorship of the Ross Institute, following a review of the department's future by the School's Policy Committee. Its recommendations favoured continuing a department 'broadly based on disease control and health services management problems in developing countries rather than on basic biology', and eventual upgrading of the DTPH teaching to an M.Sc. course. Another recommendation, that the department should work in association with the Ross Institute, was neatly solved by the double responsibilities of Bradley. Bradley's connection with the School went back to his early years as a zoology student, when an interest in snails had led him to wander into the School and on to its 3rd floor, where P.L.LeRoux, Reader in Medical Parasitology, was then working on schistosomiasis. Later, as a clinical student at UCH, he became influenced by the work of George Macdonald; and after qualifying, and intermittently doing the DTM&H, he joined a unit set up by Macdonald to begin field studies of schistosomiasis in Tanzania, where at the time Gerald Webbe was deputy director of the East African Institute for Medical Research. After years on the African continent – Uganda as well as Tanzania – and a spell in Oxford, Bradley returned to Keppel Street, Tropical Hygiene, and the Ross Institute. It was a happy choice for the School; less happy initially for Bradley, who became heir to a number of problems not diminished in scope since the days of Macdonald and Garnham: friction with other departments with interests in malaria and epidemiology of tropical diseases. Bruce-Chwatt and Garnham's successor, W.H.R.Lumsden, had quarrelled continuously over who was in charge of the Malaria Reference Laboratory. Now it took both firmness and tact in negotiation to settle the problems; although some were never entirely solved until opposing parties either retired or left for positions elsewhere, and a new era dawned in the 1990s.

Within the Department of Tropical Hygiene itself, the outlook was happier. Teaching was developed during the 1970s, by which time the DTPH course had needed a considerable amount of attention. At its inception in 1963 it had been designed as a course in control of specific tropical diseases. To this W.Barton had added an element of health services administration; but it was becoming increasingly clear that teaching of primary health care, on a level of district health care accessible to village health workers, was needed to make the course content compatible with particular needs and interests of the students. With generous ODA support, Bradley's plans for the Tropical Public Health course led to the founding of the Evaluation and Planning Centre for Primary Health Care, with Patrick Vaughan in charge of interdisciplinary staff. This group in turn spawned the Refugee Health Group referred to above (Chapter 10). These developments were in line with international concerns at a time when organisations involved with world health placed increasing emphasis on global primary health care; coincidentally a subject pursued, with particular reference to malaria, in Africa in the 1980s by the School's incoming Dean in January, 1996, Harrison C. Spencer. The DTPH course became an M.Sc. degree course in 1978, followed a year later by a new M.Sc. course in Epidemiology of Developing Countries.[58]

At the same time, the teaching staff was expanding. In 1976, Richard Feachem joined the department as Lecturer, rising through the grades to Senior Lecturer and Reader in 1982, to Professor of Tropical Environmental Health in 1987. Two years later, he succeeded Gordon Smith as Dean of the School, to preside over the radical changes to the structure of the School required for the 1990s.[59] The appointment of Feachem, trained in civil engineering and only the second Dean since Bradford Hill with no medical qualifications, was a measure of the seriousness with which the department, and ultimately the School, still views its responsibilities in sanitation in a developing world. The collaborative work with other departments which this required has been discussed above (Chapter 5), notably the involvement of B.S. Drasar, with Bradley and Feachem and others, in studies of the ecology of cholera vibrios. It was also emphasised by Drasar's joint position bridging any existing gap between the departments of Medical Microbiology and Tropical Hygiene. It was placed in further perspective when in 1979 the School's *Annual Report* specifically referred to the existing working relationship between the World Bank and the LSHTM. From the early 1970s, the School had advised the World Bank; in particular, Gerald Webbe at Winches Farm, and David Bradley at the Ross Institute had given advice on schistosomiasis in Egypt and malaria in the Philippines and Tanzania.

Among other projects involving Malaria Reference Laboratories and schistosomiasis research, and above all the successful smallpox eradication campaign, the strength of international cooperation under the umbrella of the United Nations, the WHO and the World Bank in the post-war period, has been a demonstration of the development of the power, and financial resources, of these bodies compared with the less intensive efforts of the League of Nations' Health Organisation between the wars. Then, a special course of malaria study arranged at the School, in collaboration with the League's Health Organisation, was abandoned after only a couple of years '... as no students were forthcoming'.[60]

Now in the late 1970s a major collaboration was under way between the Ross Institute and the Bank in carrying out a United Nations Development Programme project, advising governments in developing countries on low-cost sanitation. The project was 'partly a preparation for the United Nations International Drinking Water Supply and Sanitation Decade (1981–90)'.[61] Collaborative research with the World Bank regarding health aspects of excreta and wastewater management centred on the Ross Institute, but also involved the departments of Entomology, Medical Helminthology, Medical Microbiology, and Medical Parasitology. Since then, the working relationship between the Bank and the School's Tropical Hygiene department has been strengthening; Richard Feachem spent the year 1988–9 as Principal Public Health Specialist at the Bank; in 1995, he left the School, and the Deanship, for a newly created full-time position as Director of a new Public Health Department at the World Bank.

In two decades as Director of the Ross Institute and Professor of Tropical Hygiene David Bradley has carried on the department's traditions and explored new directions. Recent years have seen the 'Ross Institute' title quietly removed, and the Department of Tropical Hygiene emerge as the 'Tropical Health Epidemiology Unit' in the Department of Epidemiology and Population Sciences. At the same time, parts of the malaria, schistosomiasis, filariasis, and trypanosomiasis study groups have moved from their abandoned home at Winches Farm to newly built laboratories in Keppel Street, under the umbrella of the large Department of Medical Parasitology.[62]

Through all the changes, in London and St. Albans, the School's malaria research has continued unabated, at a time when the resurgence of malaria, in endemic areas and also as a consequence of the increased numbers of tourists from developed countries travelling to exotic locations, has aggravated problems of control as never before. Weighing up the differences between a public health transmission control approach and an 'individual risk' approach, and their relative contributions to the eradication campaigns of the 1950s and 1960s, Bradley has recently concluded that

> Eradication of malaria was treated as a military campaign; ...

MALARIA

> Malaria became, in a unique sense, the WHO's disease. It was chosen as a vehicle for developing the role of the WHO in the world and in some ways also carried over the approach of pre-1940 malariology, which has as its chief tool species sanitation. Control was very much in the public tradition, with cooperation from the community ... having a minor role. ... In the long and disorderly sorting out of policies during the decades of resurgence and 'chaos'[63] there has been a shift towards a risk approach, in several steps.

Certainly, malaria has remained a central problem for the WHO in the post-war world, as it was between the wars for the Health Organisation of the League of Nations. As a United Nations' institution, the WHO has extended and amplified the responsibilities formerly shouldered by the League of Nations, in its day-to-day workings and its interactions with tropical Schools everywhere, including London and Liverpool. The WHO Reference Laboratories, including the Malaria Reference Centre, bear witness to the LSHTM's close involvement in global health concerns today, which is also illustrated by two recent events: the School's role in producing and launching the 1993 World Development Report *Investing in Health*, accompanied by the pious hope that the WHO will overcome its 'political malaise' and so will be able to develop further 'its mandate in international health'; and the School's third Annual Public Health Forum: *Tuberculosis – Back to the Future,* held in April 1993 with 220 participants from 54 countries, and culminating in an announcement by the WHO that TB is now a Global Emergency.[64] As for malaria, 1993 also saw the publication of a volume of papers from a malaria conference whose title sums up the present state of the art in malaria research: *Malaria – Waiting for the Vaccine.* It was a conference attended by malaria experts from London and Liverpool, from WHO headquarters in Geneva, and from universities and medical research laboratories throughout the world. Also of enormous importance in the 1990s is the School's working relationship with the Overseas Development Administration (ODA), currently on nine joint programmes. One of these, as mentioned above, brings together the London and Liverpool Schools, in a joint effort to 'bring UK expertise to bear specifically upon operational malaria control programmes and bridge the transition from research to control'.[65]

WAITING FOR THE VACCINE

The title for the above conference and its report is an apt one. The wait for a malaria vaccine has been a long one, and promises to go on for longer. Even then, it would normally belong in the 'risk approach' category, protecting the immunised and 'only at high levels of coverage' substantially reducing transmission through a 'herd effect'.[66] On the development side, there are many complications. The very complexity of the life-cycle of the parasite, and the ability of both parasite and vector to develop resistance to chemical attack, suggests that highly evolved parasite mechanisms may also counteract attempts to create efficient immunological defence mechanisms. A recent conference and workshop report points up all the difficulties and at the same time summarises the possibilities and highlights the hopes. The School's involvement in the international efforts directed at vaccine development in the 1990s are reflected in recent Research Reports, on the work of the immunoparasitologists in Geoffrey Targett's group with its focus on host response to a range of infections at molecular, cellular, and population levels. Current objects of study in the unit include a number of bacteria and fungi and protozoa with intracellular lifestyles, prominent among them *Plasmodium falciparum*, and have involved cloning and sequencing of genes encoding for sexual stage specific molecules, and also synthesis of potential sexual-stage antigens. In recent years the group has collaborated with both M.E.Patarroyo in Bogota, whose claims for an effective synthetic vaccine against *P.falciparum* malaria is being tested in Africa, and with the MRC Laboratories in The Gambia, from which Brian M.Greenwood has recently returned to London as Professor of Communicable Disease Epidemiology at the School. Here his group in the Clinical Research Unit focus on studies testing whether naturally acquired antibodies against particular so-called domains of *P.falciparum* antigens are associated with protection from malaria.[67]

CHEMOTHERAPY AND MALARIA

When in 1929 Harold Raistrick was appointed University Professor and Director of the Department of Biochemistry and Chemistry as Applied to Hygiene, there to pursue his research into the biochemistry of microorganisms of medical importance, studies in the protozoology department had been concerned with chemotherapeutically active compounds of a different kind for more than two years. The School's

MALARIA

Annual Report for 1927-8 listed among activities in the Department of Protozoology the 'chemotherapy of malaria', reported by J.W.Scott Macfie and dating from December, 1927, when the department began making provision for testing 'drugs and other compounds for anti-malarial activity' in experiments with bird malaria.[68] Scott Macfie's research was initially supported by the School's Milner Fund; but it was part of a much wider scheme which, as did a number of studies in other departments, reflected the School's continuing close connections with MRC initiatives. In the case of chemotherapy, the Council cooperated with the recently established government Department of Scientific and Industrial Research: chemists serving on the MRC Committee responsible for the work were nominated by the Department; in turn, workers recommended by the Committee received grants from the Department, whereas the biological studies – the testing in animal experiments of the compounds submitted by the chemists – were supported by the Council itself.[69]

The combined work of chemists, in industry and universities, preparing synthetic compounds which *might* possess anti-malarial properties – and in the early days there were no useful leads, and compounds were submitted in a haphazard manner – and of those testing the compounds in animal models, usually canaries, involved groups all up and down the country. Not all were malaria experiments, though; in Glasgow and Leeds the focus was on substances with general antiseptic properties, and on the injections of metallic salts in attempts to treat tuberculosis. At the Liverpool School of Tropical Medicine, Warrington Yorke, who before and during World War II was to play a key role in malaria studies, was directing work on the mechanisms of action of certain arsenical and antimonial compounds in experimental trypanosomiasis, with A.R.D.Adams and Frederick Murgatroyd, whose move to the London School's clinical division in 1950 was cut short by his too early death in 1950.[70]

Most of the testing of compounds was initially carried out by Scott Macfie at the London School, and D.Keilin, with Miss Vincent and Dr.P.Tate, at the Molteno Institute at Cambridge. Testing was done on a malaria parasite of canaries, obtained from Dr.Roehl of the Bayer laboratories at Elberfeld, which in 1929 was absorbed into the larger connurbation of Wuppertal, home of much chemical industry. Scott Macfie and Keilin began by making a joint visit to Roehl and his laboratories in December, 1927; and there is a certain irony in their praises for Roehl's generosity and 'disinterested courtesy', both then and on a later visit to London, since one cannot help suspect that the MRC's sudden considerable activity in this area was sparked off by the German advances made since Ehrlich's observations of the beneficial effects of methylene blue in malaria, and of salvarsan in syphilis, at the turn of the century; and the later, wartime, German attempts to synthesise quinine substitutes with antimalarial action. Roehl had modified and standardised a technique first used by the Sergent brothers, and had developed a method of comparing the effects of new synthetic compounds with those of quinine on *Plasmodium relictum* malaria in canaries.[71] Colleagues of Roehl in the Bayer laboratories included Schulemann, Schönhofer and Wingler, whose work led to the development of plasmochin, and Kikuth who announced the synthesis of mepacrin (atebrin) by Mauss and Mietzsch in 1932. Kikuth and Shulemann were later associated with the Horton centre for a number of years.

There was a steady stream of compounds submitted for testing: from members of the Chemotherapy Committee, i.e. Robert Robinson (1885-1975) at Oxford; Dr.Hamer of Ilford's Ltd., J.B.Cohen at Leeds, Dr.Kermack, and Professor Pyman, of Messrs.Boots' Research Department. Other compounds submitted included 'a long and interesting series of thirty-five received from Dr.Ewins of Messrs.May & Baker, plant alkaloids believed to possess anti-malarial properties' and prepared by T.A.Henry of the Wellcome Chemical Research Laboratories; and from Andrew Balfour himself, a sample of coumarin, and of an exotic plant extract from San Domingo 'where it is used in the treatment of malaria'. By October 1929 a total of 257 compounds had been tested for anti-malarial activity in birds. Several showed 'anti-malarial properties of a very high order', although none matched the action of plasmochin (pamaquine), the first successful derivative of methylene blue developed in Germany in the 1920s. From the time its structure was published in 1928, work on synthetic antimalarials accelerated in laboratories throughout Europe and the United Kingdom. Mepacrine (atebrin), synthesised by Mauss and Mietzsch in 1932, came to prominence during World War II when, although toxic, it became the drug of choice in tropical theatres of war. Desowitz wrote:

> It ... turned the skin a bright yellow, caused gastrointestinal disturbances, and, most alarmingly, occasionally caused temporary insanity. Still, atebrine therapy was better than dying of malaria and during World War II it was the drug of choice – there was no other choice. ...[72]

That harsh judgement of atebrin/mepacrine ignores its importance as a suppressive drug, which became known only during World War II, when in 1943 Hamilton Fairley was appointed Chairman of the Combined Advisory Committee on Tropical Medicine, South Pacific Area, directly responsible to General MacArthur.[73] Malaria was then causing crippling losses of manpower in troops fighting in South Pacific jungles; Fairley organised two research groups in Australia, one attached to a General Hospital at Cairns, the other to another hospital further inland. In large-scale clinical trials Fairley and his teams, using his 'subinoculation' tests, were able to show that mepacrine, in daily doses of 100mg acted as a true prophylactic in *falciparum* malaria, staving off attacks indefinitely when taken regularly.[74] For Fairley, it was his 'greatest contribution to medical science, and his greatest triumph'. For the health of allied troops in the area, it meant a dramatic improvement in outlook: In December 1943 the malaria rate in Australian troops serving in hyperendemic areas had been 740 per 1,000; by November 1944, after the introduction of mepacrine in Fairley's prophylactic regime, it was down to 26 per 1,000. And at that level, administration of the drug could be continued for months and even years without serious ill effects.

Since the end of World War II, the search for new synthetic antimalarials has accelerated, as the classical ones are discredited because of unpleasant side effects, or because the parasites develop resistance. And ultimately, the efficacy of each drug depends on host-related factors as well as on its specific action on a specific parasite: the speed of absorption, the degree of its concentration in host plasma and erythrocytes, its localisation in the tissues, the rate of inactivation and excretion. Chemically, the benzene ring is the basic structure of all the classical antimalarials, as indeed in the ancestor of them all, natural quinine. Different side chains, different numbers of benzene rings, give different pharmacological properties. However rapid progress there may appear to be in malaria research currently, however great the excitement over new antimalarials and the hopes for vaccine development, there still remain vast unsolved problems.

In recent years, the search for new antimalarials in the West has been fuelled by reports from China on a natural anti-malarial compound chemically very different from quinine and its derivatives. In Chinese traditional medicine, the sweet wormwood, *Artemisia annua*, had been used for centuries as treatment for fevers including malaria. In 1971, chemists in China succeeded, by low temperatures extraction, in isolating from the leaves of the plant a substance believed to be responsible for its antipyretic and antimalarial activity. The compound, *qinghaosu* (QHS, artemisinin) is reported to have been used with success in thousands of malaria patients in China, against both chloroquine-sensitive and chloroquine-resistant strains of *Plasmodium falciparum*. Introduced into the sphere of interests at the LSHTM by Chinese students in the 1980s, this promising alternative antimalarial drug has since been studied in Medical Parasitology by Alan Fairlamb, Wallace Peters, D.C. Warhurst, and associates.[75]

For all the hard work on malaria, in chemotherapy, in epidemiology, and in parasitology, the message after a century of ups and downs from those most closely involved in the battle for control of malaria has until recently, since the failure of eradication, been somewhat downbeat; and members of the ODA supported Programme of Tropical Diseases Control at the LSHTM have been careful not to promise too much:

> Hopefully, the present decade will see a transformation from chaos to hope in malaria control.[76]

That was the message in 1991. Since then – although this barely qualifies as history yet – work at the School has brought fresh hope with a number of projects aimed at sustainable control in endemic areas, as well as treatment and basic science research. Several units in the new Department of Infectious and Tropical Diseases are involved in such studies with bearings on aspects of malaria control. Multidisciplinary research in David Mabey's Clinical Research Unit cover a wide range of programmes in developing countries, including malaria in the Gambia. Geoffrey Targett and his staff in the Immunology Unit are undertaking a range of analyses of host response and resulting immune status, at molecular, cellular, and population levels, to globally important transmissible diseases, including malaria; vaccine research, in the laboratory and in the field, remains a major interest. In fact, aspects of vaccine testing and evaluation in the field and in the laboratory link the units, including also the Infectious Epidemiology Unit. Another important factor of the Department's work has been exciting new approaches, following increasing use and knowledge of molecular and genetic techniques. These have come under particular scrutiny within Michael Miles' Pathogen Molecular Biology and Biochemistry Unit. Groups under David Baker and David Conway, respectively, are engaged in studies of enzyme and antigenic genes of *Plasmodium falciparum*. The work of Brian Greenwood's group has been referred to above.[77]

NOTES

[1] W.Odelberg and the Nobel Foundation, *Nobel The man and his prizes*, New York etc., American Elsevier, 1972, pp.161-3. For the scale of the malaria problems in Europe, even in northern Europe, see L.J.Bruce-Chwatt and J.de Zulueta, *The rise and fall of malaria in Europe,* Oxford University Press, 1980.

[2] [-], 'Sir Philip Manson-Bahr', *Trans.R.Soc.Trop.Med.Hyg.*, 1966, *60:*815-16;
on indigenous malaria see
M.J.Dobson, 'Malaria in England: a geographical and historical perspective', *Parassitologia*, 1994, *36:*35-60.

[3] H.E.Shortt and P.C.C.Garnham, 'Samuel Rickard Christophers 27 November 1873-19 February 1978 Elected FRS 1926', *Biogr.Mem.Fell.Roy.Soc.,* 1979 *25:*179-207;
P.C.C.Garnham, 'Henry Edward Shortt 15 April 1887-9 November 1987 Elected FRS 1950', *ibid.,* 1988, *34:*715-51.

[4] D.Bradley, 'Malaria - whence and whither?', in: G.A.T.Targett (ed), *Malaria - Waiting for the Vaccine,* Chichester etc., John Wiley & Sons, 1991, pp.11-29.

[5] G.Carmichael Low, 'Sir William John Ritchie Simpson', *Br.med.J., 1931, ii:*633; *Lancet,* 1931, *ii:*712;
Molly Sutphen, 'A career in Imperial Hygiene: the work of Sir William John Ritchie Simpson (1855-1931)', Ph.D.thesis, Yale, 1994.

[6] These events are covered in more detail in Chapter 10.

[7] Molly Sutphen, op.cit. note 5 above.

[8] Addendum to Mary Gibson's Ross Archives, supplied by David Bradley 1991, LSHTM.

[9] *ibid.,* letters signed by H.W.Johnston and Alec Tweedie.

[10] Mary E.Gibson's introduction to the Ross Archives, p.21;
E.R.Nye and M.E.Gibson, *Ronald Ross: malariologist and polymath: a biography*, London, Macmillan, 1997.

[11] Letter from Major H.Lockwood Stevens to Miss E.Roberts, dated Knowle, East Preston, Sussex, 23rd January, 1956.

[12] *ibid.;* [-], 'The Ross Institute and Hospital', *Nature,* 1926, *118:*124-6.

[13] Stevens's letter to Miss Roberts;
'Aldo Castellani', *Br.Med.J.,* 1971, *ii:*175; *Lancet,* 1971, *ii:*883;
'Sir Aldo Castellani', *J.Trop.Med.Hyg.,* 1971, *74:*233-7.

[14] *ibid.,* pp.235-7.
Lockwood Stevens's letter to Miss Roberts;
LSHTM *Annual Report* 1934-5, p.3.

[15] G.M., 'Sir Malcolm Watson', *Br.Med.J.*, 1956, *i:*52–3;
G.M., 'Malcolm Watson', *Lancet,* 1956, *i:*57;
John M.Gibson, *Physician to the world. The life of General William C.Gorgas,* Tuscaloosa & London, University of Alabama Press, 1989.

[16] Sir Eric Macfadyen, introduction to Watson's *African Highway,* London, John Murray, 1953;
for Watson's own accounts, see
Sir Malcolm Watson, *Some pages from the history of the prevention of malaria,* Glasgow, Alex.Macdougall, 1935;
Idem, 'Observations on malaria control, with special reference to the Assam tea gardens, and some remarks on Mian Mir, Lahore Cantonment,' *Trans.R.Soc.Trop.Med.Hyg.,* 1924, *18:*147–61;
Edmond et Etienne Sergent, *Histoire d'un marais algérien,* Alger, Institut Pasteur d'Algérie, 1947.

[17] D.J.Bradley, 'Watson, Swellengrebel, and species sanitation: environmental and ecological aspects', *Parassitologia,* 1994, *36:*137–47;
D.J.B.Wijers, 'Nicolaas Hendrik Swellengrebel 1885–1970', *Trans.R.Soc.Trop.Med.Hyg.,* 1970, *64:*315.

[18] B.Fantini, 'Anophelism without malaria: an ecological and epidemiological puzzle', *Parassitologia,* 1994, *36:*83–106.

[19] N.H.Swellengrebel, 'How the malaria service in Indonesia came into being, 1898–1948', *J.Hyg.,* 1950, *48:*148–57, p.149;
Sir Malcolm Watson, 'Malaria and mosquitoes: forty years on', *J.Roy.Soc.Arts,* 1939, *87:*482–502.

[20] Swellengrebel, op.cit. note 19.

[21] N.H.Swellengrebel, 'Report on a small experimental epidemic of benign tertian malaria started in September 1931 and followed up till January 1933', *Proc.Roy.Acad.Sci.Amsterdam,* 1933, *36:*234–9, p.234;
Swellengrebel and DeBuck, 'Prophylactic use of plasmoquine in a dosage warranting reasonable safety for routine treatment', *ibid.,* 1931, *34:*1216–20;
S.P.James, W.D.Nicol, and P.G.Shute, 'On the prevention of malaria with plasmoquine', *Lancet,* 1931, *ii:*341–2;
idem, 'A study of induced malignant tertian malaria', *Proc.Roy.Soc.Med.,* 1932, *25:*1153–81.

[22] Swellengrebel 1933, op.cit. note 21, p.239.

[23] LSHTM *Annual Report*s 1934–9, especially 1935–6, pp.52–5; 1936–7, pp.79–80; and 1937–8;
Sir Malcolm Watson, *African Highway,* London, John Murray, 1953.

[24] LSHTM *Annual Report*s 1939–40, pp.30–45; 1945–6, pp.74–83.

[25] LSHTM *Annual Report* 1938–9, p.57.

[26] G.Macdonald, 'On the scientific basis of tropical hygiene', *Trans.R.Soc.Trop.Med.Hyg.*, 1965, 59:611-20;
idem, 'Epidemiological basis of malaria control', *Bull.WHO*. 1956, 15:613-26;
idem, 'The dynamics of helminth infections, with special reference to schistosomes', *Trans.R.Soc.Trop.Med.Hyg.*, 1965, 59:489-506;
M.J.Goddard, 'On Macdonald's model for schistosomiasis', *ibid.*, 1978, 72:123-31.
[27] L.J.Bruce-Chwatt, 'Professor George Macdonald, 1903-67', in: L.J.Bruce-Chwatt and V.J.Glanville, *Dynamics of tropical disease*, Oxford University Press, 1973, pp.3-4;
H.S.Raper, 'John Smyth Macdonald 1867-1941', *Obit.Not.Fell.R.Soc.*, 1939-41, 3:853-66.
[28] 'On the scientific basis of tropical hygiene', op.cit. note 20, p.19;
G.Macdonald, 'Community aspects of immunity to malaria', *Br.med.Bull.*, 1951, 8:33-6;
George Macdonald, *The epidemiology and control of malaria*, Oxford University Press, 1957.
[29] D.Bradley, personal communication.
[30] G.Macdonald, 'Dynamic models in tropical hygiene', in: *Dynamics of tropical disease*, op.cit. note 21, pp.285-9;
idem, 'The dynamics of helminth infections ...' op.cit. note 20.
[31] D.Bradley, 'Malaria - whence and whither?', op.cit. note 4; personal communications D.Bradley and Paul Fine, cf.also Chapter 5;
G.Macdonald, 'Community aspects of immunity to malaria', *Br.med.Bull.*, 1951, 8:33-6.
[32] LSHTM *Annual Reports* 1945-6, 1946-7, 1950-1 and 1951-2.
[33] *Biogr.Mem.Fell.R.Soc.*, 1979. 25: op.cit. note 3;
MRC *Annual Report* 1931-2, p.110.
LSHTM *Annual Reports* 1931-2, pp.29-30; 1932-3, p.35.
[34] Bibliography in *Biogr.Mem.Fell.R.Soc.*, 1979, 25, op.cit. note 3 pp.199-207.
[35] LSHTM *Annual Reports* 1933-4 to 1938-9.
[36] LSHTM *Annual Report* 1937-8, p.77.
[37] Patrick Buxton, *The louse*, London, Arnold, 1939;
idem, The natural history of tsetse-flies, LSHTM Memoir No.10 London, Lewis and Co., 1954.
[38] L.J.Bruce-Chwatt, 'Quantitative epidemiology of tropical diseases', in: *Dynamics of tropical disease*, op.cit. note 21, pp.8-17.
[39] G.Macdonald, *The epidemiology and control of malaria*, op.cit. note 28, p.4;

P.C.C.Garnham, *Malaria parasites and other haemosporidia,* Oxford, Blackwell Scientific Publications, 1966, p.xv.
also quoted in part in Preface to above.
[40] L.J.Bruce-Chwatt, 'P.C.C.Garnham Master Mentor Friend', in: Elizabeth U.Canning (ed), *Parasitological Topics,* publ. by Society of Protozoologists, 1981.
LSHTM *Annual Report*s 1946–7, p.82; 1967–8, p.18.
R.Lainson and R.Killick-Kendrick, 'Percy Cyril Claude Garnham, CMG 15 January 1901–25 December 1994', *Biogr.Mem.Fell.Roy.Soc.* 1997, *43:*171–92.
[41] R.S.Bray, *Studies on the exo-erythrocytic cycle of the genus Plasmodium,* LSHTM Memoir No.12, London, H.K.Lewis, 1957.
[42] S.P.James and P.Tate, 'New knowledge of life cycle of malaria parasites', *Nature,* 1937, *139:*545;
idem, 'Exo-erythrocytic schizogony in *Plasmodium gallinaceum* Brumpt 1935' *Parasitology,* 1938, *30:*763–9.
[43] Robert S.Desowitz, *New Guinea tapeworms and Jewish grandmothers,* New York and London, W.E.Norton, 1981, p.12.
[44] H.E.Shortt, P.C.C.Garnham and B.Malamos, 'The pre-erythrocytic stage of mammalian malaria', *Br.med.J.,* 1948, *i:*192–4;
H.E.Shortt and P.C.C.Garnham, 'Demonstration of a persisting exo-erythrocytic cycle in *Plasmodium cynomolgi* and its bearing on the production of relapses', *Br.med.J.,* 1948, *i:*1225–8.
[45] *Nobel The man and his prizes,* op.cit. note 1, p.187;
Magda Whitrow, *Julius Wagner-Jauregg (1857–1940),* London, Smith-Gordon, 1993;
Sir Gordon Covell, 'Some aspects of malaria therapy', *J.Trop.Med.Hyg.,* 1956, *59:*253–61;
Eli Chernin, 'The malaria therapy of neurosyphilis', *J.Parasit.,* 1984, *70:*611–17.
[46] C.M.Wenyon, 'Warrington Yorke 1883–1943', *Obit.Not.Fell.Roy.Soc.,*1942–4, *4:*523–45;
S.R.Christophers, 'Sidney Price James 1870–1946', *ibid.,* 1945–8, *5:*507–23, pp.514–15;
Henry R.Rollin, 'The Horton Malaria Laboratory, Epsom, Surrey (1925–75)', *J.med.Biogr.,* 1994, *2:*94–7;
W.Yorke and J.W.Macfie, 'Observations on malaria made during treatment of general paralysis', *Trans.R.Soc.Trop.Med.Hyg.,* 1924, *18:*13–33; 1925, *19:*108–22.
S.P.James, W.D.Nicol, and P.G.Shute, 'A study of induced malignant tertian malaria', *Proc.R.Soc.Med.,* 1932, *xxv:*1153–81.

[47] Rickard Christophers, 'John Alexander Sinton 1884-1956', *Biogr.Mem.Fell.R.Soc.*, 1956, 2:269-90;
A recent analysis of original records for patients from Horton Hospital may be found in:
Judy R.Glynn, 'Studies on the influence of infecting dose on the severity of disease', Ph.D.thesis, University of London (Department of Epidemiology and Population Sciences, LSHTM), October 1993;
LSHTM *Annual Reports*, 1972-3, pp.29-30, and 1975-6, p.45.
[48] H.E.Shortt, P.C.C.Garnham, G.Covell, and P.G.Shute, 'The pre-erythrocytic stage of human malaria, *Plasmodium vivax*', *Br.med.J.*, 1948, i:547.
[49] H.E.Shortt, N.Hamilton Fairley, G.Covell, P.G.Shute and P.C.C.Garnham, 'The pre-erythrocytic stage of *Plasmodium falciparum*', *ibid.*, 1949, ii:1006-8;
D.Bradley assures us that the mosquitoes *were* duly counted — by Garnham and other celebrated protozoologists in person.
[50] Sir Philip Manson-Bahr, *History of the School of Tropical Medicine in London (1899-1949)*, LSHTM Memoir No.11, London, H.K.Lewis and Co.Ltd., 1956, pp.243-52;
P.C.C.Garnham, R.S.Bray, W.Cooper, R.Lainson, F.I.Awad and J.Williamson, 'The pre-erythrocytic stage of *Plasmodium ovale*', *Trans.R.Soc.Trop.Med.Hyg.*, 1955, *49*:158-67;
R.S.Bray, *Studies on the exo-erythrocytic cycle in the genus Plasmodium*, LSHTM Memoir No.12, London, H.K.Lewis & Co.Ltd., 1957;
LSHTM *Annual Report* 1963-4, p.14;
P.C.C.Garnham, 'The continuing mystery of relapses in malaria' *Protozool.Abstracts*, 1977, *1*:1-12;
A.J.Knell (ed.for the Wellcome Trust), *Malaria*, Oxford University Press, 1991, p.48;
In his preface to *Malaria parasites ...*, op.cit. note 39, Garnham 'cannot express too deeply the debt he owes to the late William Cooper, friend, consummate technician, gifted artist and gallant volunteer; ... The illustrations are largely the work of William Cooper and Audrey Besterman; ...'
W.A.Krotoski, D.M.Krotoski, P.C.C.Garnham, R.S.Bray, R.Killick-Kendrick, C.C.Draper, G.A.T.Targett, and M.W.Guy, 'Relapses in primate malaria: discovery of two populations of exo-erythrocytic stages. Preliminary note', *Br.med.J.* 1980, i:153-4.
[51] P.C.C.Garnham, *Progress in Parasitology*, The University of London, Athlone Press, 1971, p.125. [authors' italics]
[52] *ibid.*, p.126.

[53] Wellcome CMAC, pp/PCG, A.1;
R.Lainson in Garnham obituary, *Trans.R.Soc.Trop.Med.Hyg.*, 1995, *89:*129–31, p.130.
[54] Wellcome CMAC as above, B.28, c1966–7, 'with R.B.Heisch';
R.Killick-Kendrick in Garnham obituary as above, p.131;
J.D.Gillett, personal communication.
[55] LSHTM *Annual Reports* 1954–5, p.60; 1955–6, p.76; 1956–7, p.66; the DTM&H course came into existence in 1950, LSHTM *Annual Report* 1949–50, p.16;
the DTPH course was introduced in October 1963, LSHTM *Annual Reports* 1963–4, pp.84–5; 1964–5, pp.85–6.
[56] LSHTM *Annual Report* 1988–9, p.10.
[57] Bradley op.cit. note 4, p.20;
L.J.Bruce-Chwatt (ed), *Chemotherapy of Malaria,* revised 2nd ed., Geneva, WHO, 1986;
James R.Busvine, *Disease Transmission of Insects,* London etc., Springer Verlag, 1993.
R.S.Bray, personal communication, June 1998.
[58] Appendix 1, LSHTM Policy Committee, Board of Management Minutes, 22 March 1973;
LSHTM *Annual Report* 1978–9, p.24;
D.Bradley, personal communication;
D.J.Bradley, G.S.Nelson, M.G.Taylor and J.S.Weiner, 'Schistosomiasis in the Sudan', LSHTM AR 1977–8, pp.50–6;
Dan C.O.Kaseje and Harrison C.Spencer, 'The Saradidi, Kenya, Rural Health Development Programme', *Ann.trop.Med.Parasit.,* 1987, *81:*1–12;
Harrison Spencer *et al.*, 'Changing response to chloroquine of *Plasmodium falciparum* in Saradidi, Kenya, from 1981 to 1984', *ibid.,* pp.98–104.
[59] LSHTM *Annual Report* 1988–9, pp.2–10.
[60] LSHTM *Annual Report* 1927–8, p.6.
[61] LSHTM *Annual Report* 1978–9, p.27;
D.Mara and R.Feachem, 'Technical and public health aspects of low cost sanitation programme planning', *J.Trop.Med.Hyg.,* 1980, *83:*229–40;
D.J.Bradley, 'British tropical medicine for today: policy and financing-international', *Trans.R.Soc.Trop.Med.Hyg.,* 1981, *75:*suppl 35–8.
[62] LSHTM *Annual Reports* 1980–1 – LSHTM *Research Reports* 1990–3.
[63] Bradley op.cit. note 4, Table 4, p.20.
[64] LSHTM *Annual Report* 1992–3, pp.3 and 24–5;
World Development Report 1993: *Investing in Health,* Oxford University Press for the World Bank, 1993.

[65] *Malaria – Waiting for the Vaccine,* op.cit. note 4;
LSHTM *Research Report,* 1993, p.46.
[66] Bradley, op.cit. note 4, p.16.
[67] LSHTM *Research Report* 1993, p.56;
K.N.Mendis, 'Malaria vaccine research – a game of chess', in: *Malaria. ...,* op.cit. note 4, pp.183–96;
M.E.Patarroyo *et al.,* 'A synthetic vaccine protects humans against challenge with a sexual blood stage of *Plasmodium falciparum* malaria', *Nature,* 1988, *332:*158–61;
G.A.T.Targett, 'Malaria: drug use and the immune response', *Parasitology,* 1992, *105:*S61–S70;
Geoffrey A.T.Targett, 'Malaria – advances in vaccines', *Current Opinion in Infect.Dis.,* 1995, *8:*322–7.
[68] LSHTM *Annual Report* 1927–8, pp.13–15.
[69] MRC *Annual Report* 1927–8, p.107.
[70] *ibid.,* pp.107–8;
Murgatroyd obituaries, Chapter 10, note 69;
C.M.Wenyon, op.cit. note 40.
[71] L.J.Bruce-Chwatt (ed), op.cit. note 51, pp.11–14;
G.Covell, op.cit note 45, p.259.
[72] LSHTM *Annual Reports* 1927–8, pp.13–15; 1928–9, pp.27–8;
R.S.Desowitz, *The malaria capers,* New York and London, W.W.Norton & Co., 1991, pp.204–5.
[73] Sir John Boyd, 'Neil Hamilton Fairley 1891–1966', *Biogr.Mem.Fell.R.Soc.,* 1966, *12:*123–41.
[74] *ibid.,* pp.135–8;
N.Hamilton Fairley, 'Sidelights on malaria in man obtained by subinoculation experiments', *Trans.R.Soc.Trop.Med.Hyg.,* 1947, *40:*621–76.
[75] D.L.Klayman, 'Qinghaosu (artemisinin): an antimalarial drug from China', *Science,* 1985, *228:*1049–55; this article already quotes papers by Z.L.Li, H.M.Hu, D.C.Warhurst and W.Peters published in 1983 and 1984;
LSHTM *Research Report* 1992, pp.50–1;
The Role of Artemisinin and its Derivatives in the current Treatment of Malaria (1994–5), Report of an Informal Consultation convened by WHO in Geneva 27–9 September 1993, Malaria Unit, Division of Control of Tropical Diseases, Division of Drug Management and Policies, UNDP/World Bank/WHO Special Programme for Research and Training in Tropical Diseases, World Health Organization, Geneva, 1993 (we are indebted to D.C.Warhurst for loan of this document).

[76] Bradley, op.cit. note 4, p.29.
[77] LSHTM *Annual Reports* 1995–6, and 1996–7.

12

TOWARDS THE MILLENNIUM: BACK TO THE FUTURE

As the world braces itself for extensive millennium celebrations, the LSHTM reviews past achievements, and present and future policies, at the time of its own centenary, due just 3 months short of January 1st, 2000. It opened its doors to students on October 1st, 1899, founded in a world where politics were the politics of Empire, and medical concerns mostly centred on infectious diseases at home and abroad. With identification of specific disease agents then in its infancy, anti-microbial compounds yet to come, and development of vaccines in its early stages, morbidity and mortality rates were high for common childhood infections at home, and malaria, trypanosomiasis, etc., abroad. After a century of unprecedented progress in epidemiology and in biomedical sciences, human life expectancy has been rising steadily in developed as well as developing countries. Over the years, the London School has played a not inconsiderable role in such advances. When implementation of the Reid Report began during the academic year 1989–90, the year in which the medical virologist Gordon Smith was succeeded as Dean by the sanitary engineer Richard Feachem, major rearrangement of the School's infrastructure was undertaken to an extent not seen since the mid-1920s. Then it had been a question of restructuring Manson's initial tropical school, designed for the needs of Victoria's British Empire, for it to emerge as a national and international School of Public Health for a rapidly changing world; a world in the process of post-war development, which would eventually leave it with maps and political structures almost beyond recognition.

By now, in the last decade of the twentieth century, it is a world in which, at least on paper, politicians and policy makers in the Western World profess to pay less attention to nationalism and to be increasingly committed to global concerns and the furtherance of understanding of the problems, political and medical, of developing nations. Within the London School, changing attitudes in the world outside have been reflected in its teaching and research not so much in the actual subjects under scrutiny as in the methodology of, and the approach to, studies of diseases, their prevention and their general impact on public health problems existing since the opening of Manson's School and before.

Public Health as an academic discipline, with its own complement of teaching and research, arrived at the LSHTM in 1929, when Wilson Jameson was appointed Professor of Public Health. Since then, its common concerns with epidemiology, extending from infectious to chronic non-transmissible diseases, have gradually moved from the Western World to include the wider sphere of the tropics and the developing world, taking on the mantle of a truly global approach in tune with the School's avowed national and international commitments. The penultimate restructuring, following the Reid Report at the beginning of the last decade of the twentieth century, saw the School's multiple units, making up four major departments, focusing on 3 major areas which, each with its sub-divisions, can be roughly defined as:

The 'New' Public Health
Infectious Diseases, Old and New
Chronic non-infectious Diseases

All 3 categories rely more and more on interdisciplinary approaches, and are increasingly perceived in a global context. Within such a framework, 'Public Health' at the School now includes a number of disciplines and services unheard of when Public Health was first introduced at the LSHTM in 1929. In a world preoccupied with economic analysis, in a school with equal concern for developing countries and for the richer, industrialised nations at home on its doorstep, its health care research is as concerned with evaluation and planning in less developed countries as with analysis of proper use of resources at home. The application of expensive treatments and medical procedures to best advantage needs economic analysis, and economists figure prominently among the School's staff in the 1990s. The head of the Department of Public Health and Policy until 1997 was an economist by training; the present head is a physician with health sciences research responsibilities. Of the growing list of professors in the department only half have medical qualifications, and few of its readers are medically qualified. An increasing dependence on economics, statistics, and sociology, is reflected in the department's working units which include Environmental Epidemiology, Health Policy, Health Promotion Sciences, Health Services Research and Human Nutrition – the latter moved to the Department of Epidemiology and Population Health in the latest restructuring. The department had come into existence in the wake of a Government White Paper which recognised the need for 3 major public health functions: surveillance of the health of the population; the promotion of maintenance of health; and the evaluation of health services, particularly important in the context of Government strategies intent on replacing public ownership with central government controls, by private and independent ownership (of water and electricity authorities, hospitals, etc.), and controlled by public bodies such as the Audit Commission. The White Paper was followed in June 1991 by a Green Paper, *The Health of the Nation*, effectively defining national targets for health promotion and disease prevention, focusing in particular on improvements in terms of incidence, prevalence, and effects of disease. The School's Health Promotion Sciences (now 'Research') Unit, set up six months prior to publication of the Green Paper, has pursued much the same overall goals both nationally and internationally, helped at home by ESRC grants, and in Brazil, Africa, and India by ODA (DfiD) funding.

Research into, and teaching of, infectious diseases at the School goes back to the beginning of Manson's tropical school; it also straddles a number of disciplines and techniques, old and new. Today, some of the diseases studied are 'new', such as HIV infections and AIDS, and emerging virus diseases. Others are 'new' in the context of LSHTM concerns, such as tuberculosis as a concomitant in HIV and AIDS; but many more have been subjects of both research and teaching since the beginning of the century. At the School, hookworm research may be of less relevance today than in 1913, when it was instrumental in establishing the 'Rockefeller/hookworm connection', ultimately responsible for the School's transformation, in the 1920s, to a national and international school of public health (Chapter 3). Malaria on the other hand has continued as a subject of intense study and interest throughout the twentieth century. The Royal Society's first commission on malaria began work in 1898, when Ross had been studying its transmission since consulting Manson in 1895. Ross's epidemiological studies emphasised the importance of destruction of the mosquitoes' breeding sites; fifty years later, following World War II, the advent of DDT held out hopes of eradication of the mosquito vector, until development of insecticide resistance firmly dashed such hopes.

Today malaria, after waxing and waning and waxing again as a public health problem throughout the twentieth century, is now studied not only in terms of epidemiology, parasitology, and entomology, but has been given new dimensions by vaccine field trials and testing of immune responses involving, as do modern laboratory sciences, molecular techniques. In the case of malaria these techniques are applied also in the long-term studies of the development of the parasite and relevant enzyme systems, studies which aim to define specific targets for vaccines and drugs. Subjects of other applications include new diagnostic methods and mechanisms of drug resistance relevant to the ongoing analysis of investigations in the field. Similar studies of other infectious agents in the department also involve the molecular basis for pathogenesis, the whole representing the passage from molecule to population which forms such an important constituent in research at the School. The impact of use of the above techniques is also reflected in studies on schistosomiasis, leishmaniasis, leprosy, viral hepatitis, persistent herpes virus infections, and human malignancies of Epstein-Barr virus origin.

In the 1990s the emphasis is on vaccination strategies and new drug combinations, work which requires extensive field studies of immune responses in patients, coupled with highly developed laboratory techniques. It is a long-term project, with immune responses under intense scrutiny as crucial factors for the development of resistance to infection. In the meantime, what is hailed as an important advance in vector control, saving lives and preventing clinical malaria, is a method with ancient roots: the use of bednets. Today they are impregnated with various pyrethroids (some of which are also beginning to induce resistance); additives serve to make the insecticidal effect washproof. Apart from that insecticide impregnation, and the fact that current field trials are overseen by a WHO section, the use of bednets would not have surprised anybody at the time of the School's opening a century ago. Even malaria control has to some extent come full circle; the LSHTM *Annual Report* for 1994–5 had this to say:

> Undoubtedly the control measures [against malaria] most likely to have a significant effect on transmission, mortality and morbidity is the use of insecticide-impregnated bednets, and the School staff are directing or collaborating on numerous trials of their effectiveness.

A WHO diagram of the currently most important infectious transmissible diseases in terms of morbidity and mortality, published in 1995, serves also to reflect current global impact of other diseases which have been studied at the School since its inception in 1899, and which continue to be among its prime concerns in work with regional focus in central and eastern Europe, Africa, Asia, and Latin America. Diarrhoea as a cause of childhood morbidity and mortality in the developing world, and its causal relations with malnutrition, lack of breast feeding, poverty and poor hygiene, is a subject of interdisciplinary study units in Public Health and Policy, and Epidemiology and Population Health.

Unlike investigations of acute infectious diseases, their causes, epidemiology, and control, studies of chronic diseases have been building up only slowly in the twentieth century. At the LSHTM, during the second half of the century, particular emphasis has been on the epidemiology, prevention, and control of cancers and of cardiovascular disease. Studies of environmental cancers have been part and parcel of work at the School since the major pioneering investigations, by Bradford Hill and Richard Doll, of links between smoking and lung cancer in the years following the end of World War II. More recently, other environmental factors have joined an expanding list of cancer risks: radiation, radiotherapy and chemotherapy, industrial pollution, Radon in houses, residence near electricity transmitters. All are presently studied in various units within the School. In addition, the Health Promotion Sciences Unit has made observations on relative mortality rates for cancer and ischaemic heart disease in meat eaters and vegetarians (the title of the School's 6th Annual Health Forum held in April, 1966 was *Diet, nutrition and chronic disease*). In all such environmental studies today dietary factors are considered to play a major role. Viruses, long known as possible causes in some cancers, are currently under investigation in viral pathogenesis.

Studies of the epidemiology and prevention of cardiovascular disease became a focal point for work in the Public Health department when J.N.Morris took over as its head in 1967-8, bringing with him his MRC 'Social Medicine Unit'. Throughout the 1970s work in the Unit and in Epidemiology and Medical Statistics was closely linked, when Morris, G.A.Rose and D.D.Reid were all involved in-depth studies of cardiovascular disease problems (Chaps 4 & 6). Since then the field has widened. Although a number of current studies still cover problems in Britain and in Europe, there is a growing tendency to include observations on populations in, or from, developing countries. The Wandsworth Heart and Stroke Study compares differences in vascular morbidity in ethnic groups (Asians from the Indian sub-continent and from East Africa, Afro-Caribbeans, and Caucasians).

WORKING IN PARTNERSHIP WITH OUTSIDE AGENCIES

In a tight economic climate, support from and collaboration with major outside organisations has become an increasingly important part of the School's research programmes. The Wellcome Trust has long been a major benefactor, a connection which goes back to the interest taken in the old Tropical School by Henry Wellcome himself and by Andrew Balfour. The creation of the Wellcome Chair in Clinical Tropical Medicine at the end of World War II, when its first incumbent was Hamilton Fairley, augured in a second period of increasingly generous support, which in the

1990s covers both laboratory-based research at home, and fieldwork abroad, on a number of infectious disease problems. A major focus is AIDS studies, and related observations of the impact of HIV on tuberculosis prevalence in Africa, backed up by a research programme in London focusing on three major groups of opportunistic infections: mycobacterial (tb and leprosy) and cryptococcal diseases, and cryptosporidiosis. Also in London, The Wellcome Trust supports work in tropical diseases, in studies on schistosome and malaria vaccines in the Immunology Unit, and on molecular chemotherapy and genetics of resistance to infection, in other units.

A long-term association maintained at the School since the end of World War II is with the WHO. The WHO Malaria Reference Centre had had its origins in the Horton Malaria Laboratory, and came to the LSHTM in 1973, joining four other international reference centres (Chapter 11). Lately the School's Environmental Epidemiology Unit has been designated a WHO Collaborating Centre for Research, Training and Co-ordination in Environmental Epidemiology. With members of the School's staff serving on 12 of the WHO's Steering Committees, and with links to its Environmental Health division and its special programme for Research and Training in Tropical Diseases, the close working relationship between the WHO and the LSHTM promises to flourish into the next century, backed at reference level by the School's Library, which has been designated a WHO Public Reference Point.

Within the European Union, staff members at the School are involved in a number of programmes funded by the European Commission. By 1995, more than 40 EC grants supported work at the LSHTM. One multi-centre study, involving colleagues in Europe and overseas, concerned gene mutations in the malaria parasites, in an attempt to develop methods allowing evaluation of the spread of resistance to chloroquine. Other collaborations include studies of pathogenesis of tuberculosis using DNA fingerprinting, and programmes of infections with *Entamoeba histolytica* and *E.dispar*. A major EC project is concerned with the epidemiology and control of visceral leishmaniasis in north-eastern Brazil, a problem of long standing.

The School's growing interest in the economics of health care was reflected in its involvement in the preparation, and launch in the UK, of the World Bank's World Development Report, the Bank's first major statement of development policy to be devoted to world health, in 1993. Two years later the School's then Dean, Richard Feachem, resigned from the LSHTM to head a new World Bank Department of Public Health.

In the last decade of the twentieth century, working units at the

School have placed growing emphasis on close involvement with the Overseas Development Administration (ODA now DfiD), two decades after the then Ministry of Overseas Development first began creating new posts at the Liverpool and London Schools in an attempt to stem the tide of post-colonial decline in British involvement in tropical medicine abroad. From the beginning of the 1990s, nine major programmes have been undertaken with ODA funding, for which the LSHTM provides multidisciplinary manpower and expertise in areas representing a number of the School's special concerns in applied and social, as well as clinical and epidemiological, sciences. Recently an ODA funded **Malaria Consortium** was formed as a joint project of the Liverpool and London Schools, to oversee operational malaria control programmes with a view to bridging transition from laboratory research to control in the field.

The ODA programmes as well as other LSHTM-based research focus, as has been and will continue to be the School's tradition in prevention, therapy and control, on regional needs. In the 1990s and for the foreseeable future into the twenty-first century, that means continent-wide involvement: in Africa focus on economics of health care, on Gambian trials of impregnated bednets and chemoprophylaxis in malaria control, on Guinea worm eradication programmes in Niger and Nigeria, and on childhood diarrhoea and schistosomiasis control; in Asia, particular focus on work of the **Malaria Consortium**; in Latin America focus on leishmaniasis and *Trypanosoma cruzi* infections; and closer to home, on European health sector reforms.

Heading for the millennium, and for its own second century, the London School's overall aims and objectives have undergone no radical changes; but their scope and the manner of their execution have changed in ways which could not have been predicted in 1899. On the eve of its centenary the expanded, and still expanding, School has undergone another reorganisation following the Report of the committee on its future structure chaired by B.S.Drasar. Challenges to which the School needs to be responsive as the twentieth century comes to a close have been identified: first is the realisation that current major problems in public health and tropical medicine can be tackled only if a number of disparate disciplines are brought to work together within an established interdisciplinary framework. Second, it is necessary that some attention is paid to demands by certain funding agencies that research in public health and tropical medicine should be evaluated in terms of applicability in the field, and consequent impact of such applications on human health.

Third, awareness of the changes in Government policy with respect to universities which has been expressed in its research assessment exercise and the expanded participation at an undergraduate level. In response, the School has embarked on the final reorganisation of the century, with implementation taking place under its present American Dean, Harrison Spencer, himself a tropical health specialist with long experience of parasitic diseases in tropical environments, working with the now retiring Chairman of the Board of Management, Sir Joseph Smith, former Director of the PHLS, and the acting Chairman, John H. Smith, former Governor of the Gilbert and Ellice Islands. The frame of the latest reorganisation is the intention to enhance the School's strengths in innovative interdisciplinary research, and to safeguard teaching in public health and tropical medicine (or medicine in the tropics) in the future: the School is the sole remaining institution in the UK exclusively concerned with these areas.

After a hundred years of teaching, the School has acquired an extensive body of alumni, and has formed an alumni association enabling a unique network of specialists in public health and tropical medicine with a common background to meet and plan improvements in health worldwide. Hence, as a result of continued focus on health of populations in all parts of the world the School's influence in now out of proportion to its size. Through its growing numbers of alumni, many in commanding positions in international organisations such as the World Health Organization, the World Bank, Save the Children Fund, etc., and others in positions in Ministries of Health throughout the world, it has a continual impact on global public health. Through its alumni the School will see its mission fulfilled, at a time of looking back on a century of unique advance in attempts to combat disease. New threats and challenges may emerge, e.g. AIDS and other emerging viruses, and lately spongiform encephalopathies, but there is hope and strength in past achievements and future promising lines of research. Advances in epidemiology are furthering analysis and better understanding of chronic, non-infectious diseases, providing clues to aetiology on which molecular and cell biology may build to shape future preventive strategies and therapeutic measures.

Throughout the twentieth century the LSHTM has moved confidently with the times and with developments in medical science, within and without, which over the past century have built on unprecedented advances in methodologies and techniques. In recent years the School, along with other institutions academic and otherwise, has adopted for itself, and introduced in its report, a Mission Statement as a definition for students and other interested bodies of its aims, objectives, and hopes and plans for the future:

MISSION STATEMENT

The mission of the London School of Hygiene and Tropical Medicine is to contribute to the improvement of health worldwide through the pursuit of excellence in research, postgraduate teaching, advanced training and consultancy in international public health and tropical medicine. To achieve this mission the School will enhance its role as:

Britain's national school of public health,
A leading institution in Europe for research and postgraduate education in public health and tropical medicine and
an international centre of excellence in public health and medicine in developing countries.

REFERENCES: LSHTM *Annual Reports*, 1988-9 to 1996-7. B.S.Drasar, G.A.T.Targett, M.G.Taylor, and Peter Smith personal communications.

BIOGRAPHICAL APPENDIX A

Late former Members of Staff of the School

ALCOCK, ALFRED WILLIAM (1859–1933); FRS 1901

First Professor of Medical Entomology in the University of London and head of the School's Department of Entomology from its inception in 1907 until retirement in 1925.

Of the many unorthodox paths to a career at the LSHTM in its early days, Alcock's was among the most unusual. His school years at Westminster cut short by his father's financial difficulties, he was sent to India at the age of 17, to relatives in the coffee trade. For five years he tried out a number of jobs, including schoolmastering; during this time he became interested in science, helped by Michael Foster's physiology textbook. In 1881 a brother-in-law, an officer in the Indian Civil Service, offered to help him to a medical education, which he completed at Aberdeen in 3½ years graduating MB, CM in 1885. Adding a course in tropical medicine at Netley to his qualifications, Alcock then spent another 20 years in India, in the IMS, as Surgeon-Naturalist to the Indian Marine Survey, with the Indian Museum in Calcutta, and keeping in touch with medicine at the Medical College Hospital. On his return to London Patrick Manson recruited him, in 1907, to head a new medical entomology department, to join Leiper's helminthology and Wenyon's protozoology at the School of Tropical Medicine at the Albert Dock. He was the author of the first comprehensive textbook of *Entomology for Medical Officers* in 1911; in 1921 he became the first Professor of Medical Zoology in the University of London.

W.T.C., S.W.K., and P.M.-B, 'Alfred William Alcock 1859–1933', *Obit.Not.Fell.Roy.Soc.*, 1932–5, *i:*119–26.

AYKROYD, WALLACE RUDDELL (1899–1979)

Senior Lecturer in Human Nutrition LSHTM, 1960–6.

From the Ley's School in Cambridge Aykroyd went to Trinity College Dublin where, with the added distinction of having been Vice-Chancellor's Prizeman in English Prose, he graduated MB, M.Ch. in 1924, taking the MD in 1928. His interest in malnutrition was kindled when, as house-surgeon in Newfoundland, he described beri-beri in Labrador fishermen. In 1930 his appointment to the health section of the League of Nations made him one of its first international civil servants, with responsibility for international work in nutrition. In India from 1935, he witnessed the appalling effects of the Bengal famine in 1943 which the India Office, with a famous understatement, had referred to as a 'food shortage'. The experience was a fitting introduction to his post-war relief work with UNRRA and his role in the administration of FAO's campaigns for prevention of worldwide malnutrition. Retiring from FAO in 1960, he spent 6 years, until final retirement in 1966, as senior lecturer in the LSHTM's Department of Human Nutrition.

Obituary by T.P.E.[Eddy], *Br.med.J.*, 1979, *i*:544.

BALFOUR, SIR ANDREW (1873-1931)

Director of the LSHTM 1923-30.

A native of Edinburgh, Balfour graduated MB CM in 1984 and MD (Gold Medal) in 1898 at Edinburgh University. At Cambridge he gained the DPH in 1897 and, before serving as a surgeon in the South African War (1900-1), he took the Edinburgh B.Sc. in public health in 1900. His choice of career was then influenced by his fellow Scot Patrick Manson: tropical medicine became his life's work when he was appointed director of the new Wellcome Tropical Research Laboratories at Khartoum, and local MOH. His research work was published in 4 Reports from the Wellcome Research Laboratories (1904-11). In 1913 he returned to England to head the Wellcome Bureau of Scientific Research. After important organisational work in the RAMC during the Great War he was in 1923 appointed director of the LSHTM during its transitional period. The pressure of this work brought on a recurrence of serious strain of overwork which this physically robust, athletic man had first experienced years before in Khartoum. This time it proved fatal, and he died in tragic circumstances in a fall from a window in a nursing home in Kent on New Year's Day, 1931. Like Ronald Ross and others at the turn of the century he indulged himself by novel writing, which did not match in importance or readability his writings on tropical diseases and tropical public health.

Obituary in *J.Trop.Med.Hyg.*, 1931 (16 Feb.), *34*:63-4; DNB 1931-40, pp.33-4.

BIOGRAPHICAL APPENDIX A

BARNARD, CYRIL C. (1894–1959)

The School's first professional librarian, 1921–59.

As the School's first professional librarian Barnard organised and catalogued the collections of the old Tropical School when appointed in 1921. He came to the School after appointments at the Reform Club Library, the Library of the RSM, and the Wellcome Historical Medical Museum. Once settled at the School he took an external BA (London) degree, and also obtained a diploma in Librarianship. When the School Library moved into its new quarters in Keppel Street in 1929, Barnard built up the collections and laid the foundations for its present high standards. He was killed in a road accident only 6 months before he was due to retire.

LSHTM *Annual Report* 1958–9, p.15.

BASSETT-SMITH, SIR PERCY (William) (1861–1927)

Among the initial intake of 11 students at Manson's School in 1899.

Born at St. Albans, Bassett-Smith qualified in medicine at Middlesex Hospital. After obtaining MRCS and LRCP diplomas he joined the Navy as a surgeon in 1883 and served it for 38 years until retirement in 1921. He was appointed lecturer on tropical medicine and bacteriology at Haslar Royal Naval Hospital in 1900, having attended the very first course at Manson's School. In 1905 he took the Cambridge Diploma in Tropical Diseases, and in 1907 was awarded the London School's Cragg's prize for original research work. In 1912 he was appointed Professor of Clinical Pathology and Lecturer on Tropical Diseases at the newly inaugurated Naval Medical School at Greenwich. During the Great War Bassett-Smith, now in his fifties, devoted himself to research and development of measures for disease prevention in the Navy including preparation of vaccines.

Obituary by T.B.Shaw, *Trans.Roy.Soc.Trop.Med.Hyg.* 1927–8, *21:*435–8.

BERTRAM, DOUGLAS SOMERVILLE (1913–88)

Reader in Entomology, LSHTM, 1948–56, and Professor of Medical Entomology and Director of the Department of Entomology, LSHTM, 1956–76.

Educated in Glasgow, Bertram first became interested in medical entomology in the University's zoology department, moving to the Liverpool School of Tropical Medicine in 1938 and establishing its insectary for insect colonies. Joining the RAMC at the outbreak of war he was captured in Crete in 1941, and spent the rest of the war years as POW in Germany. After a short period as entomologist at the Army School of Hygiene at Mytchett, he returned to Liverpool doing research and teaching medical and veterinary entomology before joining the LSHTM in 1948 as Reader in the Department of Entomology under Buxton, whom he succeeded in 1956. Having continued research on mites and rat filariasis he later became interested in wasps parasitising the reduviid bugs transmitting Chagas' disease in South America, continuing work well after official retirement in 1976. He established the School's Electron Microscopy Laboratory and originated its research on mosquito-borne viruses in 1955.

LSHTM *Annual Report* 1988–9, pp.9–10.

BROTHERSTON, SIR JOHN (Howie Flint), (1915–85)

Senior Lecturer and subsequently Reader in Public Health, LSHTM, 1951–5.

The son of distinguished parents – his father was an Edinburgh Writer to the Signet, his mother one of Scotland's pioneer women doctors who developed its Maternity and Child Welfare Services – Brotherston was born and educated in Edinburgh, graduating MA (with history and political economy as special subjects) in 1935, and MB, M.Ch. in 1940, obtaining the MD in 1950. A DPH (London) was added in 1947, and a doctorate in public health at Johns Hopkins in 1952. His London years included lectureships in Social and Preventive Medicine at Guy's Hospital Medical School and the LSHTM from 1948 to 1951, before he became Senior Lecturer and subsequently Reader in Public Health at the LSHTM 1951–5. In 1955 he returned to the University of Edinburgh, as Professor of Public Health and Social Medicine 1955– 64, and Dean of the Faculty of Medicine 1958–63. His influence on developments in the Public Health Department of the LSHTM in the post-war years was considerable; even greater was his impact, after his return to Edinburgh as Chief Medical Officer, on Scottish Health Services in general, and on the University Department of Community Medicine at Edinburgh in particular.

'Epilogue: Tribute to Sir John Brotherston', by G.McLachlan, in: Gordon McLachlan (ed), *Improving the common weal,* Edinburgh University Press, 1987, pp.613–16.

BRUCE-CHWATT, LEONARD JAN (1907–89)

Professor of Tropical Hygiene and Director of the Ross Institute, LSHTM 1969–74.

Bruce-Chwatt came late to the LSHTM, after a long career in international malariology. Polish born, he obtained a doctorate in medicine at the University of Warsaw in 1930. In Paris he obtained the French diploma in tropical medicine before enlisting in the Polish Army Medical Corps in France at the outbreak of war in 1939. Taken prisoner by the Vichy forces he escaped to Britain where in 1942 he joined the RAMC. Appointed entomologist to a malaria field laboratory in Nigeria he gained his first experience of malaria. In the Colonial Medical Service he worked first on yellow fever, and from 1946 in the Nigerian Medical Service as malariologist. From the mid-1950s to the late 1970s he was, as a member of the WHO's malaria panel and of the WHO staff, prominent in the advances and reversals of the malaria eradication and control campaigns. He retired as chief of malaria research in 1967 and was, until final retirement in 1974, Professor of Tropical Hygiene and Director of the Ross Institute at the LSHTM after George Macdonald's death. In retirement he was associated with the Wellcome Museum of Medical Sciences and the Wellcome Tropical Institute, devoting himself to historical research.

Obituary, by J.H., *Br.med.J.* 1989, *298*:1576;

LSHTM *Annual Report* 1988–9, p.10.

BUCKLEY, JOHN JOSEPH CRONIN (1904–72)

In Leiper's department from 1927, Buckley eventually became Reader in medical parasitology before succeeding Leiper in the Julien Courtauld Chair of Helminthology in 1946.

Educated at University College Dublin Buckley graduated B.Sc. in 1924, M.Sc. in 1925, and D.Sc. in 1935. With an Irish travelling studentship he went in 1927 to the LSHTM, where he was to spend the rest of his career, beginning as demonstrator in helminthology and eventually progressing to reader in medical parasitology. When Leiper retired in 1946 Buckley succeeded him in the Julien Courtauld Chair of Helminthology. Successfully combining his teaching duties at the School with countless expeditions abroad, he made many contributions to the knowledge of life-cycles of parasites of medical and veterinary importance, notably those of river blindness in Kenya during World War II, and before that of the related parasite *Onchocerca gibsoni* and its vector in cattle in Assam and Malaya. His contributions to taxonomy included the creation of the new genus *Brugia*, separate from *Wuchereria*. His selfless use of his own body as 'anonymous volunteer' seriously affected his health in later life; partially paralysed he continued working until his death at 67.

Obituary by G.S.N. [George Nelson], *Br.med.J.* 1972, *i*:355.

BUXTON, PATRICK ALFRED (1892–1955); FRS 1943

Head of Department of Entomology, LSHTM, 1927–55.

Born in London and educated at home until the age of ten, Buxton was early influenced by his father's family tradition (an old Quaker custom) of spare time nature study, less so by his mother's family's insistence on classical languages – she was a Jex-Blake, sister of the Mistress of Girton College, Cambridge, and of the Principal of Lady Margaret Hall, Oxford. At Trinity College, Cambridge, Walter Fletcher encouraged Buxton's studies in the Natural Sciences Tripos, and during the Great War he also qualified in medicine at St.George's, and then spent his time in the RAMC collecting insects in Mesopotamia and Persia. During the 1920s he gradually equipped himself for his future role as an eminent medical entomologist, working in Cambridge, London and abroad, until he was appointed head of the department of entomology in the new LSHTM then under construction. With V.B.Wigglesworth he built up the study and teaching of insect physiology and medical entomology in the School. His studies of lice (*The louse*, 1939, 1947) involved students, friends, and family members as incubators and have become legendary; according to Wigglesworth his crowning achievement was *The natural history of tsetse-flies*, 1954.

V.B.Wigglesworth, 'Patrick Alfred Buxton 1892–1955', *Biogr.Mem.Fell.Roy.Soc.* 1956, 2:69–84.

CAMERON, THOMAS WRIGHT MOIR (1894–1980)

Lecturer in the Department of Helminthology, LSHTM, 1925–9.

Born in Glasgow and educated at Edinburgh University and the Royal (Dick) Veterinary College, Cameron came to London after wartime service in the HLI and the RAF, to become Senior Research Assistant when Leiper was setting up the Institute of Agricultural Parasitology in 1923; from 1925 to 1929 he was lecturer in the Department of Helminthology, before he returned to lecture at Edinburgh and the Dick Veterinary College. In 1932 he went to Canada, where as Professor of Parasitology at McGill University he established courses in tropical medicine and founded the Canadian Institute of Parasitology of which he was Director until he retired in 1964.

M.-B., p.231.

CANTLIE, SIR JAMES (1851–1926)

Surgeon at the Albert Dock Hospital from 1896, and on the staff of Manson's School from its inception.

Born in Banffshire, Cantlie graduated in natural science at Aberdeen in 1871 and qualified from Charing Cross Hospital in 1873. In 1877 he obtained the FRCS and also the DPH of the Royal Colleges. Between 1887 and 1889 he was Manson's partner in his practice in Hong Kong, and together they founded the College of Medicine in Hong Kong, where Cantlie served as Dean for 7 years. A member of the Egyptian Cholera Expedition in 1883 Cantlie also studied leprosy distribution in the East Indian and Pacific Archipelago. Back in London from 1896, he became surgeon to the Albert Dock Hospital and a valued teacher at Manson's School. He was a founder member of the (Royal) Society of Tropical Medicine and Hygiene in 1907; in 1898 he brought out, with W.J.Ritchie Simpson, the first issue of the *Journal of Tropical Medicine*.

Obituary in *Lancet* 1926, *i:*1121–2;

Jean Cantlie Stewart, *The Quality of Mercy: the lives of Sir James and Lady Cantlie,* London, George Allen and Unwin, 1983.

CASTELLANI (Sir) ALDO (1877–1971)

Director of Mycology and Mycological Diseases LSHTM (Ross Institute) 1934–40.

Born and educated in Florence, Castellani qualified in medicine there in 1899, and after working in Bonn came to London to Manson's School in 1901. Through Manson's recommendation he joined the Royal Society Commission on Sleeping Sickness as its bacteriologist, and left London for Entebbe with G.C.Low and Cuthbert Christie in 1902. His early observation of a trypanosome in the cerebro-spinal fluid of a sleeping sickness sufferer without initially realising its importance gave rise to a famous controversy involving Sir David Bruce and others. With Ritchie Simpson he began a movement to establish the Ross Institute, again not avoiding controversy. When the Institute became part of the LSHTM in 1934, Castellani became Director of Mycology and Mycological Diseases in the School, before his enthusiasm for Royal and politically eminent patients (including Mussolini) further clouded his reputation. He finally followed the Queen of Italy into exile in Portugal and ended his long life as Professor at Lisbon's Institute of Tropical Medicine.

Obituary, *J.Trop.Med.Hyg.* 1971, *74:*233–7;

Sir John Boyd, 'Sleeping sickness: the Castellani-Bruce controversy', *Notes and Records Roy.Soc.* 1973, *28:*93–110.

CHARLES, SIR HAVELOCK (HENRY RICHARD) (1858–1934)

Dean of the London School of Tropical Medicine 1916–24.

Born in Co.Tyrone, Havelock Charles was educated at Queen's College,

Cork and University College London, before entering the IMS in 1882. He served with the Afghan Boundary Commission from 1884-6, and afterwards was Professor of Anatomy, first at Lahore Medical College and from 1896 at the Calcutta Medical College. After more than 20 years in India he retired in 1908, and eventually became the second Dean of Manson's School when Sir Francis Lovell died in 1916.

Obituaries: *Lancet* 1934, *ii:*1015-16; *Br.med.J.* 1934, *ii:*838-9.

CHAVE, SIDNEY (1914-85)

Joined staff of the LSHTM as a 'lab-boy' in the Department of Chemistry as Applied to Hygiene in 1929, and retired after 50 years' service to the School in 1979.

Born in the year of the outbreak of the Great War, Chave was only 3 when his father was killed in France in 1917. Having joined the LSHTM in the year of its official opening, he was seconded to the EPHLS in Oxford during World War II. On his return to the School in 1946 he became Senior Technician and six years later, having graduated in psychology at Birkbeck College, was appointed to the academic staff in the Department of Public Health. Increasingly interested in health education Chave then gained a doctorate with a study of mental health in the 'new town' of Harlow (published in book form with Lord Taylor in 1964), and 5 years later became senior lecturer in J.N.Morris's Department of Community Health. He retired in 1979 as Emeritus Senior Lecturer in Public Health, an unusual distinction.

'An appreciation of Sidney Chave', *in: Recalling the Medical Officer of Health. Writings by Sidney Chave,* M.Warren and H.Francis (eds), King Edward's Hospital Fund for London, [1987].

CHRISTOPHERS, SIR (Samuel) RICKARD (1873-1978); FRS 1926

Professor of Malaria Studies in London University at the LSHTM, 1932-8.

Christophers was one of a great triumvirate of twentieth-century malariologists associated with the LSHTM: H.E.Shortt, Christophers and P.C.C.Garnham, all distinguished in addition to their scientific achievements by exceptionally long lives. Born and educated in Liverpool, of a Cornish family, Christophers graduated MB, Ch.B. from University College Liverpool in 1896, his scientific bent already shaped by the teaching of Charles Sherrington. His life-long fascination with the tropics also began before the turn of the century when he travelled, as medical officer, on the first ocean steamer to traverse the upper reaches of the Amazon. Soon afterwards he was appointed to the Malaria Commission of the Royal Society and the Colonial Office 1898–1902, an experience which led straight to the IMS and a career in its Research Department. From Mian Mir to the Central Research Institute in Kasauli, in war and in peace, Brevet Colonel Christophers served the IMS for almost 30 years until he retired in 1931. He then resumed research in London and Cambridge, from 1932 to 1938 as Leverhulme Fellow of the MRC and Professor of Malaria Studies at London University, working in a special Malaria Unit at the LSHTM. His written studies culminated, as late as 1960, with the publication of *Aedes aegypti* (L.): *the yellow fever mosquito*.

H.E.Shortt and P.C.C.Garnham, 'Samuel Rickard Christophers', *Biogr.Mem.Fell.R.Soc.* 1979, *25:*179–207;

'Tribute to Sir Rickard Christophers on his 100th birthday', *Trans.Roy.Soc.Trop.Med.Hyg.* 1973, *67:*729–54.

CHRISTOPHERSON, JOHN BRIAN (1868–1955)

Assistant surgeon to the Albert Dock Hospital 1896–1902.

Born in Yorkshire, son of the late rector of Falmouth, Christopherson – 'Christo' to family and friends – went to Caius College Cambridge and qualified from St.Bartholomew's Hospital in 1893. After further studies in Vienna he became assistant surgeon to James Cantlie at the Albert Dock Hospital in 1896. His London career was interrupted by service in the South African War, after which he joined the newly formed Sudan Medical Services in the Sudan, a position in which he was closely associated with the Wellcome Laboratories at Khartoum and Andrew Balfour. When he discovered the parasite of the local relapsing fever, a dispute over nomenclature (which he eventually won), soured his hitherto friendly relations with Balfour. Interested in leishmaniasis (kala-azar), schistosomiasis, and leprosy, his most notable discovery was accidental. Treating patients, with tartar emetic as recommended by Leonard Rogers, he was surprised to find that as the kala-azar regressed, the treatment also killed the eggs of *Schistosoma haematobium*. After retirement from the Sudan, Christopherson headed the bilharzia clinic of the Ministry of Pensions and eventually, in the 1920s, developed an interest in pulmonary diseases as physician to the London Chest Hospital.

Obituaries in *Lancet* 1955, *ii:* 255–6; *Br.med.J* 1955, *ii*:327–8.

COOPER, WILLIAM (1900–64)

Technician in protozoology, LSHTM, 1919–64

At the age of 16 Cooper came straight from school to work, with a War Office grant, with John Gordon Thomson and his brother David, in War Office research laboratories. In 1919 he worked as technician with special knowledge of malaria at the Shoreham Malarial Concentration Camp; and in November of that year he joined John Gordon Thomson's protozoology department at the Albert Dock. He was a mainstay of the department both in London and on expeditions abroad, and after World War II became Chief Technical Assistant to the Department of Parasitology. He was artistically gifted and his illustrations grace papers and textbooks. His services as a volunteer, with others, in Garnham's *Plasmodium* experiments in 1954 were heroic as well as enthusiastic, and contributed much to their success.

M.-B., pp.246–7; LSHTM *Annual Report* 1963–5, p.14.

CROWDEN, GUY PASCOE (1894–1966)

At LSHTM Lecturer in Applied Physiology 1929, Reader in Industrial Physiology 1934, and Professor of Applied Physiology 1946–62.

Brought up in Wisbech where his father was in general practice, Crowden's medical studies at University College London were interrupted by the Great War. With the King's Own Yorkshire Light Infantry he served in France where experience with the Gas Brigade at Ypres, Somme, and Passchendale shaped a growing interest in the physiology of work and stress. In 1924 he became an assistant in the University College physiology department, and in 1929 he was appointed lecturer in applied physiology at the LSHTM. His research interests ranged from fatigue and recovery in muscular work to effects of heat and cold in nutrition. In 1934 he became Reader in Industrial Physiology at the School and finally, after service in the RAMC during World War II, he was appointed Professor of Applied Physiology in 1946. He retired in 1952. His connections with firms interested in industrial welfare work were to prove a link to the School's later involvement with occupational health.

Obituaries: *The Times,* 5 Aug. 1966; *Lancet* 1966, *ii:*1257-8.

CRUICKSHANK, JOHN CECIL (1899-1956)

First came to the LSHTM as a student in the Dip.Bact. course in 1932, and stayed on as demonstrator and later lecturer; in 1945 he became Reader, and two years later Professor of Bacteriology as Applied to Hygiene.

A Scot educated at George Watson's College, Edinburgh during the Great War, Cruickshank served with the Gordon Highlanders for a year at the end of the war before going on to study medicine at Edinburgh, graduating MB, Ch.B. in 1921. After house posts in Sheffield and Chesterfield he obtained the Dip.Trop.Med. at Liverpool in 1923, then joined the West African Medical Service in the Gambia until 1930. Returned to Britain he spent a short period in general practice before deciding on a career in bacteriology, taking the Dip.Bact. and staying on at the LSHTM, where he became a lecturer in 1937. Like others in the department he followed Topley and Wilson into the EPHLS during World War II. In 1945 he returned to the School as Reader; and 2 years later, when Graham Wilson left to head the peacetime PHLS, Cruickshank succeeded him as Professor of Bacteriology as Applied to Hygiene. He was outstanding both in teaching and research, and was mourned by students and staff when he died at the age of 57.

Obituaries: *Lancet* 1956, *ii:*1001-2; *Br.med.J* 1956, *ii:*1061; 1121-2.

CULPIN, MILLAIS (1874-1952)

Lecturer in Industrial and Medical Psychology, LSHTM 1930; University Chair of Medical Industrial Psychology, LSHTM, 1931-9.

Trained at the London Hospital where he eventually became ophthalmic surgeon and surgeon registrar, Culpin turned to neurology and clinical psychology during the Great War, influenced by his war experiences. He later wrote *Psychoneuroses of Peace and War* (1920) and *Recent Advances in the Study of the Psychoneuroses* (1931). Brought into the field of industrial psychology by collaboration with Major Greenwood in the IHRB he became lecturer in industrial and medical psychology at the LSHTM in 1930, and was appointed to a new University Chair in Medical Industrial Psychology at the LSHTM in 1931.

Obituaries: *Lancet* 1952, *ii:*643; *B.med.J.* 1952, *ii:*727–8; 955–8; 1207.

DANIELS, CHARLES WILBERFORCE (1862–1927)

Nominated by Manson to the Royal Society's Commission on Malaria in 1898, Daniels worked with Ross, Christophers and Stephens until joining the Tropical School in 1900 as its second superintendent, retiring from this post in 1910 to become physician to the Albert Dock Hospital and continuing to lecture on tropical medicine.

Born in Manchester, Daniels was lucky in his early instruction in science in its famous grammar school, which led to a scholarship to Trinity College, Cambridge, and a Cambridge MB at the London Hospital in 1886. After 4 years in the Colonial Medical Service in Fiji he was transferred to British Guiana, where his work on filariasis attracted the attention of Patrick Manson. In 1898 Manson nominated Daniels as a member of the Royal Society Commission on Malaria, working first with Ross in Calcutta and subsequently with Stephens and Christophers in Nyasaland. Some of his preparations made in Africa were included in the teaching collections at the Albert Dock when on his return to England in 1900 he joined the School, succeeding D.C.Rees as superintendent. After 2 years in Kuala Lumpur from 1903 to 1905 he rejoined the School as Director for 5 years. In 1910 he was appointed physician to the Albert Dock Hospital in charge of beds while continuing to lecture to students on tropical medicine until, during the Great War, he showed the first signs of the slow progressive illness which was to kill him, after a valiant fight, in 1927.

Obituary by A.W.Alcock in *Trans.Roy.Soc.Trop.Med.Hyg.* 1927–8, *21:*249–53.

DAVIDSON, GEORGE (1917-97)

LSHTM: Ross Institute 1946-80; Professor of Entomology as Applied to Malaria 1980-3.

Having graduated B.Sc. in the summer of 1939, Davidson went straight into the RAMC, joining a Field Malaria Unit first in North Africa and then in Italy. His knowledge of pre-war discoveries of 'anophelism without malaria' and the *Anopheles maculipennis* complex enabled him to give valuable advice on the sitting of base camps away from habitats of particularly dangerous *Anopheles* species. Back in England – after 5 years he was evacuated with a severe attack of malaria – he was recruited to the Ross Institute by George Macdonald immediately after the war, and sent to test new synthethic insecticides in the Belgian Congo. After a period in Tanganyika Davidson returned to Keppel Street, producing important work on insecticide resistance in colonies of *Anopheles* mosquitoes, and discovering the complex of species constituting what had hitherto been regarded as a single species, *An.gambiae*. Among Davidson's malaria vectors among the anophelines stand out.

Chris Curtis and Simon Miles. 'George Davidson (1917-97) *Parassitologia* 1997, *39*:1.

DELAFIELD, MAX EVERARD (1886-1974)

Professor of Chemistry as Applied to Hygiene LSHTM 1929-49.

Educated at Merchant Taylors School, London, and Jesus College, Cambridge, Delafield qualified at St.Thomas's Hospital before holding lectureships at University College Hospital Medical School and University College, London. He then became Head of the Department of Hygiene and Bacteriology at Queen Elizabeth College London, and finished his career as the LSHTM's first – and last – Professor of Chemistry as Applied to Hygiene in Raistrick's biochemistry department from 1929 until retirement in 1949.

LSHTM *Annual Report* 1974-5, p.33.

EDDY, TREWAVAS PEARCE (1908-92)

Senior Lecturer, LSHTM Department of Human Nutrition 1959-73.

T.P.Eddy – TP to his friends – came to the LSHTM only after retiring as Director of Medical Services in Sierra Leone in 1959. He had gained his medical education at Exeter College Oxford and the Middlesex Hospital Medical School, and had worked in colonial medical services in Nigeria and the Gambia before coming to Sierra Leone. In the LSHTM's human nutrition department under Platt he at first worked on a survey of food in hospitals commissioned by the Nuffield Provincial Hospitals Trust. Subsequently his research included aspects of nutrition of the elderly and of immigrant Asian children. Another of his interests was the effect of environmental factors on health. A man of many parts, he was very musical and built a harpsichord of his own; his paintings were hung at the Medical Art Society's shows.

Obituary by J.C.Waterlow *Br.med.J.* 1993, *306:*512-13; LSHTM *Annual Report* 1992-3, p.29.

EDSALL, GEOFFREY (1908-1980)

Professor and Head of the Department of Microbiology, LSHTM, 1972-5.

Having graduated MD at Harvard University in 1934, Edsall served as intern at Massachusetts General Hospital before beginning a career with parallel appointments at Harvard and in the Massachusetts Public Health Laboratories, culminating in the simultaneous appointments as Professor of Applied Microbiology at Harvard 1960-72, and superintendent of the State Laboratory Institute 1960-72. In 1972 he joined the LSHTM for 3 years as Professor of Microbiology. He was a member of the WHO's expert panel on immunology 1963-80.

LSHTM *Annual Report* 1980-1, p.21.

BIOGRAPHICAL APPENDIX A

EVANS, DAVID GWYNNE (1909-84); FRS 1960.

Professor of Bacteriology and Immunology, LSHTM, 1961-71.

Born near Manchester of Welsh parents Evans graduated B.Sc. in physics and chemistry in 1934 (M.Sc. the following year) from Manchester University. At the time H.B.Maitland in the bacteriology department needed a chemist to help in the public health laboratories and Evans was selected, entering by chance the field of bacteriology and immunology where he was soon to make his mark. Maitland introduced him to work on the toxins of *Bordetella pertussis* and related organisms: the basis was laid for his later work on whooping cough immunisation and other vaccine work, including standardisation of vaccines and antisera. In 1940 Evans joined the Department of Biological Standards under Percival Hartley at the NIMR. Although he continued to work on pertussis vaccines, the demands of the war years included studies of spore-bearing anaerobes causing gas gangrene, and the production of standard antitoxins against their toxins. Returning to Manchester in 1947 Evans became Reader in the bacteriology department and a much valued teacher and researcher before returning to head the Biological Standards Control Laboratories in 1955, becoming Director of the department at the NIMR 3 years later. In 1961 Evans was appointed to the Chair of Bacteriology and Immunology at the LSHTM, succeeding E.T.C.Spooner who had become Dean. Ten years later he left the School for the directorship of the new National Institute for Biological Standards and Control of the MRC. He retired in 1976, the year the National Biological Standards Board was established to take over from the MRC responsibility for managing the Institute.

A.W.Downie, C.E.Gordon Smith and J.O'H.Tobin, 'David Gwynne Evans' *Biogr.Mem.Fell.Roy.Soc.* 1985, *31:*173-96.

FAIRLEY, SIR NEIL HAMILTON (1891-1966); FRS 1942

Assistant Physician, Hospital for Tropical Diseases, and Lecturer, LSHTM, 1929-40; Wellcome Chair of Tropical Medicine 1946-50.

Born in Australia, one of 4 surviving sons, all with medical qualifications, of a family originally from Lanarkshire, Neil Hamilton Fairley qualified at Melbourne University in 1915. At Melbourne

Hospital in 1916 he witnessed an alarming, and well-nigh uncontrollable, outbreak of meningococcal meningitis in the armed forces, before sailing for Egypt with the 11th Australian General Hospital. There his wartime experiences included outbreaks of typhus fever and schistosomiasis, before in 1919 he left Cairo for London and the Lister Institute under C.J.Martin using his stay in England to gain the DPH, Cambridge, and the MRCP, London. Back in Australia in 1920 Fairley worked at the Walter and Eliza Hall Institute in Melbourne, interrupted by 3 years in Bombay, where he returned to schistosomiasis studies. In Bombay he also investigated cases of guinea-worm disease and tropical sprue, the ultimate case being his own, which forced him to return to Melbourne in 1925. In 1929 he resigned his appointments in Australia to join the LSHTM and the Hospital for Tropical Diseases. World War II saw Fairley's most distinguished contributions to medical science and to malaria research in the field: the setting up of research groups at Cairns, and convincing both authorities and serving personnel of the need for regular, daily, doses of atebrin as preventive medication. Back in London in 1946 Fairley took up the newly created Wellcome Chair of Tropical Medicine at the LSHTM, but was forced by illness to resign in 1950. Never recovering fully, he died at Sonning in 1966.

Sir John Boyd, 'Neil Hamilton Fairley 1891–1966', *Biogr.Mem.Fell.Roy.Soc.* 1966, *12:* 123–41.

FULTON, FORREST (1913–71)

Reader in Bacteriology and Immunology, LSHTM, 1949–59, when the title of Professor of Virology – the first in Britain – was conferred on him by the University of London.

Forrest Fulton came to medicine in an unorthodox way, having switched at Oxford from law to animal physiology, and then completed his education at the London Hospital graduating BM, B.Ch. in 1939. Joining the EPHLS he served his traineeship at Oxford and in 1942 became part of the staff of the NIMR at Hampstead. In 1949 Fulton was appointed to a readership in bacteriology and immunology at the LSHTM where, after vaccine work at the NIMR, he turned to the new discipline of virology, producing distinguished work on influenza and polio, particularly in the methodology of studies of the antigenicity and cytopathology of influenza and polio viruses. He was a gifted and conscientious teacher, appreciated by his students, but privately a lonely and withdrawn bachelor. His early untimely death was a loss to the School and to virology.

Brit.med.J. 1972,: 116; Lancet 1972, *i:*155.

GARNHAM, PERCY CYRIL CLAUDE (1901–94); FRS 1964

Reader in Medical Parasitology, LSHTM, 1947, then succeeding H.E.Shortt in Chair of Medical Parasitology and Head of Department in 1952. Retired as Professor Emeritus 1968.

Born in London, P.C.C.Garnham graduated MB BS from St.Bartholomew's Hospital in 1923, adding the DPH (London) the following year. He then joined the Colonial Medical Service and remained with it in Kenya, eventually as Provincial Medical Officer, for more than 20 years until 1947. His particular interests there ranged from the viral aetiologies of Rift Valley Fever and of Nairobi Sheep Disease, studied in cooperation with the service's Veterinary Department, and through bird malaria to monkey and human malaria. It was examination of a monkey liver there which first suggested to him the liver as the site for the exo-erythrocytic stages in human malaria which he later explored so successfully at the LSHTM. To his students and staff he could seem stern and detached, but his enthusiasm and encouragement never failed them – as witnessed by the career of R.Killick-Kendrick, who under his guidance rose through the ranks from junior technician in 1949 to research assistant, Ph.D. student, and finally colleague and friend. At the LSHTM his most notable research achievement was the elucidation of the pre-erythrocytic and exo-erythrocytic cycles in human malaria. His classic *Malaria Parasites and other Haemosporidia* was published in 1966. After final 'retirement' in 1980 Garnham, always fascinated by mysticism, worked on a book on Edgar Allan Poe which was nearing completion when he died on Christmas Day, 1994.

Obituary, *Trans.Roy.Soc.Trop.Med.Hyg.* 1995, *89:* 129–31, by J.R.Baker, P.E.C.Manson-Bahr, R.Lainson and R.Killick-Kendrick;

R.Lainson and R.Killick-Kendrick, 'Percy Cyril Claude Garnham CMG. 15 January 1901–25 December 1994', *Biogr.Mem.Fell.Roy.Soc.* 1997, *43:* 171–92.

GILLETT, JOHN DAVID (1913-95)

Laboratory assistant, LSHTM, 1930-6; Senior Research Fellow, 1978-93.

J.D.(David)Gillett's unorthodox career began when he left Grammar School in Walthamstow at the age of 17 with no qualifications, but with an abiding interest in insects, instilled in him by his father. Through membership of the London Natural History Society he was introduced to Buxton and to a lowly job tending the department's insect colonies, at 75 pence a week. From there he rose to work with Wigglesworth, and eventually on to important work in Uganda's Medical Department for 26 years. In 1962 Gillett returned to Britain, appointed to the Chair of Applied Biology at Brunel University. After retirement from Brunel in 1978, he worked as Senior Research Fellow, with MRC support, back at the LSHTM, until shortly before his death.

'Biography of John David Gillet, OBE, D.Sc.', *Mosquito Systematics* 1984, *16*:317-28;
The Times obituary, 10 November 1995.

GREENWOOD, MAJOR (1880-1949); FRS 1928

First Professor of Epidemiology and Vital Statistics, LSHTM, 1927-45; Acting Dean 1943-5.

The 3rd generation and only surviving son in a family of East End General Practitioners, Major Greenwood was expected to follow suit, but was rescued for medical research by the physiologist Sir Leonard Hill, father of Bradford Hill. Trained in the laboratories of Hill, and instructed in biometry and statistics by Karl Pearson, Greenwood developed – 'humanised' it has been said – Karl Pearson's rigorous mathematical logic in a way which made medical statistics acceptable to a previously hostile and uncomprehending medical profession. In 1910 he became medical statistician to the Lister Institute; after the end of the Great War, working for the MRC, he was appointed the first senior medical statistician to the new (1919) Ministry of Health. Having already collaborated with W.W.C.Topley on MRC sponsored studies in experimental epidemiology, their collaboration continued when, in 1927, both men were appointed to new chairs in the new LSHTM, where singly and together they left their marks on the School, its teaching and its research between the wars.

Obituary by Lancelot Hogben in *Obit.Not.Fell.Roy.Soc.* 1950–1, 7:139–54.

HAMILTON, PATRICK JOHN SINCLAIR (1934–88)

Joined D.D.Reid's epidemiology department at the LSHTM in 1966 and became Head of the new Tropical Epidemiology Unit in 1971–5; after experience with the WHO in Trinidad he returned to the LSHTM as Head of the new large Department of Community Health 1982–8.

Having studied at Cambridge and Edinburgh Patrick Hamilton graduated in medicine in 1958 and early acquired an interest in tropical medicine during military service in Nepal. Having worked in a leprosy hospital in West Bengal and lectured in medicine at Makerere, Uganda, he came to the LSHTM and Donald Reid's department in 1966, soon demonstrating his talents for epidemiology and for organisation of research in the realisation of the Whitehall study of cardio-respiratory disease. In 1971 he became the first Head of the new Tropical Epidemiology Unit at the School, followed in 1975 by his appointment to the WHO's first Caribbean Epidemiology Center in Trinidad. From there he returned to the LSHTM in 1982, as Professor of Community Health and Head of the Department of Community Health; among his achievements here were moves to revitalise the School's links with the NHS. His untimely death at the age of 53 occurred in West Africa where he had gone, against medical advice, to honour a commitment to the WHO Onchocerciasis Control Programme.

Obituaries: *Lancet* 1988, i:1469; *Br.med.J.* 1988, ii:297; 550.
LSHTM *Annual Report* 1987–8, p.8.

HILL, SIR AUSTIN BRADFORD (1897-1991), FRS 1954

Reader in Epidemiology and Vital Statistics, LSHTM, 1933-45, Professor of Medical Statistics, LSHTM, and Honorary Director of the MRC's Statistical Research Unit, 1945-61; 'acting' Dean, then Dean, LSHTM, 1955-7.

The 3rd son of the physiologist Sir Leonard Erskine Hill, FRS, Austin Bradford Hill was destined for the study of medicine when, as a pilot in the Great War, he was invalided out of the forces with near fatal tuberculosis while serving at Gallipoli in the Dardanelles campaign. Recovering at home against the odds, he took an external London degree in economics and, encouraged by the family friend Major Greenwood, began statistical studies for the MRC in 1923. Moving with Greenwood to the new LSHTM in 1927, he became Reader in Epidemiology and Vital Statistics in 1933. In 1937 was published the first edition of his *Principles of Medical Statistics,* a textbook which has influenced generations of medical statisticians and epidemiologists at home and abroad, and left its mark on the development of medical science in the 2nd half of the twentieth century, as have his seminal studies on carcinogenic effects of smoking (with Sir Richard Doll), and on the use of randomisation in clinical trials of new drugs.

Obituary by Sir Richard Doll in *Biogr.Mem.Fell.Roy.Soc.* 1994, *40:*129-40.

HINDLE, EDWARD (1886-1973); FRS 1942

Milner Research Fellow, LSHTM 1924-5. While Regius Professor of Zoology at Glasgow taught D.B.Bertram and W.H.R.Lumsden who both later held chairs at LSHTM.

Born in Sheffield and largely educated at home by his mother, Hindle won a scholarship to the Royal College of Science (Imperial College) in 1903, graduating in zoology in 1906. After a year at Liverpool School of Tropical Medicine he spent a couple of years in California, obtaining a Ph.D. at Berkeley in 1910, and back home adding the Natural Science Tripos at Cambridge. Active in both world wars, Hindle was early committed to tropical research since his work at Liverpool on trypanosomes, also the subject of his thesis at Berkeley and his work at

Cambridge under G.H.F.Nuttall. After service in the Royal Engineers in the Great War Hindle was appointed Professor of Biology at the School of Medicine in Cairo followed by a year as Milner Research Fellow, LSHTM 1924-5, and subsequently leading the Royal Society's Kala-Azar Commission in China. His last venture into active research, before he became enmeshed in administration as Regius Professor of Zoology at Glasgow, saw him change in 1928 to virus research at the Wellcome Bureau of Scientific Research, whose director was then C.M.Wenyon. Here he made fundamental discoveries on yellow fever vaccine in monkeys and man, less than 10 years later developed in mouse tissue culture by Max Theiler.

P.C.C.Garnham, 'Edward Hindle 1886-1973', *Biogr.Mem.Fell.Roy.Soc.* 1974, *20:*217-34.

HINDS, STUART WILLIAM (1916-83)

Reader in Public Health LSHTM 1956-67.

Born in what was then Northern Rhodesia, Stuart Hinds was educated at the King's School, Canterbury, and qualified from Guy's Hospital in 1939. In World War II he served with the RAF in North Africa. After the war he was lecturer in Child Health at, successively, Hammersmith Hospital and Bristol. A great interest in preventive medicine led to an appointment as Reader in Public Health at the LSHTM in 1956; work which he enjoyed, although he was perhaps happier in his friendly relations with overseas postgraduate students than in day-to-day exchanges with colleagues within the department, where his relations with W.S.Walton steadily deteriorated. In 1960 he was seconded to WHO, reporting on conditions and health services in Eastern Turkey. Retiring from the School in 1967 he left for appointments in child health and public health at the Universities of Michigan and Texas.

Lancet obituary 1983, *i:*136.

JAMESON, SIR (WILLIAM) WILSON (1885-1962)

First Professor of Public Health and Director of the Division of Public Health, LSHTM, 1929-40; simultaneously Dean of the School following the death of Balfour.

Educated at Aberdeen University and University College London Wilson Jameson graduated in arts at Aberdeen in 1905 and qualified MB Ch.B. at Marischal College in 1909. After resident posts in London Hospitals he obtained the DPH in 1914. Henry Kenwood, on the lookout for talent for his department as Professor of Hygiene at UCL appointed him assistant lecturer in the same year; the two men then shared academic and wartime duties throughout the Great War. Jameson served in France, Italy, and at Aldershot as Specialist Sanitary Officer in the RAMC, deputising in between in teaching duties and the running of the department for Kenwood during the latter's absences serving with the Army Medical Advisory Board. Demobilised in 1919, Jameson then spent almost 10 years as MOH in Finchley and St.Marylebone, and writing *Synopsis of Hygiene* (1st ed. 1920). Appointed to the new Chair of Public Health at the LSHTM with effect from January 1st, 1929, he managed his new responsibilities as Professor, Head of the Division, and Dean of the School with the consummate skill and tact needed within the new School, until World War II called him to other duties as Chief Medical Officer to the Ministry of Health in 1940. His further very distinguished career included decisive influence on the creation of the NHS through his links with the Ministry of Health and the Ministry of Education.

Neville M.Goodman, *Wilson Jameson, Architect of National Health*, London, Allen and Unwin, 1970.

KILPATRICK, SIR JAMES (MacCONNEL), (1902-60)

Dean of the LSHTM 1957-60.

Born and educated in Belfast, Kilpatrick graduated MB from Queen's University in 1924, and joined the RAF the following year, an obvious candidate for its medical branch. Working at home and abroad, he was interested in pathology and tropical medicine, and eventually turned to physiological aspects of aviation medicine. During World War II his work contributed substantially to improved hygiene and sanitary practices at RAF units everywhere; in the later stages of the war he successfully reduced incidence of disease in West Africa as RAF principal medical officer. In 1951 he was appointed Director-General of the RAF's medical services, a position he held until he was called to be the Dean of the LSHTM in 1957, following Topping's death in office and Bradford Hill's temporary deanship. Unhappily Kilpatrick himself died in office after only 3 years, respected by staff and students but denied the time to make a lasting impression as Dean.

Obituaries: *Lancet* 1960, *i*:884–5; *Br.med.J.* 1960, *i*:1211–12.

LEIPER, ROBERT THOMSON (1881–1969); FRS 1923.

Helminthologist, London School of Tropical Medicine 1905–24 (Wandsworth Scholar 1912–14); University Professor 1920, and Courtauld Professor of Helminthology and Director of the Department of Parasitology LSHTM, including Winches Farm, 1924–46.

Born in Kilmarnock where Leipers had farmed for generations, R.T.Leiper moved with his family to Warwick at an early age. The death of his father from tuberculosis, when no therapy was available when Robert Leiper was 14, affected him greatly and by his own admission turned him to medical science rather than clinical practice. He showed great promise in his medical studies at Glasgow and in 1902 was awarded 2 resident scholarships before graduating MB, Ch.B. (Glasgow) in 1904. A year later Patrick Manson recruited him as helminthologist for his new Tropical School. Until his death 64 years later Leiper was connected with the School, before and after 'retirement', playing an important role in the politics of transformation of Manson's School into the LSHTM both before and after World War I. In the early years at the School he travelled extensively, making essential contributions to the knowledge of a number of helminths and their life-cycles, and in 1923 he founded the *Journal of Helminthology* and began planning the Institute of Agricultural Parasitology at Winches Farm near St.Albans. Active long after normal retirement age Leiper was acknowledged by colleagues as the man who put helminthology on the map in the twentieth century.

P.C.C.Garnham, 'Robert Thomson Leiper 1881–1969', *Biogr.Mem.Fell.Roy.Soc.* 1970, *16:* 385–404;

Sheila Willmott, 'Centenary biographical note: Robert Thomson Leiper, 1881-1969', *Internat.J.Parasit.* 1982, *11*:423-4.

LOVELL, SIR FRANCIS (HENRY), (1844-1916)

First Dean of the London School of Tropical Medicine 1903-16.

Born in Bedfordshire and educated at St.Bartholomew's Hospital, Francis Lovell became MRCS in 1865 and LSA 2 years later. From 1873 to 1878 he was colonial surgeon in Sierra Leone, and from 1878-93 chief medical officer and president of the General Board of Health in Mauritius. He was then appointed surgeon-general of Trinidad and Tobago, serving there until retirement from the Colonial Service in 1901. Back in London he became involved with Manson's new School, travelling far and wide raising funds in cash and subscriptions throughout the Far East and Canada. In 1903 he was elected Dean of the School; and by a felicitous mixture of modesty and courtesy with force of character he continued to serve the School's development and its fund-raising activities with success until his death.

Obituaries: *Lancet* 1916, *i*:319; *Br.med.J.* 1916, *i*:221-2.

BIOGRAPHICAL APPENDIX A

LOW, GEORGE CARMICHAEL (1872–1952)

Associated with Manson's School from November, 1899, Low was among the 2nd intake of students in January, 1900. He was Cragg's Research Scholar 1901–2, Superintendent of the School 1903–5. In July, 1910, he became lecturer at Manson's School and from 1912 Assistant Physician, then full physician and finally Senior Physician to the Albert Dock Hospital. After the Great War he moved with the Hospital for Tropical Diseases to Endsleigh Gardens and became Director of the Division of Tropical Medicine, LSHTM, until retirement in 1937.

One of the many younger fellow Scots who joined Manson at the London School, Low was among the second batch of students gaining the diploma in 1900. As Manson's research associate he demonstrated the passage of filariae along the mosquito proboscis and their entry into the human host via the bite. He took part in the crucial Roman Campagna demonstration in the Ostia mosquito-proof hut where *Plasmodium vivax* malaria was endemic. Travelling widely in the Caribbean and in Africa, on London School and Royal Society expeditions, Low made very considerable contributions to tropical medicine, always in close touch with Manson in the early years. A founder member of the (Royal) Society of Tropical Medicine and Hygiene in 1907, and superintendent, and later senior physician at the Hospital for Tropical Diseases, Low played a key role in both the Society, the HTD, and the School. As physician in ordinary to George V he was present as the King's life was 'moving peacefully to it's close', and possibly assisted in cutting short the painful last hours.

G.C.Cook, 'George Carmichael Low FRCP: twelfth President of the Society and underrated pioneer of tropical medicine', *Trans.Roy.Soc.Trop.Med.Hyg.* 1993, *87:*355–60;

N.H.F., 'George Carmichael Low', *Trans.Roy.Soc.Trop.Med.Hyg.* 1952, *46:*571–3.

MACDONALD, GEORGE (1903-67)

Professor of Tropical Hygiene and Director of the Ross Institute, LSHTM, 1945-67.

The son of J.Smyth Macdonald, professor of physiology, George Macdonald graduated MB, Ch.B. at Liverpool in 1924, and adding the DPH in the same year; from 1925 to 1929 he was then research assistant at the Sir Alfred Lewis Jones Laboratories in Freetown, Sierra Leone, followed by 2 years as research officer to the Malaria Survey of India. He returned to England in 1931 to take his MD (Liverpool) and the DPH (London) in 1932; he then moved back to India as Principal Medical Officer to the tea estates of the Mariani Medical Association in Assam. His work there caught the attention of Sir Malcolm Watson, who recruited him as Assistant Director of the Ross Institute in 1937, an appointment which involved serving in Ceylon (Sri Lanka) as malariologist to the Malaria Control Scheme of the tea and rubber estates. At the outbreak of war in 1939 his commission in the RAMC led to command of the 1st Malaria Field Laboratory in the Middle East. Later he was adviser to Montgomery during the allied armies' advance through North Africa and Sicily into Italy. In 1945 he returned to teach tropical hygiene at the Ross Institute, where in 1947 he succeeded Watson (who had retired in 1942) as Director. At the same time he was appointed the first Professor of Tropical Hygiene (University of London) at the LSHTM. A member of the WHO expert panel on malaria, Macdonald's strong character and convictions made him an uncompromising opponent in scientific discussions, and he had his enemies within the School; but he was internationally respected and commanded affection as well as loyalty from his own staff. Even during his last year of advancing illness he carried on with research and teaching until his death in December, 1967. His classic book *Epidemiology and Control of Malaria* was published in 1957.

L.J.Bruce-Chwatt, 'Professor George Macdonald, 1903-67', *in: Dynamics of Tropical Disease,* L.J.Bruce-Chwatt and V.J.Glanville (eds), Oxford University Press, 1973, pp.3-4.

BIOGRAPHICAL APPENDIX A

McDONALD, WILLIAM ARTHUR (1895-1941)

Laboratory Assistant to Alcock, 1912-15; then with Leiper in Egypt and chief technician in helminthology and parasitology until 1941.

Came as laboratory assistant to A.W.Alcock 1912-15; then as Sergeant, RAMC, assisting Leiper in Egypt 1915-16, and staying on as Leiper's chief assistant and technician in helminthology and parasitology, at home and on expeditions, until his sudden and unexpected death in 1941. He developed the McDonald pipette, used universally in parasitological laboratories.

P.Manson-Bahr's *History of the School of Tropical Medicine in London*, pp.245-6.

MACKAY, DONALD MILLER (1920-81)

Principal of the East Pakistan branch of the Ross Institute 1959-73; Senior Lecturer and Deputy Director of the Ross Institute, LSHTM, 1973-81.

Born and educated in Glasgow MacKay graduated in 1943 as the year's most distinguished graduate. A year later he entered the Colonial Service in Northern Rhodesia, moving to Ghana in 1954, there combining duties of Government medical officer with those of medical officer to a large gold mine. Another move in 1959 took him to East Pakistan (Bangladesh), where he became principal of the local branch of the Ross Institute. In 1973 he returned to London as senior lecturer and deputy director of the Ross Institute at the LSHTM. His wide range of work also included editorship of 3 medical journals, and involvement in the Royal Institute of Public Health and Hygiene's own diploma course in public health.

Obituaries: *Lancet* 1981, *ii:*482-3; *Br.med.J.* 1981, *283:*738.

MACKAY, ROBERT (1885-1928)

Manson's 'lab-boy' at the Albert Dock, 1899-1928.

A 'cockney waif of remote Scottish ancestry thrown up by the back streets of London' (according to Sir Philip Manson-Bahr), dwarfed and a hunchback, but highly intelligent, Robert MacKay became Manson's indispensable 'lab-boy' in 1899. In time he became more of a homegrown personal assistant and technician, an expert with the microtome and a superior microscopist. When the School moved to Endsleigh Gardens in 1920 (after Manson's retirement), he carried on alone in the laboratory at the Albert Dock until, in 1928, he was killed in an accident at the gates of the Albert Dock Hospital.

Manson-Bahr's *History of the School....,* pp.243-5.

MACKINTOSH, JAMES MACALISTER (1891-1966)

Professor of Public Health LSHTM 1944-56; Dean 1945-50.

Born in Kilmarnock, J.M.Mackintosh graduated MA from Glasgow University in 1911, before his subsequent medical studies were interrupted by service in France with the 6th Cameron Highlanders in 1914. Wounded, he returned to Britain to graduate MB Ch.B. in 1916. Back in France he then served as Captain in the RAMC from 1917 to 1920. Having obtained the DPH he then began what the *Lancet* called 'the peripatetic career pattern of the health officer of those days': Assistant Health Officer for Dorset, 1920-4; Burton-on-Trent, 1924-6; Leicestershire 1926-30 (in 1929 he somehow found the time to qualify as a barrister at Gray's Inn). Between 1930 and 1937 he was County MOH for Northamptonshire, where he pursued his abiding interest in sanitation and social problems related to rural housing, always much in demand with his gift for public speaking. Appointed Chief Medical Officer in the Scottish Department of Health in 1937, he found life as a civil servant a disappointing experience, and it was with a measure of relief that he accepted the Chair of Public Health in his old university at Glasgow in 1941. In 1944 he moved south to the University of London to fill the Chair of Public Health at the LSHTM, vacant since Wilson Jameson's wartime departure for the Ministry of Health in 1940, and to take over the deanship of the School. It then fell to him to rebuild the Department of Public Health, its fabric ruined by enemy bombs, its teaching having been in abeyance throughout the war. This he did with consummate skill, liked and respected within and without the School, and also abroad for his work for the WHO.

Obituaries: *Br.med.J.* 1966 *i*:1118–19; *Lancet* 1966, *i*:988–90.

MANSON, SIR PATRICK (1844–1922); FRS 1900

Founder of the London School of Tropical Medicine at the Albert Dock, and of Tropical Medicine as an academic discipline.

Born into a large well-to-do family near Aberdeen, Patrick Manson's practical skills and family connections led to apprenticeship in a firm of ironmasters when he left school. But heavy manual labour proved too much for a not robust physique, and Manson took up the study of medicine at Aberdeen University, graduating in 1865. The following year he became MO for Formosa (Taiwan) in the service of the Chinese Imperial Maritime Customs, arriving at Takao (Kaohsiung) in June 1866. For 5 years there, and subsequently 3½ years at Amoy on mainland China, his light duties allowed him to work in local missionary hospitals, in contact with Chinese patients and their diseases – becoming distressingly aware of the shortcomings of British medical training when faced with tropical diseases. Armed with a microscope acquired on leave in London in 1875, he was able to extend his painstaking studies of filarial larvae and the mosquitoes transmitting the infections. Seminal papers were published in 1877 and 1878. In 1883 Manson left Amoy and the Imperial Customs Service for private practice in Hong Kong, where he was joined 4 years later by James Cantlie. Inspired by Manson's 'applied science in the practice of medicine' Cantlie also saw the need for a medical college in Hong Kong to train young Chinese in 'Western' medicine. With the help of Manson, who was trusted by both the Chinese and the European communities, the College – forerunner of the University of Hong Kong – opened in 1887. By then Manson's health was deteriorating, and in 1889 he sailed for home and retirement. Only a year later he was thrust back into action when what had seemed a comfortable retirement fortune was decimated by a sharp fall in the value of the Chinese dollar. Manson went back to practice in London; became physician to the Seamen's Hospital Society; medical adviser to Chamberlain's Colonial Office; and spokesman for education in tropical medicine. In 1899 the Liverpool and London tropical schools opened. From then on Manson worked, nominally as Lecturer but in reality as the founder and prime mover within the London School until, again in poor health, he retired in 1912. But he never ceased to take an interest in the life of the School, and in the development of the academic discipline of tropical medicine and its sub-disciplines which he had founded. He died in 1922, a week after he had given his final blessing to his School's imminent transformation into the LSHTM.

Sir Ian A.McGregor, 'Patrick Manson 1844–1922: the birth of the science of tropical medicine', (3rd Manson Oration), *Trans.Roy.Soc.Trop.Med.Hyg.* 1995, *89:*1–8;

P.H.Manson-Bahr and A.Alcock, *The life and work of Sir Patrick Manson,* London, Cassell & Co.Ltd, 1927.

MANSON-BAHR, SIR PHILIP (HENRY), (1881–1966)

Lecturer at Manson's School at the Albert Dock from 1919, and Senior Physician to the HTD in Endsleigh Gardens and Director of Clinical Studies, LSHTM, 1937–47.

Philip Henry Bahr was born in Liverpool and educated at Rugby and Trinity College, Cambridge, where he specialised in zoology. Having qualified at the London Hospital in 1907 he married Manson's daughter, changed his name to Manson-Bahr, and devoted the rest of his career to tropical medicine. Having studied filariasis in Fiji at the instigation of Manson, he worked on malaria and sprue – a life-long interest – in Ceylon (Sri Lanka) before 1914. In the Great War he served with the RAMC in the Middle East and Egypt, where with Hamilton Fairley he worked on schistosomiasis. He was also instrumental in establishing Malaria Diagnosis Stations in forward areas during the war. After demobilisation he was appointed lecturer at Manson's School, and later Senior Physician at the HTD and Director of Clinical Studies at the LSHTM 1937–47. Up until his death he also worked tirelessly as editor of successive editions of *Manson's Tropical Diseases,* work later followed up by his eldest son, Clinton Manson-Bahr.

Obituaries: *Lancet* 1966, *ii:*1198–9; *Br.med.J.* 1966, *ii:*1332; 1397; 1461; *Trans.Roy.Soc.Trop.Med.Hyg.* 1966, *60:*815–16.

MICHELLI, SIR (PIETRO) JAMES (1853–1935)

Secretary to the Seaman's Hospital Society, Greenwich, 1887–1927,

and to the London School of Tropical Medicine 1899–1924.

Born and brought up in Ireland in a continental family settled in Cork, where his father was Austrian Consul, James Michelli became involved in hospital administration in London as Secretary to St.Mary's Hospital between 1882 and 1887. In 1887 he transferred to the Seamen's Hospital Society at Greenwich, where his contributions gave new life to the Society's development and its responsibilities for its hospital and the branch hospital across the Thames at the Albert Dock. In this capacity he was of invaluable help to Manson and Chamberlain in the development of the London School; he was Secretary to the School from 1899–1924, when the School and the Seamen's Hospital parted ways. In the early days Michelli was responsible for raising funds for the Chamberlain and the Milner scholarships at the School.

Obituaries: *Lancet* 1935, *i:*874; *Br.med.J.* 1935, *i:*808.

MURGATROYD, FREDERICK (1902–51)

Lecturer in Clinical Tropical Medicine, LSHTM, and assistant physician, HTD, 1937–9; 1950–1 Professor of Clinical Tropical Medicine and Director of Department, LSHTM.

Having graduated MB Ch.B. at Liverpool in 1926 Murgatroyd was persuaded by Warrington Yorke to turn to tropical medicine. He was appointed lecturer in protozoology at the Liverpool School in 1927. Working closely with Warrington Yorke on the action of drugs against sleeping sickness he was seconded to the Gambia as the MRC's first senior research fellow in tropical medicine in 1936. The following year he was appointed lecturer in clinical tropical medicine at the LSHTM, and physician to the HTD, serving also the Albert Dock Hospital and the Dreadnought Hospital at Greenwich. During World War II he served in the RAMC in France and West Africa. Returning to London he found clinical facilities reduced during the war years. He was determined to restore them to former standards and lived, but only just, to see the fruits of his labours when, succeeding Hamilton Fairley as Professor of Clinical Tropical Medicine in 1950 he could move his unit into the new HTD at St.Pancras. His tireless and many-sided work in tropical medicine took its toll when, only 14 months after taking over the Chair, he collapsed and died in December 1951.

Obituaries: *Lancet* 1951, *ii*:1229; *Br.med.J.* 1951, *ii*:1586-7.

NAIRNE, SIR PERCEVAL ALLEYN (1841-1921)

Chairman of the Seamen's Hospital Society and the London School of Tropical Medicine in its early days.

As Chairman of the Seamen's Hospital Society Nairne played an essential part in the planning and later in the management of the London School of Tropical Medicine. By profession a prominent solicitor, Nairne as a bachelor with a strong sense of duty and dedication to charitable causes concentrated his energies on the Seamen's Hospital Society (SHS) and Manson's School. The Nairne family has a long association with the SHS: Sir Perceval Nairne's father, Captain Alexander Nairne, RN, became a member of its Committee of Management in 1836; the present Chairman, since 1978, is Sir Patrick Nairne.

Manson-Bahr's *History ....*, pp.125-6.

NEWHAM, HUGH BASIL GREAVES (1874-1959)

Director and Superintendent of the Tropical School from 1910; after the School's move to Endsleigh Gardens and eventually to Keppel Street, Director of the Museum and its teaching collections until retirement in 1938.

Born in Winslow, Bucks., where his father was a practising family doctor, Basil Newham qualified from St.Thomas's Hospital in 1898. Interested in the emerging specialty of tropical medicine after clinical experience in the Far East and in British Guiana, he joined Manson's School at the Albert Dock in 1906. In 1910 he succeeded his friend C.W.Daniel as director and superintendent, working hard at administration and teaching. During the Great War he served as consultant in East Africa. After the war he moved with the School to Endsleigh Gardens, and eventually to the LSHTM in Keppel Street as director of the museum and its teaching collections. He retired in 1938.

Obituary: *Lancet* 1959, *ii*:978; 1096.

BIOGRAPHICAL APPENDIX A

PARKINSON, GEORGE SINGLETON (1880-1953)

Assistant Director, Department (Division) of Public Health 1928-40; 'acting Dean' and then Dean, 1940-3.

From Bath College the young Parkinson went to fight in the South African War. Qualifying at Bristol in 1906 he joined the RAMC, taking the DPH in 1913, and serving in France and Belgium during the Great War. Via Gibraltar and the Royal Army Medical College he came to Wilson Jameson's department at the fledgling LSHTM in 1928, where according to Jameson he was a 'tower of strength' to staff and DPH students alike. At the outbreak of World War II he again joined the RAMC, thus earning the distinction of having served in 3 major wars. He served as dean from 1940 to 1943, when he was appointed director of the Public Health subcommission in North Africa.

Obituaries: *Br.med.J.* 1953, *ii:*513-14; *Lancet,* 1953, *ii:*457.

PLATT, BENJAMIN STANLEY (1903-69)

Professor of Nutrition and Head of Department of Human Nutrition LSHTM 1946-69.

A Yorkshireman educated at Liverpool, B.S.Platt graduated B.Sc. in chemistry in 1923 and, after a period working in medical research, MB Ch.B. in 1930. In 1932 he went to the Henry Lester Institute for Medical Research in Shanghai, where his work with G.D.Lu had important results for the understanding and treatment of beri-beri. In 1938 he joined the scientific staff of the MRC, and directed the nutrition survey unit in Nyasaland 1939-40. In 1944 he was appointed director of the MRC's new human nutrition research unit, which went with him when, as professor of nutrition and head of the department of human nutrition he came to the LSHTM in 1946. During World War II and after, Platt's passionate concern for those suffering from malnutrition in all parts of the world gave him a central position in international policy making within the UN, the WHO, and FAO.

Obituaries: *Br.med.J.* 1969, *ii:*243; 364; *Lancet* 1969, *ii:*224; 276.

RAISTRICK, HAROLD (1890-1971); FRS 1934

London University Chair of Biochemistry and Director of Division (Department) of Biochemistry and Chemistry as Applied to Hygiene LSHTM 1929-56.

Born in the West Riding of Yorkshire, Raistrick graduated in chemistry from Leeds University in 1912. The following year he was granted a 3-year Board of Agriculture and Fisheries Research Scholarship. Prevented by the outbreak of war from spending part of the time in Emil Fischer's laboratories in Berlin, and not eligible for war service because of physical disability, Raistrick worked until the end of 1920, with an added MRC grant, on the products of bacterial action under Gowland Hopkins. With a D.Sc. from Leeds in 1920, Raistrick was appointed in 1921 to lead a new department of applied biochemistry at the Ardeer factory of Nobel's Explosives Co. Here he began his studies of the microfungi, or moulds, and their products. His appointment as director of a new division of biochemistry and chemistry as applied to hygiene at the LSHTM in 1929 was largely a research position. Here Raistrick was able to continue his promising research on moulds, alas missing out on penicillin, in a department which also missed the opportunity of cooperation with other departments with biochemical interests. In the end he did, however, act as scientific adviser to the Ministry of Supply on penicillin production from 1944 to 1947. He was elected FRS in 1934, retired from the School in 1956, and died in 1971.

J.H.Birkinshaw, 'Harold Raistrick 1890-1971', *Biogr.Mem.Fell.Roy.Soc.* 1972, *18*:489-509.

REES, DAVID CHARLES (1868-1917)

First superintendent and Medical Tutor of the London School of Tropical Medicine, 1899 -1901.

D.C.Rees qualified from the Charing Cross Hospital Medical School and obtained the Conjoint Board Diploma in 1895; he then went to Nigeria with General Lugard's Frontier Force. He returned to London just as Manson's School was about to open, and was recruited by Manson to organise the course when the School's first session began on October 1st, 1899. He did this so capably that he was much missed by fellow teachers when at the end of 1901 he resigned in order to take up the post of district surgeon and port health officer at Port Elizabeth. Here he dealt with outbreaks of plague and smallpox until, ironically, he died of typhus fever while trying to stamp out the disease, in 1917.

Br.med.J. 1917, ii:469-70; Lancet 1917, ii:549.

REID, DONALD DARNLEY (1914-77)

Lecturer in Epidemiology LSHTM 1945-8; Reader in Epidemiology and Vital Statistics 1948-59; Professor or Epidemiology 1959-77; Director of Department of Medical Statistics and Epidemiology 1961-77.

Born in a Scottish fishing village, D.D.Reid qualified in medicine at Aberdeen in 1937. Joining the Royal Air Force Volunteer Service, he was drafted to Bomber Command in September 1939. Like many others, Reid was profoundly influenced by his war experience; in his case the psychological illnesses of aircrews sent on dangerous missions. His work in this area came to the attention of Bradford Hill, who after the end of the war recruited him to his department at the LSHTM, where he eventually succeeded Hill in 1961. His research ranged widely, from early psychiatric epidemiology to the cardio-respiratory disease epidemiology which occupied so many able minds at the School in his time. He was also outstanding as a teacher, training epidemiologists who flocked to the School from near and far. He worked hard and travelled widely, and his too early death at 63 was a loss to the School, and to the science and teaching of epidemiology.

Geoffrey Rose, 'Professor D.D.Reid', In: Donald Darnley Reid 1914-77, a memorial volume, LSHTM, 1979, pp.1-2; and J.Epid. & Community Health 1978, 32:229-30.

RENWICK, JAMES HARRISON (1926-94)

LSHTM: Reader in Human Genetics 1968-79; Professor of Human Genetics and Teratology 1979-91, and Head of Preventive Teratology Unit 1977-91.

Renwick qualified MB Ch.B. at St.Andrews in 1948, and obtained a Ph.D. at UCL in 1956, having begun work on genetic effects of the Hiroshima bomb while serving in the RAMC during the Korean war of 1950-3. He returned to his Scottish roots in the department of Human Genetics at the University of Glasgow in 1959, eventually as Professor of Human Genetics. In 1968 he moved to the LSHTM, where he became Head of a new Preventive Teratology Unit in 1977. His great interest in prevention of human congenital malformations led him in the late 1970s to enthusiastic pursuit of a favourite hypothesis linking congenital malformations to potato blight, a connection which has never been proved. Emeritus Professor since retirement in 1991, Renwick died in September 1994.

LSHTM *Annual Report* 1993-4, p.26; *The Times,* 18 October 1994.

ROGERS, SIR LEONARD (1868-1962); FRS 1916

Extra Physician to the HTD and Lecturer at the School 1921-31.

Born near Plymouth Hoe of Cornish parents, Leonard Rogers qualified in medicine from St.Mary's Hospital, London, in 1891 and entered the IMS in 1893. For nearly 30 years he remained in India. His contributions to research and innovations in therapy were many and wide ranging; in early years he cooperated with the veterinary services in controlling an outbreak of rinderpest. He introduced emetine as a treatment for amoebic dysentery, and famously, intravenous infusions of hypertonic saline (later with added sodium bicarbonate) in cholera. His work on kala-azar in Assam between 1896 and 1914 was stronger on epidemiology than on aetiology; in 1915 he showed the value of tartar emetic treatment against the disease, narrowly preceded by an Italian publication the previous February. The treatment of leprosy was also a life-long interest, and he founded the British Empire Leprosy Relief Association. His lasting monument is the School of Tropical Medicine in Calcutta which he built up, in the face of difficulties, over a period of 10 years; it opened in Calcutta in the year of his retirement from the IMS.

J.S.K.Boyd, 'Leonard Rogers 1868-1962', *Biogr.Mem.Fell.Roy.Soc.,* 1963, 9:261-85.

BIOGRAPHICAL APPENDIX A

ROSS, SIR RONALD (1857-1932); FRS 1901

Only peripherally connected to the School, through the early Manson connection and his nominal position as Director-in-Chief of the Ross Institute and its Hospital until his death, following which the Institute became part of the LSHTM.

Born in Nepal, 3 days after the outbreak of the great Indian Mutiny, Ross came of a family with a long history of service in India. Sent back to England for his education at the age of 8, he showed some artistic talent; but on leaving school he entered St.Bartholomew's Medical School at his father's express wish. Having qualified in 1881, he took a course at Netley and then immediately sailed for Bombay and the IMS. His interest in malaria research grew over the years, stimulated by Manson, and on August 20th 1897 ('Mosquito Day') he found 'pigmented cysts' in the gut wall of an *Anopheles* mosquito fed on malaria blood. His subsequent career included inspired work in mathematical epidemiology, acrimonious disputes with Manson and with Italian researchers, a Nobel Prize, and work for the Liverpool School. After the opening of the Ross Institute Ross himself was no longer in good health, suffering a stroke after a long Eastern tour. He never fully recovered, and was wheelchair bound in later years.

G.H.F.N.[Nuttall], 'Sir Ronald Ross 1857-1932', *Obit.Not.Fell.Roy.Soc.* 1932-5, *i*:108-15; *Br.med.J.* 1932, *ii*:609-11; *Lancet* 1932, *ii*:695-7.

SAMBON, LOUIS WESTENRA (1865-1931)

Associated with Manson from the early days of the Tropical School as its parasitologist, Sambon kept up the connection after Manson's death, lecturing at the LSHTM until his sudden death in Paris at the age of 65.

A colourful character of mixed European parentage, Sambon was educated at St.Bartholomew's Hospital and the University of Naples, where he graduated MD in 1891. By then he had already had experience, as a student, of control measures in a severe outbreak of cholera at Naples in 1884, which for him was an introduction to a lifetime's epidemiological studies of acute and chronic diseases. Settling in London he became a friend of Patrick Manson, and joined his School as parasitologist. With G.C.Low and the Italian artist Enzio Terzi he took part in the famous malaria experiment in the Roman Campagna at the turn of the century. An enthusiastic teacher and researcher, the results of his later attempts to prove parasitic origins of such different diseases as pellagra and cancer could not be established, although Sambon himself never lost faith in his theories. He died suddenly on a visit to Paris in August, 1931.

Obituaries: *Br.med.J.* 1931, *ii:*514–15; *Lancet* 1931, *ii:*613.

SANDWITH, FLEMING MANT (1853–1918)

Lecturer at Manson's School and Senior Physician to the Albert Dock Hospital, 1904–14.

Educated at Charterhouse and St.Thomas's Sandwith qualified in 1876 and added the LRCP in 1877. He served as ambulance-surgeon in the Turco-Serbian war of 1876, and in the Russo-Turkish campaign of 1877–8. In 1883 he was in Egypt helping to combat a cholera epidemic, and stayed on as vice-director of the Public Health Department of the Egyptian Government until 1885, when he was appointed Professor of Medicine in the Egyptian Medical School and physician to the Kasr-el-Ainy Hospital in Cairo. In 1900 he went as Senior Physician to the Imperial Yeomanry Hospital at Pretoria, where he served throughout the South African war. Subsequently settled in London he lectured on tropical diseases at St.Thomas's, and was recruited by Manson to his new School, as Senior Physician to the Albert Dock Hospital, in 1904. Maintaining a special interest in hookworm disease since his days in Egypt he became, with R.T.Leiper, an important influence in the School's interactions with the Rockefeller Foundation, which grew out of a shared concern with hookworm problems worldwide, and which ultimately led to the founding of the LSHTM. Never quite recovering from wartime stresses and strains in Africa, he died in enforced retirement in the South of England in 1918.

Obituary in *Br.med.J.* 1918, *i:*273.

BIOGRAPHICAL APPENDIX A

SCHILLING, RICHARD SELWYN, (1911–97)

LSHTM: Reader, then Professor of Occupational Health and Director of Unit 1956–76; Director, TUC Centenary Institute 1968–76.

Educ. St.Thomas's Hospital MS.
After house posts at St.Thomas's and Addenbrooke's Hospital, Cambridge, Schilling began his career in occupational health as Asst.Industrial MO at ICI (metals) in Birmingham, and became Medical Inspector of Factories 1939–42. During World War II he served as Captain in the RAMC in France and Belgium 1939–40, and as Secretary to the Industrial Health Research Board of the MRC 1942–6. From 1947 he was Reader in Occupational Health at Manchester University until he joined the LSHTM in 1956.
Publications: (ed) *Modern Trends in Occupational Health* 1960; (ed) *Occupational Health Practice* 1973, 2nd ed. 1980; etc.

SHORTT, HENRY EDWARD (1887–1987); FRS 1950

Appointed Reader in Medical Parasitology, LSHTM, 1938; after war interruption Professor of Medical Parasitology and Director of Department of Parasitology 1945–51. In 'retirement' continued working at Winches Farm.

Born in India of Scottish/Cornish parentage Shortt, like most expatriate children of that era, was sent home for schooling at an early age. When he was 9 his father died, and he was educated at the Inverness Royal Academy and the University of Aberdeen, where he qualified in 1910. A year later he passed into the IMS, serving it until 1939. On arrival in India he was posted to Benares in 1912, then on to Cawnpore and Kasauli where he met S.R.Christophers, with whom he was to collaborate in the Mesopotamia Expeditionary Force during World War I, and later at the Central Research Institute at Kasauli and at the Malaria Bureau. In 1935 Shortt was appointed Director of the King Institute of Preventive Medicine in Madras, responsible for the province's water supply, smallpox control, supply of antiserum against snake bite, etc. During this period he also worked on avian malaria, especially the wild reservoir of *Plasmodium gallinaceum* which tied in with his later contributions in his collaborations with Garnham. Another research interest was satisfied in his study of *Babesia canis,* begun with Christophers in India and continued in retirement at Winches Farm. His greatest achievements were his observations on the life-cycles of the parasites of leishmaniasis and of malaria. Having suffered and survived attacks of dysentery, ankylostomiasis, malaria and even bubonic plague in his early years in Mesopotamia and India, Shortt died at the age of 100 in 1987.

P.C.C.Garnham, 'Henry Edward Shortt 1887–1987', *Biogr.Mem.Fell.Roy.Soc.* 1988, *34:*715–51.

SIMPSON, SIR WILLIAM (JOHN RITCHIE) (1855–1931)

Lecturer on Tropical Hygiene at Manson's School 1899–1923; with Castellani campaigned to found the Ross Institute and its Hospital which opened at Putney in 1926.

Of Scottish descent, Simpson was orphaned at an early age and sent to school in Jersey. He graduated MB CM at Aberdeen in 1876 (MD 1880), and obtained the DPH at Cambridge. After a period as MOH in Aberdeen, Simpson became Calcutta's first MOH in 1886, and in 1898 was appointed to the Chair of Hygiene at King's College, London; he also lectured at Manson's School from its opening in 1899 until retirement from both appointments in 1923. Between 1923 and 1926 he worked with Castellani to found the Ross Institute at Putney. In addition to his academic appointments Simpson worked hard abroad, becoming an expert at control of epidemics, from dysentery, enteric fever, and bubonic plague in South Africa to plague and other public health problems from Singapore to Africa's Gold Coast. An admirer of Ross and his malaria control policies, Simpson was a tireless and unselfish partner in his and Castellani's efforts to found the Ross Institute.

Sir Ronald Ross, 'Sir William John Ritchie Simpson', *J.Trop.Med.Hyg.* 1931, *34:* 333–4; also *DNB* 1931–40, pp.812–13.

SMITH, CHARLES EDWARD GORDON (1924–91)

LSHTM: Senior Lecturer in Bacteriology 1957–61; Reader in Virology 1961–4; Dean 1971–89.

Born in Fife, Gordon Smith qualified MB Ch.B. at St.Andrews in 1947 and entered the Colonial Medical Service in 1948. He held clinical appointments in Malacca and Kuala Lumpur 1949–51, and became virologist at the Kuala Lumpur Institute for Medical Research 1952–7. He then moved to London and the LSHTM as Lecturer in Bacteriology, promoted to Reader in Virology in 1961. From 1964 to 1970 he served as Director of the Microbiological Research Establishment at Porton Down, before returning to the LSHTM as Dean. From 1972–89 he was also Chairman of the Board of the PHLS. His research was initially on leptospirosis in the tropics, and later particularly on tropical viruses transmitted by arthropods, within the rapidly growing field of arbovirology. As Dean Gordon Smith saw the School through modernisation and restructuring in the early 1970s and, in the 1980s, through a second restructuring, under heavy financial pressure. He retired in 1989, and died in August, 1991.

LSHTM *Annual Report* 1900–91; *The Times*, 10 August 1991.

SPOONER, EDWARD TENNEY CASSWELL (1904–95)

LSHTM: Professor of Bacteriology and Immunology 1947–60; Dean 1960–70.

Born in Dorset and educated at Clare College Cambridge and St.Bartholomew's, Spooner qualified in 1927 and spent 2 years as a Commonwealth Fellow, 1929–31, at Harvard University, working with Zinsser in Bacteriology. He returned to Cambridge and the Department of Pathology in 1931. During World War II Spooner did outstanding work in the RAMC's Medical Research Section, particularly on streptococcal infections, until he was released to become Director of the EPHLS in Cambridge in 1943. In 1947 he was appointed Professor of Bacteriology and Immunology at the LSHTM, where he became Dean in 1960. As a member of the MRC from 1953 to 1957 he served on a number of its committees on viral diseases, among them poliomyelitis, polio vaccine, and trachoma. He also chaired the Colonial MRC's subcommittee on leprosy, and edited the *Journal of Hygiene* from 1949 to 1955.

The Times, 15 September 1995.

THOMSON, JOHN GORDON (1878-1937)

Professor of Protozoology and Director of the Department, LSHTM, 1918-37.

Born in Linlithgowshire, John Gordon Thomson graduated MA from Edinburgh University in 1903, and 5 years later qualified in medicine. After house appointments he went to Liverpool as research student in tropical medicine in 1910, becoming in 1912 pathologist to the Royal Southern Hospital and research fellow at the Liverpool School. With a Beit Memorial research fellowship he came to the London School as lecturer in 1914. In 1915 he went to Egypt with the RAMC; later in the war he and his brother, Dr.David Thomson, who had both enjoyed the patronage of Ronald Ross when they first came to Liverpool, worked at the War Office malaria research laboratories. After the war he was appointed to the Chair of Protozoology at the London School where he was a gifted teacher, maintaining a collection of cultures of trypanosomes and other pathological organisms and blood films for teaching purposes. At the same time he travelled abroad, on visits and expeditions, on malaria surveys and for the League of Nations.

Obituaries: *Br.med.J.* 1937, *ii:*394-5; *Lancet* 1937, *ii:*473.

TOPLEY, WILLIAM WHITEMAN CARLTON (1886-1944); FRS 1930

Professor of Bacteriology and Immunology, LSHTM, 1927-44.

Born in Lewisham, Topley graduated BA at St.John's College, Cambridge, in 1907, and qualified MB B.Ch. from St Thomas's Hospital in 1911. By then he was already an assistant director of the pathology department at Charing Cross Hospital. Always keen on research, wartime experience of a severe epidemic of typhus in Serbia turned his mind to epidemiology, and in 1922 he was appointed professor of bacteriology in the University of Manchester. By then, Topley was developing the study of experimental epidemiology, in which he came to rely on the statistical contributions of Major Greenwood; in 1927 both men were appointed to new chairs at the new LSHTM. Their collaboration and friendship continued throughout their time at the School, until the threat of war catapulted Topley into organising the EPHLS. With his younger friend and associate, Graham Wilson, Topley published in 1929 the first of many editions of their classic text, *Principles of Bacteriology and Immunity*. In 1941 he took over as Secretary to the Agricultural Research Council. War-time stress and a family history of coronary disease caused his sudden death in February 1944, 2 days after his 58th birthday.

M.Greenwood, 'William Whiteman Carlton Topley 1886–1944', *Obit.Not.Fell.Roy.Soc.* 1944, *4:* 699–712.

TOPPING, ANDREW (1890–1955); FRSE 1938

First full-time Dean of the LSHTM, 1950–5.

Born in Scotland, Andrew Topping took an MA degree at Aberdeen in 1911 and qualified MB Ch.B. on the eve of the Great War. Entering the RAMC he served in France, Gallipoli, and Mesopotamia, and after the war as senior medical officer with the Anglo-Persian Oil Co. at Abadan. Back in Britain he added the MD and DPH to his qualifications in 1923, and embarked on a career in public health and preventive medicine, first at Woolwich and then Lancashire, followed by a short but impressive period as MOH for Rochdale in 1930–2. In London from 1932 he served the LCC and its laboratory service, and during World War II was in charge of the ambulance service while lecturing on public health at Charing Cross. Later in the war he served as European Director of UNRRA. In November 1947 Topping was appointed Manchester's first professor of preventive and social medicine; 3 years later he returned to London as the LSHTM's first full-time Dean. In the few years left to him, he made innovations in teaching programmes in public health, introducing extensive fieldwork with outside communities and local authorities. His keen interest in the work of students past and present also led to the formation of the students' association, with regular reunions of former students from near and far. In 1954 Topping, as a member of the Colonial Medical Advisory Service, was seriously injured in a road accident in Africa. He never fully recovered, and died in August 1955.

Obituaries: *Br.med.J.* 1955, *ii:* 622–4; *Lancet* 1955, *ii:* 511–13; 568–9; LSHTM *Annual Report* 1954–5, p.15.

WALTON, WILLIAM STANLEY (1901-79)

Professor of Public Health, LSHTM, 1956-67.

The son of a headmaster of Gateshead Grammar School, Walton qualified in medicine at Durham in 1925. After public health appointments at Middlesbrough, Plymouth, and West Bromwich, he distinguished himself during World War II by conducting the evacuation of the West Bromwich and District Hospital under heavy assault from the air with incendiary and high explosive bombs. From 1946 he was MOH for Newcastle upon Tyne and lecturer in charge of the department of public health at Durham University. In 1956 he moved south to the London University chair of public health at the LSHTM. During a decade at the School, while not entirely happy personally within the department, Walton was popular with students and initiated a short course in medical administration for staff of regional hospital boards. His special interests were in child health; he served on WHO expert committees, and as adviser to schools of public health abroad.

Obituaries: *Br.med.J* 1979, *i:*1224; 1575; *Lancet* 1979; *i:*451; LSHTM *Annual Report* 1978-9, p.35.

WATSON, SIR MALCOLM (1873-1955)

Director, The Ross Institute of Tropical Hygiene, LSHTM, 1933-42.

Scottish born, Malcolm Watson graduated MB Ch.M. at Glasgow in 1895. After qualifying he set out for South Africa, Australia, Singapore, and the Philippines, and returned home with an abiding interest in tropical areas. Having gained the Cambridge DPH he joined the Malayan Medical Service in 1900. There he pioneered control measures based on Ross's recent discoveries in combating the then devastating malaria epidemics of the country. Within a few years Watson's policy succeeded in immeasurably improving the situation and Watson left Government service for tea estate practice. In 1928 he returned to London as director of the malarial control department of the Ross Institute at Putney, and between 1928 and 1929 created the Institute's India branch, an important part of its concerns, with new techniques for malaria control on tea estates and in other problem areas. When after Ross's death the Institute moved to the LSHTM, Watson remained its director and was appointed director of the School's Department of Tropical Hygiene. Here he built up the department while continuing to apply his principles of malaria control abroad, especially in the developing Rhodesian copper belt. Watson's *Prevention of Malaria in the Federated Malay States* was first published in 1911, and *Rural Sanitation in the Tropics* in 1915. *African Highway* is scientifically autobiographical.

Obituaries: *Br.med.J.* 1959, *i:*52–3; *Lancet* 1956, *i;* 57.

African Highway (1953) is a look back on past achievements.

WEINER, JOSEPH SIDNEY (1915–82)

LSHTM: Demonstrator, Department of Applied Physiology, 1940–1; Director of MRC Environmental Physiology Unit, 1963–80, and Professor of Environmental Physiology 1965–80.

Born in South Africa, Joseph Weiner read physiology, anatomy, and anthropology for a B.Sc. in 1934 at Witwatersrand University, and physiology for an M.Sc. in 1936. The following year he moved to Britain, joining the LSHTM's department of applied physiology 1940–1, and for the rest of the war the MRC unit at Queen Square. In 1947 he qualified MRCS, LRCP from St.George's, and was appointed reader in physical anthropology at Oxford. In 1963 he moved back to the LSHTM as director of the MRC Environmental Physiology Unit, and 2 years later he was appointed professor of environmental physiology, establishing links with Occupational Health. He also had a hand in setting up 2 new degrees at London University: an M.Sc. in ergonomics, and subsequently the M.Sc. in human and applied physiology.

Obituary: *Br.med.J.* 1982, *285:*982–3; LSHTM *Annual Report* 1981–2, pp.25–6.

WENYON, CHARLES MORLEY (1878–1948); FRS 1927

Head of Protozoology, London School of Tropical Medicine, 1905–14.

Born in Liverpool, C.M.Wenyon at the age of 2 went with his family to China, where his father was a pioneer medical missionary who established a hospital near Canton. Ten years later he was, with two siblings, sent back to school in Bath. On leaving school he studied zoology and physiology first at Leeds and later, from 1899, at UCL under E.A.Minchin and E.H.Starling, graduating B.Sc. with honours and entering Guy's Hospital Medical School with a scholarship in 1901. At Guy's he qualified in medicine, with honours and a Gold Medal in bacteriology in 1904. A year later he was appointed head of a new protozoology department at Manson's School. For the best part of 10 years Wenyon served the School in teaching, and in research carried out on expeditions abroad, in the Sudan, Baghdad, Syria, Malta, etc. On the eve of war in 1914, Wenyon resigned from his post at the School to join his old friend from days in the Sudan, Andrew Balfour, at the new Wellcome Bureau of Scientific Research. He was to continue this association for the rest of his life: in 1924 he succeeded Balfour as Director-in-Chief of the Wellcome Bureau for 20 years, retiring in 1944 but remaining a consultant until his death in October 1948.

Cecil A.Hoare 'Charles Morley Wenyon 1878–1948', *Obit.Not.Fell.Roy.Soc.* 1948–9, 6:627–42.

WIGGLESWORTH, SIR VINCENT (BRIAN) (1899–1994); FRS 1939

LSHTM: Lecturer in Medical Entomology 1926; Reader 1936–44.

A scholar at Caius College, Cambridge, Wigglesworth (V.B.W.), after a double first in the Natural Sciences Tripos, qualified in medicine at St.Thomas's in 1926, having just been offered a post as entomologist in Buxton's department at the LSHTM. Within a year he was off on an expedition to Nigeria, Ghana, and Sierra Leone, travelling by canoe in search of malaria, sleeping sickness, plague and finally yellow fever at the British Station in Accra. Having had 2 mosquitoes named after him, he went in 1935 to the Far East, and was present in Sri Lanka during the devastating malaria epidemic of 1935. At the School he was a model lecturer and, being ambidextrous, a particularly nimble insect physiologist at the microscope. By 1934 he had published *Insect Physiology*; 5 years later appeared the first of many editions of *Principles of Insect Physiology*. During World War II Wigglesworth was made Director of the Agricultural Research Council Unit of Insect Physiology; in 1945 he moved with it to Cambridge, as Reader in Entomology in the University. In 1952 he was appointed Quick Professor of Biology, retiring from the Chair in 1966, but continuing active in College and University for another more than 20 years.

Michael Locke, 'Sir Vincent Brian Wigglesworth 1899–1994', *Biogr.Mem.Fell.Roy.Soc.* 1996, *42:*539–53.

WILCOCKS, CHARLES (1896–1977)

Director, Bureau of Hygiene and Tropical Diseases 1942–61; Heath Clark Lecturer 1960; Member of Court of Governors, LSHTM, 1963–71.

A graduate of Manchester University Wilcocks served in the Great War in Egypt and the Palestine Campaign 1915–19 (wounded at Gaza 1917). Graduating MB Ch.B. in 1924 he then joined the East African Medical Service in 1927, becoming Tuberculosis Research Officer in Tanganyika in 1930. At the Bureau of Hygiene and Tropical Diseases (he took the DTM&H in 1941) from 1938, Wilcocks was its Director from 1942 to 1961. Closely involved with the School, he furthered friendly cooperation between School and Bureau in his time.

LSHTM *Annual Report* 1976–7, p.25.

WILSON, SIR GRAHAM (SELBY) (1895–1987); FRS 1978

LSHTM: Reader in Bacteriology 1927–30; Professor of Bacteriology as Applied to Hygiene, 1930–47.

Born in Newcastle upon Tyne, Graham Wilson moved south to Surrey with his family at the age of 6, and was educated in London, at King's College and Charing Cross Hospital Medical School, earning Gold Medals from both the University of London and Charing Cross in addition to his MB BS. He served with the RAMC 1916–20, and then embarked on an academic career, working under W.W.C.Topley both at Charing Cross and at Manchester. When Topley moved to the LSHTM in 1927 he took Wilson with him, insisting he be given a readership as they had then already embarked on the writing of their lasting classic *Principles of Bacteriology and Immunology* ('Topley and Wilson'), after many editions and changes of editors still in print as *Principles of Bacteriology, Virology and Immunity.* In 1930 Wilson was appointed to a personal chair of Bacteriology as Applied to Hygiene. During World War II he became involved, again with Topley, in the EPHLS; and in 1947 he left the School, but maintaining friendly relations, to concentrate on the Directorship of the post-war PHLS. His research ranged widely, from salmonellosis and brucellosis to human and bovine tuberculosis, milk hygiene, control of diphtheria, and typing of staphylococci. Elected FRS, in 1978, he died nine years later, at the age of 91.

E.S.Anderson and Sir Robert Williams, 'Graham Selby Wilson 1895-1987' *Biogr.Mem.Fell.Roy.Soc.* 1988, *34:*887-919.

WOODRUFF, ALAN WALLER (1916-92)

Senior Lecturer in Clinical Tropical Medicine, LSHTM 1948-52; Physician, HTD, and Wellcome Professor of Clinical Medicine LSHTM 1952-81.

Born in Scotland, A.W.Woodruff qualified MB BS from Durham University in 1939 (MD 1941). After House appointments in Newcastle upon Tyne he served in the RAFVR as MO and Medical Specialist in World War II. In 1946 he took the DTM&H at the School, and after another 2 years in Newcastle upon Tyne was ready to devote himself to tropical medicine at the LSHTM and the HTD, until he retired in 1981. During this time he also held a number of visiting professorships at universities in Egypt, Libya, Iraq, Uganda and Sudan. At home he became best known to the general public for his fierce denouncement of dogs in public parks, on the well-justified grounds of the danger of transmission, through dog faeces, of *toxocara* worms to playing children; the worms cause eye lesions and blindness in humans. His research interests also included anaemia, malaria and other parasitic diseases, and sprue. He published, with S.Bell, *A Synopsis of Infections and Tropical Diseases* in 1968 (3rd edition with S.G.Wright, 1987) and edited other texts. Immediately after retirement from the LSHTM Woodruff left to become professor of medicine at the University of Juba, Sudan, where he died of a heart attack in Khartoum in October, 1992.

Obituaries: *Trans.Roy.Soc.Trop.Med.Hyg.* 1993, *87:*129; *The Times,* 20 October 1992.

Current and recently retired Members of Staff of the School.

ACHESON, ROY MALCOLM, b.1921

LSHTM: Sen.Lect. then Reader, in Social and Preventive Medicine (jointly with Guy's HMS) 1959-62; Director, Centre for Extension in Community Medicine 1972-6.

Educ. Trinity College Dublin, then Brasenose College and Redcliffe Infirmary, Oxford; clinical and research posts, Oxford. Lecturer in Social Medicine, University of Dublin 1955-9; Assoc.Professor, then Professor of Epidemiology, Yale University 1962-7; and after LSHTM Professor of Community Medicine, University of Cambridge 1976-88.
Publications: *Seminars in Community Medicine* (joint ed) 1971 and 1976; *Health, Society and Medicine: an introduction to community medicine* (with S.Hagard) 1985; etc.

ARMITAGE, PETER, b.1924

LSHTM: MRC Statistical Research Unit 1947-61; Professor of Medical Statistics 1961-76.

Educ. Trinity College, Cambridge (Wrangler 1947).
Joined Ministry of Supply 1943-5, then National Physics Laboratory 1945-6. Left LSHTM to become Professor of Applied Statistics (formerly of Biomathematics) in the University of Oxford from 1976 until retirement in 1990.
Publications: *Sequential Medical Trials* 1960, 2nd ed.1975; *Statistical Methods in Medical Research* 1971, 3rd ed. 1994; etc.; papers in professional journals.

BLACK, NICHOLAS ANDREW, b.1951

LSHTM: Sen.Lect. in Public Health Medicine 1985-93; Head, Health Services Research Unit, Dept of Public Health and Policy 1988-93; Reader 1993-5; Professor of Health Services Research 1995-

Educ. Birmingham University and Medical School.

After house appointments in hospitals in Stafford, Warwick and Sheffield, Nick Black served for a year as MO for Save the Children Fund in Nepal, returning as registrar and then Senior Registrar in Community Medicine in Oxfordshire and the University of Oxford, before joining the LSHTM in 1985.

Publications: has written and edited a number of monographs, among them *The biology of health and disease 1985*, and *Caring for health: dilemmas and prospects,* 1985, as well as a number of chapters in edited works and numerous papers on aspects of health care and policy.

BRADLEY, DAVID JOHN, b.1937

LSHTM: Research for George Macdonald/Ross Institute in Africa in the 1960s; Professor of Tropical Hygiene and Director of the Ross Institute 1974–

Educ. Selwyn College, Cambridge, and UCHMS.
Bradley served for 3 years as Med.Res.Officer at the Ross Institute's Bilharzia Research Unit in Tanzania 1961–4, then lectured at Makerere University, Uganda, 1964–9. Back in England he spent 5 years in tropical research at Oxford (Sir William Dunn School of Pathology and Exeter College) before joining the LSHTM. He has served and serves as Director, WHO Collaborating Centre for Environmental Control of Vectors 1983– ; Member, WHO Expert Advisory Panel on Parasitic Diseases 1972– ; Technical Advisory Group, Diarrhoea Programme 1979–85; Panel of Experts on Env.Managem., 1981– ; External Review Group on Trop.Disease Programme, 1987; etc. Publications: (jointly) *Drawers of Water* 1972; *Sanitation and Disease* 1983; *The Impact of Development Policies on Health* 1990; etc.; and numerous papers in professional journals.

BRASS, WILLIAM, b.1921

LSHTM: Professor of Medical Demography 1972–88, and Director, Centre for Population Studies 1978–88 (Reader, Medical Demography 1965–72; Director of Centre for Overseas Population Studies 1974–8; Head, Department of Medical Statistics and Epidemiology 1977–82).

Educ. Edinburgh University.
Served as Scientific Officer, Royal Navy Scientific Service, 1943–6, then

in the East African Statistical Department of the Colonial Service 1948–55; Lecturer, then Sen.Lect., Aberdeen University 1955–64, before joining the LSHTM.
Publications: *The Demography of Tropical Africa* 1968; *Methods of Estimating Fertility and Mortality from Limited and Defective Data* 1975; *Advances in Methods for Estimating Fertility and Mortality from Limited and Defective Data* 1985; etc.

BUSVINE, JAMES RONALD, b.1912

LSHTM: Lecturer 1946; Reader 1954; Professor of Entomology as Applied to Hygiene 1964–76, Emeritus 1977.

Educ. Eastbourne College and Imperial College, London. Following three years with ICI and work on MRC grants 1940-2 became Entomological Adviser, Min.of Health, 1943–5 before joining the LSHTM in 1946. Member of WHO Panels on Insecticides and Pest Resistance.
Publications: *Insects and Hygiene 1951* (3rd ed.1980); *A Critical Review of the Techniques for Testing Insecticides* 1957 (2nd ed. 1971); *Arthropod Vectors of Disease 1975; Insects, Hygiene and History* 1976; *Discovery of Disease Transmission by Arthropods and 90 Years of Attempts to stop it* 1993; many papers in professional journals.

CAIRNCROSS, SANDY, b.1948

LSHTM: Res.Fell. 1976–7; Sen.Lect. in Trop.Health Engineering 1984–92; Reader in Environmental Health 1995– (from 1990 heading ODA funded Tropical Environmental Health Programme).

Educ. Cambridge University.
In 1974 Cairncross began a long period of involvement in environmental health projects in Africa teaching at the Min.of Works Technician Training School in Lesotho and as the Ministry's Resident Engineer for Water Supplies Construction. In 1982 he moved to Mozambique as Chief of the Studies and Projects Department of the Water Supply and Sanitation Management Board before returning to the LSHTM in 1984. From 1992 to 1995 he was Senior Project Officer for the UNICEF/WHO Dracunculiasis Eradication Programme, now within reach of a successful

conclusion.

COOK, GORDON CHARLES, b.1932

LSHTM: Sen.Lect. in Clinical Sciences and Hon.Consultant, HTD and UCL Hosp.s 1976-97.

Educ. Royal Free Hospital Sch.Med., London University.
After hospital appointments at the Royal Free, Hampstead General, Royal Northern, Brompton, and St.George's, 1958-63, Cook, commissioned RAMC, was seconded to the Royal Nigerian Army 1960-2. From 1963 to 1969 he was a Lecturer at the Royal Free HSM and Makerere University College in Uganda, subsequently serving as Professor of Medicine and Consulting Physician to the Universities of Zambia 1969-74, Riyadh 1974-5, Papua New Guinea 1978-81 (Sen.MO, MRC 1975-6). Other appointments include Hon.Sen.Lect.in Med., UCL, 1981-.
Publications: *Communicable and Tropical Diseases* 1988; *Parasitic Disease in Clinical Practice* 1990; *From the Greenwich Hulks to Old St.Pancras: a history of tropical diseases in London* 1992; *Manson's Tropical Diseases* (ed.), 20th ed., 1996, etc.; papers in professional journals (including historical).

CRAWFORD, DOROTHY HANSON, b.1945

LSHTM: Professor of Microbiology in Department of Clinical Sciences 1990-6.

Educ. St.Thomas's Hospital Medical School.
At UCHMS 1980-5 and at the RPGMS at Hammersmith 1985-90, Dorothy Crawford pursued an early and lasting interest in cell response to Epstein-Barr virus(EBV), pioneering along the way the production of clinically useful monoclonal antibodies such as the antibody to the Rhesus D antigen. She moved to the RPGMS in 1985 with a view to exploring molecular techniques used in the department of virology and applying them in her research. At the LSHTM she heads a number of groups studying EBV infection in immunocompromised hosts; herpes virus persistence in normal individuals; sources of EBV latency; and the use of the scid mouse model in such studies.
To her many papers on all these subjects in professional journals she has

recently added more popular articles in the *New Scientist* and elsewhere.

CURTIS, CHRIS F, b.1939

LSHTM: Research Fellow, Sen.Res.Fell., Ross Institute 1975–80, then moved to Dept. of Entomology with Davidson; Reader in Entomology 1988, Professor 1992.

Educ. University of Edinburgh.
With an early – and abiding – interest in chromosome translocation and the possibilities of genetic control of insect vectors, Curtis worked after graduation first in the tsetse research laboratories at Langford, and then with the ICMR in India, before joining the Ross Institute in 1975. Working closely with George Davidson, he moved with him to Entomology in 1980. His pioneering work in vector control of malaria – genetic control, impregnated bednets, and the detection and management of growing malaria vector resistance to the pyrethroids used – continues to date in field work in Asia and Africa (Tanzania).
Publications: *Appropriate Technology in Vector Control* 1989; a number of chapters in edited volumes, and numerous papers in professional journals.

DENHAM, DAVID, b.1937

LSHTM: Res.Fellow, Lecturer, Sen.Lect., 1968–81; Reader 1982–95.

Educ. Birkbeck College, University of Cambridge School of Veterinary Science.
Joining the Ministry of Agriculture at Weybridge as Asst.Scientific and Asst.Experimental Officer at the age of 17 in 1954, Denham studied part-time at Birkbeck, graduating with a First in zoology in 1962. He proceeded to Cambridge where he gained a Ph.D. in 1967 – George Nelson was the external examiner, and a year later recruited him to head a research group studying lymphatic filariasis at the LSHTM, where ever since he has taught and worked enthusiastically on immunological aspects of filarial infections, with a special interest in *Brugia pahangi* in animal hosts.
Publications: *Counting and identifying microfilariae. A laboratory manual* 1978; chapters (jtly) in: *Animal Models in Parasitology* 1982;

Helminth Zoonoses 1987; *Chemotherapy of Tropical Diseases* 1987; research papers in professional journals.

DOLL, SIR (WILLIAM) RICHARD (SHABOE), b.1912, FRS 1966

LSHTM: MRC appointment to work with Bradford Hill in first smoking and lung cancer studies.

Educ. St.Thomas's Hosp.Med School.
Appointments with the MRC 1946–69: Member of its Statistical Res.Unit 1948– , Deputy Director 1959, Director 1961–9. From 1963 to 1969 Doll taught Medical Statistics and Epidemiology at UCHMS, then becoming Regius Professor of Medicine at Oxford 1969–79 and, in 'retirement' Hon.Consultant, Imp.Cancer Res.Fund Cancer Studies Unit, Radcliffe Infirmary, Oxford, 1983– .
Publications: *Prevention of Cancer: pointers from epidemiology*, 1967; (jtly) *Causes of Cancer* 1982; etc.; numerous papers in professional journals.

DRASAR, BOHUMIL SAWDON, b.1943

LSHTM: Lecturer, Microbiology 1976; Sen.Lect.Med.Microbiol.1978; Reader, Bacteriology 1981; Head, Bacterial Molecular Genetics Unit 1990–3; Academic Coordinator 1990–6; Acting Dean, 1995; Professor of Bacteriology 1990– .

Educ. Universities of Birmingham and London.
Drasar began his career in bacteriology as research assistant in the Bacteriology Department at St.Mary's HMS 1964–8; then as a Member of the MRC's Gastroenterology Unit from 1967 to 1976 he remained for another 5 years in the Bacteriology Dept. at St.Mary's followed by 3 years in the PHLS's Bact.Metabolism Res.Lab., before joining the LSHTM in 1976, having spent 1971 in the Anaerobe Lab. at Virginia Polytech.Inst. & State Univ. of Virginia, USA.
Publications: 5 books and numerous scientific papers on the many and varied aspects of bacteriology in which Bo Drasar has been and continues to be involved.

ELLIS, DAVID STUART, b.1921

LSHTM: Res.Asst., then Asst.Electron Microscopist, EM Unit, 1966–74; Asst.Electron Microscopist, Dept.Protozool. 1975–82; Sen.Lect. and Academic Head of Electron Microscopy Lab. 1982–7. Emeritus Leverhulme Res.Fell. 1989–91; Hon.Sen.Res.Fell., Clinical Studies, 1987– .

Educ. University of Oxford (Univ.Coll.) and St.George's Hosp.
After wartime education spent 20 years with the Ballet Rambert before returning to medical science in the School's Electron Microscopy Unit. Hon.Consultant Microbiologist, PHLS in association with CAMR, Porton, 1987– .
Publications: Book chapters and scientific papers on structural studies of parasites and viruses, from trypanosomes and *Brugia pahangi* to the hepatitis viruses and emerging haemorrhagic and HIV viruses and, memorably, smallpox virus identification in the 1973 outbreak at the School.

FAIRLAMB, ALAN H., b.1947

LSHTM: Research Fellow 1980–1; Sen.Clin.Lecturer 1987–90; Professor of Molecular Parasitology and Head of Biochemistry and Chemotherapy Unit 1990–6.

Educ. University of Edinburgh Medical School.
After 9 years as House Officer in Edinburgh hospitals and 9 as Research Fellow at Edinburgh, Amsterdam, and the LSHTM, Fairlamb was for 6 years Asst.Professor at New York's Rockefeller University before coming to the LSHTM. In 1996 he moved from the School to Dundee University as Wellcome Principal Research Fellow, Professor, and Head of the Division of Molecular Parasitology and Biological Chemistry.
Publications: numerous research papers, review articles, abstracts and editorials.

FEACHEM, RICHARD GEORGE ANDREW, b.1947

LSHTM: Professor of Tropical Environmental Health 1987-95; and Dean 1989-95.

Educ. University of Birmingham, University of New South Wales.
Having spent 4 years as a Res.Fellow at the Univ.of New South Wales and another two at the University of Birmingham, Feachem joined the School in 1976. From 1988-9 he was Principal Public Health Specialist with the World Bank. He left the School and the Deanship, in 1995 to become Senior Adviser on population, health and nutrition at the World Bank.
Publications: *Water, Wastes and Health in Hot Climates* 1977; (jtly) *Sanitation and Disease* 1983; *Environmental Health Engineering in the Tropics* 1983; *The Health of Adults in the Developing World* 1992; etc.; papers in scientific journals.

FINE, PAUL ELMER MORE, b.1940

LSHTM: post-doc, dept.s Stats.and Epid., and Med.Protozool.1974-5; Lecturer in Tropical Hygiene, Ross Institute, 1976-9, Sen.Lect. 1979-87; Reader in Communicable Disease Epidemiology, EPS, 1987-92; Head, Communicable Disease Epidemiology Unit, 1990-6; Professor of Communicable Disease Epidemiology, 1992- .

Educ. Princeton University, University of Pennsylvania, LSHTM.
Having acquired a taste for epidemiology and tropical hygiene as a Peace Corps Volunteer in Morocco, Paul Fine spent one year at the School and another at the University of California's School of Public Health at Berkeley before settling into Tropical Hygiene at the Ross Institute, where his multi-disciplinary background in zoology, veterinary medicine, epidemiology and medical parasitology has stood him in good stead. He has written extensively on all these subjects in a number of chapters in edited works and numerous scientific papers.

HEALY, MICHAEL JOHN ROMER, b.1923

LSHTM: Professor of Medical Statistics 1977–89.

Educ. University of Cambridge, Trinity College.
After 3 years at the Admiralty's Department of Scientific Research from 1944 to 1947, Healy pursued his interest in the application of statistical methods in biology and agriculture at Rothamsted Experimental Station between 1947 and 1965. In 1965 he was appointed head of the Division of Computing and Statistics at the MRC's Clinical Research Centre, moving closer to a more medical outlook in statistics, before concluding his career at the LSHTM.
Publications include 3 books, *Matrices and Statistics* 1986; *GLIM – an introduction* 1988; and a short multi-author work on prediction of adult height, 1975; subjects treated in papers in professional journals include analyses of statistical methodology, computation, and statistical aspects of biological investigation.

HOWARD, COLIN RONALD, b.1949

LSHTM: Research Assistant 1971–2; Lecturer in Microbiology 1972–8, Sen.Lect.in Virology 1978–84, Reader 1984–90, Professor and Head of Biochemical Virology Group 1990–1.

Educ. Universities of Durham, Birmingham, and London.
Having graduated M.Sc.(Virology) at Birmingham in 1971, Howard spent 20 years at the School, in a rapidly accelerating career in Virology, with an interval of 3 years, 1987–90, as a NATO Visiting Investigator in the Department of Immunology at Scripps' Research Institute at LaJolla, California. In 1991 he left the LSHTM to become Professor of Veterinary Microbiology and Parasitology and Head of the Department of Pathology and Infectious Diseases at the Royal Veterinary College, St.Pancras.
Publications: *The Arenaviruses* 1985; (with A.J.Zuckerman) *Hepatitis Viruses of Man* 1979; (jt ed.), *Diagnosis Methods in Viral Hepatitis* 1978; (ed), *New Developments in Practical Virology* 1982; numerous papers and review articles in journals of Virology and Immunology.

KIRKWOOD, BETTY R, b.1951

LSHTM: Lecturer in Medical Statistics 1979-86; Lect.in Communicable Disease Epidemiology 1986-8; Director of WHO Collaborating Centre for Environmental and Epidemiological Aspects of Diarrhoeal Diseases 1988- ; Sen.Lect.in Communicable Disease Epidemiology 1988-93; Reader in Maternal and Child Epidemiology 1993-4; Professor of Epidemiology and International Health 1995- , and Head of Department 1996- .

Educ. Universities of Cambridge (New Hall) and London (Imperial College).
From her second degree at Imperial College Betty Kirkwood went as Statistician to the Epidemiological Research Laboratory of the Central Public Health Laboratory 1973-7, followed by 2 years as Head of the Scientific Applications Group at Chelsea College's Computer Centre, before joining the LSHTM in 1979.
Publications: *Essentials of Medical Statistics* 1988; (jtly) *Case-Control studies of childhood diseases in developing countries* 1995; chapters in edited volumes and papers in professional journals.

LAINSON, RALPH, b.1927, FRS 1982

LSHTM: Lecturer in Medical Protozoology 1955-9; Attached Investigator, Dept.of Medical Protozoology 1962-5.

Educ. University of London.
Having been Garnham's first Ph.D. student when Garnham took over from Shortt in 1952, Lainson stayed on as Lecturer at the School until 1959, when he left to become Officer-in-Charge at the Dermal Leishmaniasis Unit in Baking-Pot, Cayo, Belize from 1959 to 1962; he was to spend the rest of his working life in South America, although never cutting his ties with Garnham and the LSHTM. From 1965 to retirement in 1992 Lainson was Director of the Wellcome Parasitology Unit at the Evandro Chagas Institute in Belém, Brazil, working on the leishmaniases, their sandfly vectors and epidemiology. He was elected to Fellowship of the Royal Society in 1982.
Publications: well over 200 papers on leishmanias and other protozoal parasites.

LUMSDEN, W.H.RUSSELL, b.1914

LSHTM: MRC Sen.Fellow in Buxton's dept. 1946-7; Chair of Medical Protozoology 1968-79.

Educ. University of Glasgow, and Liverpool School of Tropical Medicine.
Having graduated in science and medicine from the University of Glasgow Lumsden studied tropical medicine and hygiene at the Liverpool School, and worked as a research fellow in the department of parasitology and entomology. During World War 2 he served in malaria field laboratories of the RAMC, and then spent a year with Buxton before joining the Yellow Fever Research Institute at Entebbe, Uganda, where he remained until he became Director of the East African Trypanosomiasis Research Organization (EATRO) from 1957 to 1963.
Publications: W.H.R.Lumsden and D.A.Evans(eds), *Biology of the Kinetoplastida*, 2 vols, 1979; papers in professional journals, etc.

MABEY, D.C.W, b.1949

LSHTM: Sen.Lect., Dept.of Clinical Sciences 1986-94; Hon.Consultant Physician, HTD, 1986- ; Professor of Communicable Diseases 1994- .

Educ. University of Oxford and St.Thomas's Hospital Med.School.
After qualifying and hospital appointments in London Mabey spent 4 years as junior clinician at the MRC laboratories in the Gambia before returning to London to become Senior Lecturer in the Dept.of Clinical Sciences at the LSHTM. In 1994 he was appointed Professor of Communicable Diseases.
Publications: A number of chapters in textbooks and edited volumes, as well as original articles, reviews and other contributions to the literature on STDs such as AIDS and chlamydial infections in the tropics.

McADAM, KEITH P.W.J., b.1945

LSHTM: Wellcome Professor of Tropical Medicine 1984– (seconded to MRC Laboratories, The Gambia, from October 1995), and Head of Department of Clinical Sciences 1988–94; Consultant Physician HTD 1984– .

Educ. University of Cambridge (Clare College), and Middlesex Hospital Medical School.
After hospital posts at Middlesex, Royal Northern, Brompton and the National Hospital for Nervous Diseases 1969–73, McAdam was Lecturer in Medicine at the Inst. of Med.Res. at Goroka, Papua New Guinea, 1973–5, and MRC Travelling Fellow 1975–6. For another year he then worked as Visiting Scientist in the Immunology Branch of the Nat.Cancer Inst. at Bethesda, followed by appointments as Asst.Prof. and Assoc.Professor at Tufts University School of Medicine from 1977 until he joined the LSHTM in 1984. McAdam has written extensively on immunology and tropical medicine, with particular reference to amyloidosis, acute phase proteins, leprosy, tuberculosis, AIDS, inflammation, etc.

McMICHAEL, ANTHONY JOHN, b.1942

LSHTM: Professor of Epidemiology 1994– .

Educ. Adelaide and Monash Universities, Australia.
His undergraduate career sealed by a year as full-time President of the Australian National Students' Union, McMichael spent a year in general practice in Melbourne before becoming a Res.Fell. at Monash Univ. while preparing his Ph.D. thesis 1969–72; from 1972–6 he taught in the School of Public Health in North Carolina, USA; back in Adelaide, he worked for 10 years as Res.Scientist in the Division of Human Nutrition of the CSIRO as Head of its Epidemiol. Res.Program. From 1986 to 1993 McMichael was Professor of Occupational and Environmental Health in the Univ.of Adelaide before being appointed Professor of Epidemiology at the London School.
Publications: *Planetary Overload: global environmental change and the health of the human species* 1993, 1994, 1995; with B.S.Hetzel, *The LS Factor: lifestyle and health* 1987, 1988, 1989 (Chin.ed.1994); jt.ed.of monographs on aspects of cancer risks and public health problems;

chapters in edited books, and papers and articles on aspects of community health and epidemiology.

McPHERSON, KLIM, b.1941

LSHTM: Res.Asst., Dept.Med.Stats & Epid. 1966-9; Prof.of Public Health Epidemiology, and Head of Health Promotion Sciences Unit, PHP, 1991- .

Educ. University of Cambridge (Christ's College).
After 2 years as Res.Scientist in industry and a summer investigating 'immigrants in industry' in Tower Hamlets for the Institute of Race Relations, McPherson was for 3 years Res.Asst. in Medical Statistics and Epidemiol. at the LSHTM. He then worked at the MRC's Clin.Res.Centre 1969-76 (1 year in the Dept. of Preventive and Social Med. at Harvard Med.School) before becoming Univ.Lect.in Med.Stats at Oxford 1976-90 (Fellow of Nuffield College 1977-90). On sabbatical leave in the spring of 1984 he lectured in the Dept.of Community Med. at Harare Med.School, Zimbabwe, and another sabbatical in 1989 was spent at the Univ.of Otago in New Zealand. He was appointed to the LSHTM in 1991.
McPherson's publications have focused in particular on Breast Cancer studies and Prevention of Coronary Heart Disease in women, and on ethical aspects of randomised controlled trials, patient choice, and consent.

MILES, MICHAEL ALEXANDER., b. 1947

LSHTM: Lecturer in Med.Protozool. 1971-81; Wellcome Trust Sen.Lect 1981-9; Head of Wolfson Unit of Molecular Med.Microbiol.and Parasitology 1984-7; Head of Applied Molecular Biology & Diagnostics Unit, and Sen.Lect. in Med.Parasitol. 1990-3; Professor of Med.Protozoology 1993- .

Educ. UCL and LSHTM.
Having completed his Ph.D. thesis on *Trypansoma cruzi* research, M.A.Miles joined the Wellcome-Harvard Scheme, on secondment to Bahia, Brazil 1971-5, then to the Wellcome Parasitology Unit in Belém, Pará, Brazil 1976-81, carrying out research on Chagas' disease and

leishmaniasis. Back at the LSHTM since 1981 his research interests continue to focus on *T.cruzi* and the *Leishmania donovani* and *L.braziliensis* complexes and their molecular epidemiology, as well as genetic exchange, reservoir hosts, recombinant vaccines, and immunodiagnosis of giardiasis in Chile and the UK.

Publications: numerous papers in professional journals on all these subjects, and in chapters in edited volumes.

MORRIS, JEREMY NOAH, b.1910

LSHTM: Professor of Public Health 1967-78; Hon.Res.Officer 1978-.

Educ. University of Glasgow, UCH, LSHTM.

Having qualified in 1934, Morris spent the pre-war years in hospital residencies and general practice. At the beginning of World War II he was Asst.MOH for Hendon and Harrow 1939-41, after which he joined up in the RAMC as Med.Specialist 1941-6 (when he took part in the care of troops in the evacuation from the Far East). After a year as Rockefeller Fellow in preventive medicine Morris then was appointed Director of the MRC's Social Medicine Unit 1948-75, and Professor of Social Medicine at the London Hospital until moving, with his MRC Social Medicine Unit, to the LSHTM in 1967.

Publications: *Uses of Epidemiology* 1957, 3rd ed.1975; papers on coronary heart disease and exercise, and on health and preventive medicine.

NELSON, GEORGE, b.1923

LSHTM: Reader in Med.Parasitology 1963-7; Professor of Helminthology and Head of Dept.of Helminthology 1967-80.

Educ. University of St.Andrews (grad.1948 having won medals for anatomy, physiology, medicine, and pathology).

After a year as house physician at Dundee Royal Infirmary Nelson returned to St.Andrews as Jun.Lecturer in Pathology, before entering the Uganda Med.Service as MO in charge of the West Nile District 1950-6; here he also found time for research on leprosy, onchocerciasis and schistosomiasis. In 1956 he transferred to the Kenya Med. Service's

Division of Vector Borne Disease (where Garnham had worked for so long until he joined the LSHTM after World War II); and in 1963 Nelson too came to the School. In 1980 he made his last move, to take up the Walter Myers Chair of Parasitology at the Liverpool School.
Publications: chapters in a number of edited books, and papers in professional journals on onchocerciasis, schistosomiasis, trichinosis, parasite transmission, and parasitic zoonoses.

NORMAND, CHARLES, b.1952

LSHTM: Professor of Health Policy 1991– ; Head of Department 1992–6.

Educ. Economics degrees at Universities of Stirling (BA) and York (Ph.D.).
Charles Normand held the Ellis Hunter Fellowship in Economics at the University of York during the academic year 1977–8, and was Principal Economist for Housing, Education, Health and Social Services in the Northern Ireland Civil Service 1982–3. This latter post he held while on leave from the University of Stirling, where he had been appointed Lecturer in Economics in 1978. From 1986 to 1988 he was at the University of York as Senior Research Fellow in Economics and Deputy Director, Health Economics Consortium. He finally moved to London and the LSHTM after 2 years as Director of the Health and Health Care Research Unit at Queens University, Belfast, 1988–90.
Publications: (with A.Weber), *Social Health Insurance: a guidebook for planning*, 1994; reports on aspects of health economics for universities and WHO; many chapters in edited volumes and papers in professional journals.

ORMEROD, WALTER EDWARD, b.1920

LSHTM: Sen.Lect., then Reader in Med.Protozool. 1954–82; Emeritus Reader 1982; Sen.Res.Fellow in Histopath.& Electron Microscop. 1988– .

Educ. Univ.of Oxford, Radcliffe Infirmary.
At Oxford during World War II, Ormerod began his career as wartime unqualified surgeon at the Radcliffe in 1943, becoming registrar 1944–5,

and then held an MRC Studentship in the Dept.of Pharmacology 1947-9, before moving on as staff member to the NIMR at Hampstead and then Mill Hill. His last appointment before joining the LSHTM as Lect.in Applied Pharmacol.at St.Mary's Hosp.Med. School in 1951-4. While at the LSHTM Ormerod was always involved in fieldwork on aspects of human trypanosomiasis in Africa and South America.
Publications: chapters in edited volumes, notably *The African Trypanosomiases* 1970 and *Biology of the Kinetoplastida* 1979; papers in professional journals, especially on trypanosomes and sleeping sickness.

PARRY, ELDRYD HUGH OWEN, b.1930

LSHTM: Sen.Res.Fellow 1990-5, and Head of Clinical Studies Unit until 1994.

Educ. University of Cambridge (Emmanuel College) and Welsh National School of Medicine.
After junior posts at Cardiff Roy.Infirmary, Nat.Heart Hospital, and Hammersmith Hosp. 1956-65, Parry embarked on a long career in Africa when he was seconded to UCH, Ibadan, 1960-3, followed by an appointment as Assoc.Professor at the Haile Selassie I University at Addis Ababa 1966-9. He then became Prof. of Medicine at Ahmadu Bello Unit. 1969-77, and Founding Dean in the Faculty of Health Sciences of the Univ. of Ilorin, Nigeria, 1977-80. From 1980-5 he served as Dean and Professor of Medicine in the School of Medical Sciences at Kumasi, before returning to the UK as Director of the Wellcome Tropical Health Education Trust.
Publications: *Principles of Medicine in Africa* 1976; papers on medicine in the tropics in medical journals.

PAYNE, PHILIP REID, b.1928

LSHTM: Res.Officer, Dept of Human Nutrition 1966-70; Sen.Lecturer 1970-4; Reader in Applied Nutrition 1974-88; Professor and Head, Dept of Public Health and Policy 1988-9; now Emeritus.

Educ. South East Essex Polytechnic.
On graduation Payne became a member of the scientific staff of the MRC's Human Nutrition Res.Unit under B.S.Platt 1951-66, before

joining Platt's department at the School, where he was to spend the rest of his academic career. In addition to ODA and FAO consultancies his interests and research have over the years focused on radioactive tracer methodology and mathematical models applied to nutritional problems, energy metabolism and obesity in young children, and the relationship between dietary protein deficiency and malnutrition and disease.
Publications: with A.Gray, *World Health and Disease: evolving patterns*, 1992; a number of chapters in edited volumes, and numerous papers in professional journals.

PETERS, WALLACE, b.1924

LSHTM: Professor of Med.Protozoology 1979–89, now Emeritus.

Educ. St.Bartholomew's Hospital.
Having served in the RAMC 1947–9, Peters practised tropical medicine in West and East Africa 1950–2. Between 1952 and 1955 he was on the WHO staff in Liberia and Nepal and then served as Asst.Director (Malariology) in the Health Department of Papua New Guinea 1956–61. Back in Europe he was Research Associate at CIBA in Basle 1961–6, before being appointed to the Walter Myers Chair of Parasitology at Liverpool University in 1966, where he was also Dean of the Liverpool School of Tropical Medicine 1975–8. From 1979 he was joint Director of the Malaria Reference Laboratory of the PHLS before moving to the LSHTM. For the WHO he has served as Chairman of the Steering Cttee on Chemotherapy of Malaria 1975–83, as Member of its Expert Advisory Panel 1967– , and on Steering Cttees on leishmaniasis.
Publications: *A Provisional Checklist of Butterflies of the Ethiopian Region* 1952; *Chemotherapy and Drug resistance in Malaria* 1970, 2nd ed.1987; *Antimalarial Drugs,* 2 vols. (ed.with R.Killick-Kendrick); *The Leishmaniases in Biology and Medicine* 1987; etc.

SMITH, PETER GEORGE, b.1942

LSHTM: Professor of Tropical Epidemiology 1989– , and Head of the Dept. of Epidemiology and Population Sciences 1990– .

Educ. City University.
P.G.Smith began his career within the MRC, with its Statistical Research

Unit 1965-7, and the Clinical and Population Cytogenetics Unit 1967-9; after 2 years in Uganda, at Makerere Univ. Medical School 1970-1, and with the WHO's International Agency for Research on Cancer 1971-2, he then joined the Cancer Epidemiology and Clinical Trials Unit 1972-9 (Dept.Epidem., Harvard School of Public Health, 1975) before coming to the LSHTM in 1979.
Publications: (ed.with R.H.Morrow) *Methods for field trials of intervention against tropical diseases* 1991; papers in professional journals; etc.

SPENCER, HARRISON C., Jr, b.1944

LSHTM: Dean and Professor of Public Health and Tropical Medicine, 1966- .

Educ. Haverford College, Johns Hopkins University Sch.Med., University of California, Berkeley.
Having completed his qualifications in medicine, internal and preventive, and tropical public health, Harrison Spencer began what became a long association with the CDC, Atlanta, Georgia, from 1972, interspersed with periods of research in South America and Kenya (malaria and community medicine), and as Sen.MO at the WHO in Geneva. In 1991 he was appointed Dean of Tulane University School of Public Health and Tropical Medicine where he has been, successively, Professor in the Dept.of Tropical Medicine, and in the Dept. of Biostatistics and Epidemiology. In 1995 he was appointed Dean of the LSHTM, a position he took up in January, 1996.
Publications: chapters in edited volumes on African trypanosomiasis, malaria and its epidemiology, dracunculiasis and amoebiasis; papers, often multi-author, on many aspects of a number of tropical diseases and tropical public health, and, jtly, *International Health and Development,* in preparation.

STEWARD, MICHAEL W., b.1940

LSHTM: Reader in Immunology 1977–81; Professor 1982– . Head, Molecular Immunology Unit 1991–3; Head, Dept.of Clinical Sciences 1994– .

Educ. University of Leeds.
Having completed his Ph.D. in Biochemistry at Leeds in 1967, Michael Steward spent 2 years as a post-doc in immunology at Duarte, California, before becoming Lecturer in Immunology at the Institute of Child Health in London; after 3 years there, and 5 years at the Kennedy Institute of Rheumatology, he was appointed Reader at the LSHTM.
Publications: *Immunochemistry* 1974; *Antibodies: their structure and function* 1984; (jt.ed) *Immunochemistry* 1978; *Laboratory tests in rheumatic diseases* 1979; and, with J.Steensgaard, *Antibody affinity: thermodynamic aspects and biological significance* 1983; chapters in edited books and papers in professional journals.

TARGETT, GEOFFREY ARTHUR TREVOR, b.1935

LSHTM: Sen.Lect.1970–6; Reader 1976–83; Professor of Immunology of Protozoal Diseases 1983– , Head of Dept. of Med.Parasitology 1988– .

Educ. Universities of Nottingham and London.
On graduation Targett went straight into the MRC's Bilharzia Research Group as Research Scientist, 1957–62, and then spent another 2 years at the NIMR, leaving in 1964 for a Lectureship in the Dept.of Natural History, at St.Andrew's University. In 1970 he left St.Andrew's to join the LSHTM, where as a leading immunoparasitologist his current work is centred on development and trials of malaria vaccines.
Publications: (ed) *Malaria: Waiting for the Vaccine* 1991; numerous papers in internat.med. and scientific journals.

TAYLOR, MARTIN GEOFFREY, b.1944

LSHTM: MRC studentship 1966–9; post-doc in helminthology 1970–2; Wandsworth Scholar 1972–4; Rockefeller and Clark Found.Res.Fell. with George Nelson 1974–6; ODMTC Lect. 1976–80;

Sen.Lect., then Reader, in Med.Helminth.1981-91; Professor 1991- ; Head, Immunology and Vaccine Design Unit 1990-3; Director, WHO Collaborating Centre for Research and Training on Schistosomiasis 1995- .

Educ. Universities of Bristol, London, and Brunel.
Apart from 1 year after graduation with Voluntary Service Overseas, under the auspices of the Min.of Agric.and Fisheries, and Wildlife of Tanzania, Taylor has spent his entire career to date at the LSHTM and its Winches Farm Laboratories. He has written extensively on schistosomes, schistosomiasis, and vaccine development, in book chapters and papers in professional journals, and edited *A brief history of virology, protozoology, and helminthology at Winches Farm 1924-92* when the laboratories closed in 1992.

VAUGHAN, JOHN PATRICK, b.1937

LSHTM: Sen.Lect.1975-83; Dir.Trop.Med.Epidem.Unit 1975-9; Reader 1983-7; Prof.of Health Care Epidemiology 1987-   ; Head, Dept.Public Health and Policy 1989-93.

Educ. Guy's HMS.
After early tropical experience, as Specialist Physician in Papua New Guinea 1966-8, and as Head of Dept.of Epidemiol.and Biostatistics at the Univ.of Dar-es-Salaam 1969-73, Vaughan was Sen.Lect. in Epidemiol.and Public Health at Nottingham Med.School from 1973 until he joined the LSHTM in 1975.
Publications: include many books, jtly & ed, on all aspects of Community Health Care at home and abroad, monographs on health and medicine, and papers on health and epidemiology.

WARHURST, D.C., b.1938

LSHTM: joined the School 1976; from Sen.Lect.became Reader 1993.

Educ. University of Leicester.
On leaving University Warhurst went straight to the NIMR and malaria research with Frank Hawkins 1963-8, then to the Liverpool School to work with Wallace Peters. His early interest in chemotherapeutic agents

in malaria, and chloroquine resistance in man and animals has led to a large volume of research carried out with increasingly sophisticated techniques and including work on giardiasis and amoebiases in addition to malaria. In recent years Warhurst's interest in antimalarials has extended to natural plant products of Chinese origin, especially artemisinin (quinhaosu) and its derivations.

Publications: a number of chapters in edited volumes, and numerous papers in professional journals on all these subjects.

WARREN, MICHAEL DONALD, b.1923

LSHTM: Sen.Lect. & Hon.Consultant in Social Med.(jtly with Royal Free HMS) 1958-64; Sen.Lect.in Social Med. 1964-7; Reader in Public Health 1967-71; Professor of Community Health 1978-80.

Educ. Guy's Hospital Med.Sch. and LSHTM.
After serving as Sqdn Leader in the Medical Branch of the RAF 1947-51, Warren was Dep.MOH for Hampstead 1952-4, and Asst.Principal MO to the LCC 1954-8. Warren left the LSHTM in 1971 to become Professor of Social Medicine, and Director of a Health Services Research Unit, at the University of Kent (briefly interrupted by 2 years back in Keppel Street in a 'caretaker' position) until he retired in 1983. He was joint editor of the *Brit.Journal of Preventive and Social Medicine* 1969-72.
Publications: (jtly) *Public Health and Social Services,* 6th ed. 1965; *Physically disabled people living at home* 1978; (ed.jtly), *Recalling the Medical Officer of Health* 1987; *The Genesis of the Faculty of Community Medicine* 1997; etc.

WATERLOW, JOHN CONRAD, b.1916, FRS 1982

LSHTM: Professor of Human Nutrition 1970-82; Emeritus 1982.

Educ. Trinity College Cambridge, London Hospital Med.College.
Having been a wartime Scientific Staff Member of the MRC from 1942, Waterlow became Director of the MRC Tropical Metabolism Research Unit at the University of the West Indies 1954-70, until he returned to London and the Chair of Human Nutrition. His research interests have centred on protein malnutrition and protein metabolism on which he has worked and written extensively.
Publications: *Protein-energy malnutrition* 1992; (jtly) *Protein Turnover in Mammalian Tissues and in Whole Body* 1978; (jt ed) *Diet and Disease: in traditional and developing societies* 1990; etc.

WEBBE, GERALD, b.1929

LSHTM: Reader in Med.Parasitology 1967-79; Scientific Director, Field Station, (Winches Farm), 1968-79; Professor of Applied Parasitology and Sub-Dean, Winches Farm, 1979-93; Head, Department of Med.Helminthology 1980-8.

Educ. University of Sheffield
Entering the Colonial Medical Service after graduation Webbe served as med.entomologist/parasitologist responsible for malaria control programmes to the Ministry of Health, Tanzania, 1952-65, and as Asst.Director of the East African Institute for Med.Res., Mwanza, Tanzania, 1962-5. From 1965 to 1967 he headed the Clinical Tropical Trials Dept.of Bayer AG's Farbenfabriken in W.Germany, conducting trials of new compounds for the treatment of amoebiasis and Chagas' disease in South America and Mexico. While at Winches Farm he served 1986-92 as Consultant Director of CAB (Commonwealth Agricultural Bureaux, International Institute of Parasitology). Now Emeritus Professor, Webbe is still active, in particular in schistosomiasis control research programmes in China.
Publications: (with P.Jordan) *Human Schistosomiasis* 1969; *Molluscicides in the control of schistosomiasis* 1974; (with P.Jordan) *Schistosomiasis: Epidemiology, Treatment and Control* 1982; (ed) *The Toxicology of Molluscicides: International Encyclopedia of Pharmacology and Therapeutics* 1987; chapters in edited volumes and papers in professional journals.

ZUCKERMAN, ARIE JEREMY, b.1932

LSHTM: Sen.Lect.in Dept.of Bacteriology and Immunology 1965-8; Reader in Virology 1968-72; Professor of Virology 1972-5; Director, Dept.of.Med.Microbiology 1975-88.

Educ. Universities of Birmingham and London.
After house appointments at the Royal Free and Whittington Hospitals Zuckerman served in the Medical Branch of the RAF 1959-62 (Tutor in Aviation Medicine, Advanced Flying School, and Epidemiological Res.Lab.PHLS). Left the LSHTM in 1988 to become Dean of the Royal Free Hospital Med.School 1989- .

PREVENTION AND CURE

Publications: *Virus Diseases of the Liver* 1970; *Hepatitis-associated Antigen and Viruses* 1972 (2nd ed. as *Human Viral Hepatitis* 1975); with C.R.Howard, *Hepatitis Viruses of Man* 1979, etc.

CHRONOLOGICAL TABLE LSHTM

1818 William Wilberforce and Zachary Macauley launch appeal for 'relief of distressed seamen' in wake of Napoleonic wars.

1821 Wilberforce's Committee becomes the *Seamen's Hospital Society (SHS)* with a hospital ship, the *Grampus*, loaned by the Admiralty.

1831 The *Grampus* replaced by the larger *Dreadnought;* this name adopted for subsequent ships and finally for the Society's on-shore hospital buildings at Greenwich, established in 1870.

1866 Patrick Manson arrives in Formosa (Taiwan) as MO to Chinese Imperial Maritime Customs and learns of tropical diseases the hard way; 1871 transfers to Amoy.

1883 Manson settles in private practice in Hong Kong, joined in 1887 by James Cantlie; launch of Hong Kong's Medical College.

1889 Manson retires to Scotland.

1890 Opening of SHS's Branch Hospital at the Albert Dock.

1892 Manson appointed physician to the Albert Dock Hospital with its incoming patients from Africa, India, and the Far East suffering from tropical diseases; attracts students keen to learn their diagnosis and treatment.

1894 Manson begins annual course of lectures to students at St.George's Hospital.

1897 Manson appointed medical adviser to Colonial Office with access to Chamberlain and H.J.Read. Lectures at St.George's 'On the necessity for special education in tropical medicine'; Read responds with memorandum.

1898 Cantlie and W.J.Ritchie Simpson found *Journal of Tropical Medicine;* Ronald Ross discovers bird malaria cycle.

PREVENTION AND CURE

1898–1902	Malaria Committee of the Royal Society (C.W.Daniels, J.W.W.Stephens and S.R.Christophers) reports from India and West Africa.
1899	Opening of Tropical Schools in Liverpool (April) and London (October).
1899–1910	Position of 'Superintendent' (Medical Tutor) revolving between D.C.Rees, Daniels, and G.C.Low ('Director' in his last year).
1899–1900	Low, Thomas Bancroft, and Manson establish passage of filarial larvae through salivary glands of mosquito into its proboscis.
1900	Low, Sambon and Terzi spend three months in mosquito-proof hut in malarial Roman Campagna, proving epidemiological point: no mosquitoes between dusk and dawn, no malaria.
1902	First Royal Society Sleeping Sickness Commission begins work in Uganda.
1903	Sir Francis Lovell appointed School's first Dean.
1905	Manson appoints first specialist lecturers (helminthology and protozoology); School admitted School of the University of London, Faculty of Medicine, in tropical medicine only; Robert Leiper establishes life-cycle of Guinea worm at Accra.
1907	Formation of the (Royal) Society of Tropical Medicine and Hygiene.
1908	Sleeping Sickness Bureau established.
1911–13	Short-lived *Journal of The London School of Tropical Medicine*.

CHRONOLOGICAL TABLE LSHTM

1913 The Rockefeller Foundation's new International Health Board under Wickliffe Rose makes early contact with the School's helminthologists to consult on hookworm disease.

1913-14 Leiper and E.L.Atkinson confirm Japanese results on life-cycle of *Schistosoma* species.

1914 C.M.Wenyon leaves School for Wellcome Bureau of Scientific Research in the Tropics; succeeded by John Gordon Thomson.

1914-18 The Great War. Teaching in abeyance; staff and hospital part of war effort. First scientific malaria survey of war carried out by S.R.Christophers and H.E.Shortt, modelled on Christophers' earlier malaria surveys in India.

1918-19 The great influenza pandemic ('Spanish' flu).

1918-20 Move of Hospital for Tropical Diseases and the London School of Tropical Medicine to Endsleigh Gardens.

1919 Creation of Ministry of Health; Christopher Addison first Minister of Health, replaced 1921 by Alfred Mond.

1919-20 Preliminary moves by Rockefeller Foundation to explore possibilities for a School of Public Health in London.

1921 Topley and Greenwood begin collaboration on experimental epidemiology;
report of Athlone Committee on Tropical Diseases with observers from the Rockefeller Foundation, June 10th-17th;
Alfred Mond as Minister of Health sets up committee to draft scheme for 'Institute of State Medicine', July;
London University adopts the degree of Ph.D.

1922 A week before his death in April Manson accepts Rockefeller proposals for School.

PREVENTION AND CURE

1923 In March the 'National Theatre Committee' accepts Rockefeller offer of £52,000 for site on corner of Gower Street and Keppel Street.
Andrew Balfour appointed Director of new School in October. Opening of Leiper's Institute of Agricultural Parasitology. Castellani and W.J.R.Simpson launch appeal for 'Ross Clinic'.

1924–5 H.Lockwood Stevens and Sir Charles McLeod revive failing Ross Appeal.

1924 Charter for School of Hygiene given Royal approval. The SHS abdicates responsibility for Tropical School followed by plans for 'Imperial Hospital for Tropical Diseases'; project shelved in 1927, when SHS decided to cooperate and not close down hospital in Endsleigh Gardens. School abandons original Diploma of Tropical Medicine and begins introducing London University Diploma of Bacteriology together with DPH(Engl.) and DTM&H(Engl.).

1925 The Horton Malaria Centre for malaria therapy opens at Epsom (later the Malaria Reference Laboratory and WHO Regional Malaria Centre for Europe).

1926 P.A.Buxton succeeds A.W.Alcock in Department of Entomology; V.B.Wigglesworth appointed Lecturer in Medical Entomology; Ross Institute and Hospital for Tropical Diseases opens at Putney.

1926–9 Building of new School (LSHTM) on Keppel Street site.

1927 J.J.C.Buckley joins Leiper's department. On Lockwood Stevens' initiative Sir Malcolm Watson is brought in to conduct Ross Institute malaria control policy. Topley and Greenwood appointed to new chairs of bacteriology and epidemiology, respectively, at LSHTM.

CHRONOLOGICAL TABLE LSHTM

1929 New LSHTM officially opened by Prince of Wales on July 18th. Wilson Jameson appointed Head of Division of Public Health. Balfour writes his last report before complete breakdown. Two main Divisions replace Old Tropical School: Medical Zoology (helminthology, protozoology and entomology); and Clinical Tropical Medicine (remaining in Endsleigh Gardens). Harold Raistrick appointed University Professor and Director of Department of Biochemistry and Chemistry as Applied to Hygiene.
Arrival at School of Neil Hamilton Fairley.
Millais Culpin joins School as Lecturer in Industrial Psychology.
G.P.Crowden appointed Lecturer in Applied Physiology.
Development of School Library and Museum collections under Barnard and Newham, respectively.

1930 G.S.Wilson appointed Professor of Bacteriology as Applied to Hygiene.
Development of DPH course to include seminars and tutorials and closer links with Epidemiology and Medical Statistics.

1931 Balfour's frozen body found in grounds of Cassell Hospital, Kent, where he was being treated for clinical depression, on January 30th; Wilson Jameson takes over as first Dean of LSHTM.
S.R.Christophers joins the LSHTM as Professor of Malaria Studies in the University of London.
Millais Culpin appointed University of London Professor of Medical Industrial Psychology at LSHTM.
Death of W.J.R.Simpson.

1932 MRC Malaria Unit under S.R.Christophers established with Leverhulme grant at LSHTM.
Death of Ronald Ross.

1933 A.Bradford Hill appointed Reader at LSHTM.

1934 Ross Institute moves under the umbrella of the LSHTM, and its hospital becomes 'Ross Ward' of the HTD.

PREVENTION AND CURE

1934–9 Watson builds up the Ross Institute as its Director until retirement in 1942.

1935 Publication of first edition of Major Greenwood's *Epidemics and Crowd Diseases*.

1935–6 Reorganisation of teaching of epidemiology, with more emphasis on textbooks and informal discussions with seminars, less on formal lectures.
MRC Special Report on experimental epidemiology by Topley, Greenwood, Bradford Hill and Joyce Wilson.
Formation of Bacteriological Warfare Subcommittee of the Committee of Imperial Defence.
Wigglesworth appointed London University Reader in Entomology at LSHTM.

1937 Existing 'Divisions' become 'Departments' by decree of the Board of Management.
Publication of first edition of Bradford Hill's *Principles of Medical Statistics*.
J.G.Thomson dies in office; helminthology and protozoology united in new single large Department of Parasitology, with readership in medical parasitology for H.E.Shortt.
George Macdonald appointed assistant director of Ross Institute.

1938 Report of the Emergency Bacteriological Services Subcommittee, chaired by Topley.
LSHTM Annual Report emphasises preparation for war, including consideration of emergency shelters on agenda in Public Health.

CHRONOLOGICAL TABLE LSHTM

1939–45 World War II. All regular courses suspended; short intensive courses in tropical medicine and hygiene for MOs about to serve in tropical areas.
Bomb damage to Malet Street wing: extensive damage to Museum's collections of teaching aids, but no personal injuries, in May 1941.
Successive changes of Dean because of wartime commitments of Wilson Jameson and Brigadier Parkinson.

1941 Topley appointed Secretary to the ARC;
G.S.Wilson becomes Director, EPHLS.

1944 Introduction of use of DDT.
Formation of MRC's Human Nutrition Unit under B.S.Platt.

1944–5 J.M.Mackintosh takes office as Professor of Public Health on October 1st, 1944, and as Dean on January 1st, 1945.

1945 V.B.Wigglesworth leaves for Cambridge with Research Unit of Insect Physiology.
Greenwood retires as Emeritus Professor of Epidemiology and Vital Statistics; succeeded by Bradford Hill as Professor of Medical Statistics.
Gradual return of staff from wartime appointments; EPHLS becomes PHLS.

1945–6 Ex-service men and women apply in unprecedented numbers for DPH courses.
Rockefeller Foundation offers fellowships for training of 'Hand-picked' students in Public Health Department.
Growing collaborations with other Schools of University: Institute of Child Health, Hammersmith Postgraduate Medical School, LSE.
Introduction of lectures on sociology and social medicine.

1946 Leiper retires, H.E.Shortt becomes Professor of Medical Protozoology and Director of Department.
Neil Hamilton Fairley takes up newly created Wellcome Chair of Clinical Tropical Medicine.
Creation of Department of Human Nutrition, LSHTM,

with Platt in the country's first Chair of Human Nutrition, and continuing as Head of MRC Unit until its closure in 1967.

1947 Graham Wilson leaves Department of Bacteriology for full-time Directorship of PHLS; succeeded by E.T.C.Spooner in Topley's chair and as head of department.
J.C.Cruickshank inherits Wilson's personal title and J.T.Duncan becomes Reader in Medical Mycology.
George Macdonald appointed first Professor of Tropical Hygiene and Director of Ross Institute.
J.H.F.Brotherston appointed Lecturer in Preventive and Social Medicine in Department of Public Health; his arrival augurs in developments in emerging 'medical sociology' and growing impact of economics on Public Health.

1948 Introduction of National Health Service (NHS) July 5th, following NHS Act of 1946 (NHS(Reorganisation) Act followed 1973).
Hamilton Fairley forced by illness to resign Wellcome Chair; Murgatroyd succeeds him but dies suddenly in December, 1951.
A.W.Woodruff then inherits Wellcome Chair.
D.D.Reid becomes Reader in Epidemiology and Vital Statistics.

1949 M.A.Delafield retires and sub-department of 'Chemistry as Applied to Hygiene' disappears.
Department of Medical Statistics re-titled Medical Statistics and Epidemiology.

1950 First preliminary report by Doll and Hill on smoking and lung cancer.
Bradford Hill fights, and wins, his case for his department to be classified as 'pre-clinical' rather than 'non-clinical'.
Andrew Topping succeeds Mackintosh as first full-time Dean.

1951 HTD moves to St.Pancras Way.

	Establishment of 'Sub-Unit of Occupational Health' linked to Industrial Health Service at Slough.
1952	H.E.Shortt retires; P.C.C.Garnham succeeds him. Publication of MRC Report on streptomycin in tuberculosis controlled clinical trial. Introduction of Applied Nutrition Research Unit, specialising in nutrition and food technology in colonial territories, funded by the CO and linked to the MRC's Gambian activities.
1953	Post-war revival of parasitology department's fieldwork at Winches Farm. M.D.Warren becomes tutor to foreign students, acting as counsellor in language and personal problems during their first term.
1954	End of the School's involvement in the MRC's Gambian projects.
1955	Buxton dies in office, succeeded by D.S.Bertram. Death of Andrew Topping; Bradford Hill 'acting' Dean, then Dean for two years.
1955–6	Sub-Unit replaced by Rockefeller Unit of Occupational Health. R.S.F.Schilling Director of Unit and University Reader in Occupational Health.
1956	J.M.Mackintosh retires, succeeded in Public Health by W.S.Walton in Chair and Stuart Hinds as Reader. Rockefeller Foundation awards School £17,000 grant to investigate protein values of tropical dietaries. Retirement of Harold Raistrick, succeeded by J.H.Birkinshaw.
1957	Sir James Kilpatrick appointed Dean.
1958	Geoffrey Rose joins epidemiology department: 'part-time' Reader 1964; 'Visiting Professor of Epidemiology and Preventive Medicine' 1970; Full Professor of Epidemiology 1977.

PREVENTION AND CURE

1959   Forrest Fulton appointed to Britain's first chair of Virology at LSHTM.
Hospital Feeding Survey (Nuffield Provincial Hospitals' Trust) under T.P.Eddy introduced in the Department of Nutrition.

1960–5   Major restructuring of facilities for library, teaching and research with support from the Wolfson Trust and Marks and Spencer; new lectureships funded by Ministry of Overseas Development.

1960   Death of Sir James Kilpatrick; E.T.C.Spooner leaves Bacteriology to become full-time Dean.
With additional grants from the Rockefeller Foundation and the Leverhulme Trust Fund the Rockefeller Unit of Occupational Health becomes a full department, and R.S.F.Schilling Professor.
FAO/WHO Expert Committee on Nutrition endorses Platt's concept of 'marasmic kwashiorkor'; W.R.Aykroyd joins nutrition department as senior lecturer after retiring from FAO, and T.P.Eddy moves to nutrition (cf 1959) from Sierra Leone Medical Services.

1961   C.E.Gordon Smith appointed Reader in Virology.
D.G.Evans takes over from Spooner in Bacteriology.
Bradford Hill retires. Peter Armitage succeeds to his Chair in Medical Statistics and D.D.Reid becomes Director of the Department of Medical Statistics and Epidemiology. Richard Doll becomes Director of the MRC Statistical Research Unit.

1962   Birkinshaw retires; 'Biochemistry' absorbed into a number of other departments with 'biochemical needs' instead of a separate department.
UNICEF provides money for special courses in applied nutrition work in developing countries.

1963   'West Block' of Winches Farm restored; George Nelson begins to rebuild experimental helminthology at the Field Station, eventually to become WFL (Winches Farm Laboratories).

CHRONOLOGICAL TABLE LSHTM

1964   LSHTM introduces Academic Postgraduate Diploma in Nutrition (becomes M.Sc. course 1971–2).
Hospital Feeding Survey published.
London University confers title of Professor of Entomology as Applied to Hygiene on J.R.Busvine.

1965   William Brass joins the Department of Medical Statistics and Epidemiology as Reader in Medical Demography (Professor 1972; Director, Centre for Overseas Population Studies, 1974–8; Head, Department of Medical Statistics and Epidemiology 1977–82; retired 1988).

1967   J.J.C.Buckley retires, succeeded by George Nelson.
Gerald Webbe joins Department of Helminthology and is appointed scientific Director of Winches Farm Field Station and eventually Sub-Dean.
Walton retires and is succeeded by J.N.Morris who replaces existing staff with his MRC Social Medicine Research Unit. Only Sidney Chave and M.D.Warren remain, easing transition from DPH to M.Sc. degree course in Social Medicine.
P.J.S.Hamilton joins Department of Medical Statistics and Epidemiology as tropical epidemiologist.
MRC Human Nutrition Unit disbanded; staff transferred to LSHTM.
Death of George Macdonald.

1967–8   Reorganisation of Public Health Department, re-establishing links with LSE and bringing in R.F.L.Logan to head 'Organisation of Medical Care Unit'. Department also to include the Ministry of Health's 'Chronic Disease Control Unit' and J.H.Renwick's 'Human Genetics Unit'.
Ongoing introduction of M.Sc. degree courses to replace diploma courses: 1967–9 M.Sc. in Medical Parasitology and M.Sc. in Medical Statistics.

1968   Report of Todd Committee.
TUC Centenary Institute of Occupational Health established with TUC funding; Schilling appointed to University Chair of Occupational Health.
Department of Parasitology divided into Medical

Helminthology at WFL under G.S.Nelson, and Medical Protozoology in Keppel Street under W.H.R.Lumsden (following Garnham's retirement). Onchocerciasis research begins at WFL, while studies on the *Brugia* species, first separated out by Buckley, continued under David Denham at Keppel Street.

1969 First M.Sc. degrees in Occupational Medicine.
Morris introduces new 2-year M.Sc. course in Social Medicine. Bruce-Chwatt appointed Professor of Tropical Hygiene and Director of the Ross Institute.
Death of B.S.Platt.
Wellcome Trust initiates international cooperative research programme between Harvard School of Public Health, the LSHTM, and South American tropical institutes.

1970 Tropical epidemiology formally incorporated in Department of Medical Statistics and Epidemiology, with support from the Wellcome Trust.
C.E.Gordon Smith replaces Spooner as Dean.
J.C.Waterlow succeeds Platt, and Wellcome Foundation provides £118,000 for new clinical and metabolic unit in the department.
Public Health department acquires Professor of Social Psychiatry (J.K.Wing) jointly with the Institute of Psychiatry.

1970-1 New M.Sc. degrees in: Medical Demography; Occupational Hygiene; Social Medicine.

1971 D.G.Evans resigns from School, and the Department of Bacteriology and Immunology becomes the Department of Microbiology (later of Medical Microbiology). New M.Sc. in Human Nutrition.

1972 Geoffrey Edsall succeeds Evans as Professor and Director of Department of Microbiology.
Death of J.J.C.Buckley.
Roy Acheson appointed Professor and Director of new Centre for Extension Training in Community Medicine; discontinued in 1978 after Acheson's departure for

Cambridge in 1976.

1973 Miss Algeo catches smallpox on duty in bacteriology laboratories; before virus identified by David Ellis two unvaccinated visitors to patient in Miss Algeo's ward at St.Mary's were infected and died. Public Inquiry has wide repercussions inside and outside the School.

1973-4 The MRC arbovirus research project at Kisumu, Kenya, moves its laboratory work, first housed at Porton Down, to new MRC laboratory at Winches Farm.

1974 Geoffrey Edsall resigns; succeeded by A.J.Zuckerman. David Bradley appointed Professor of Tropical Hygiene and Director of Ross Institute.
Major review and initiation of modernisation in face of severe financial difficulties throughout British Universities.

1975 New M.Sc.s in: Clinical Tropical Medicine and Medical Microbiology (jointly with RPMS Hammersmith).

1976 Bertram and Busvine retire; W.W.McDonald succeeds to chair and as head of entomology.
Retirement of R.S.F.Schilling, succeeded by J.C.McDonald who then resigned after 5 years to return to McGill University, there to establish new School of Public Health.

1977 Death of Donald Reid; M.R.J.Healy appointed to Chair of Medical Statistics.
Introduction of Nutrition Policy Unit financed by Ministry of Overseas Development.

1978 DTPH course replaced M.Sc. degree course.
J.N.Morris retires; M.D.Warren, Professor at Kent since 1971, reluctantly accepts Chair of Public Health, but soon returns to Kent; Dame Rosemary Rue of Oxford Regional Health Authority bridges gap until 1982; 2 year M.Sc. course reverts to 1 year duration.
Ross Institute creates Evaluation and Planning Centre for

PREVENTION AND CURE

Health Care with ODA support.

1979–80 Introduction of M.Sc. degree course in 'Epidemiology in Developing Countries'.
School's Arbovirus Research Unit revived under M.G.R.Varma, Professor of Medical Entomology.
Retirement of W.H.R.Lumsden from Medical Protozoology; succeeded by Wallace Peters moving from Walter Myers Chair at Liverpool, and George Nelson replaces him at Liverpool, leaving Helminthology at LSHTM;
W.W.McDonald leaves LSHTM after only 3 years for Chair of Medical Entomology at Liverpool.

1980 Major (ultimately less than successful) reorganisation of School, grouping existing 13 departments in 3 major Divisions.
'Microbiology' becomes 'Medical Microbiology'; B.S.Drasar becomes Reader in Bacteriology jointly with Department of Tropical Hygiene.
Title of Professor of Entomology as Applied to Hygiene conferred on George Davidson, who moved from Ross Institute to Entomology as 'caretaker' Director, retiring 2 years later.
Introduction of M.Sc. in 'Community Medicine and Epidemiology'.

1981 Title of Professor of Immunology conferred on M.W.Steward (Reader from 1977).
Refugee Health Groups within Ross/Tropical Hygiene funded by Edna McConnell Clark Foundation.

1982 J.C.Waterlow retires as Professor of Human Nutrition; post frozen until 1993. Philip Payne, Reader in Applied Nutrition, succeeds as head of department, and Famine Research Unit is established in association with International Disaster Institute.
M.G.R.Varma appointed joint Head of Entomology and the Arbovirus Unit.
Restructuring of departments brings Patrick Hamilton back from Caribbean as Director of Community Health.

CHRONOLOGICAL TABLE LSHTM

1983   G.A.T.Targett appointed Professor of Immunology of Protozoal Diseases (becomes Head of Department of Parasitology in 1988).

1984   Keith P.W.J.McAdam appointed to Wellcome Chair of Tropical Medicine and Consultant at HTD (Head of Department of Clinical Sciences 1988–94).

1986   Creation of academic initiative post for specialist in insect behaviour, with links to Imperial College and Birkbeck College.
Board of Management sets up working party under Sir John Reid to recommend plans for another restructuring of the School.

1987   Richard Feachem appointed Professor of Tropical Environmental Health.
Professorial Titles conferred: P.R.Payne, Applied Nutrition; J.P.Vaughan, Health Care Epidemiology.
Death of H.E.Shortt.

1988   Death of Patrick Hamilton and of D.S.Bertram.

1989   P.G.Smith appointed Professor of Tropical Epidemiology (Head of Department of Epidemiology & Population Sciences from 1990).
George Kazantis retires from Chair of Occupational Health; Occupational Health ceases to be separate department.
A.J.Zuckerman leaves School to be Dean of Royal Free HMS.
B.S.Drasar awarded personal Chair in Bacteriology, and Heads Bacterial Molecular Genetics Unit.
Michael Healy retires from Chair of Medical Statistics, succeeded by Stuart Pocock.
Philip Payne resigns.
Death of Bruce-Chwatt.
Wallace Peters retires from Chair of Medical Protozoology; eventually succeeded by M.A.Miles in a personal chair under the new policy of awarding personal chairs on merit, rather than filling original established

chairs.

1988–90 Gordon Smith retires as Dean in September, 1989, having supervised initial moves in final restructuring of LSHTM for the 1990s as recommended in the Reid Report, and followed up by new Dean, Richard Feachem.

Four new large departments formed by merging disciplines:

Department of Clinical Sciences now includes tropical medicine, medical microbiology, clinical nutrition, and tropical pathology.

Department of Epidemiology & Population Sciences now includes epidemiology, statistics, medical demography, tropical public health, and preventive teratology.

Department of Medical Parasitology now includes medical entomology, medical helminthology, and medical protozoology.

Department of Public Health & Policy now includes community medicine, occupational medicine and hygiene, health service planning and evaluation, and nutrition policy; Chair in Community Health to be replaced by Chairs in Health Policy and Public Health Epidemiology.

1990 A.H.Fairlamb appointed Professor of Molecular Parasitology.
Dorothy Crawford joins Department of Clinical Sciences as Professor of Microbiology, heading the Cellular and Molecular Virology Unit.
Klim McPherson appointed to Chair of Public Health Epidemiology.
Ruth McWilliam retires as Secretary of the School, succeeded by B.K.Gooch.

1991 April: 1st Annual Public Health Forum: *Malaria – Waiting for the Vaccine* (additional sponsors WHO, ODA,

World Bank, Swiss Tropical Institute).
Charles Normand appointed to Chair in Health Policy.
Retirement of G.A.Rose and of M.G.R.Varma.

1992 April: 2nd Annual Public Health Forum: *Europe Without Frontiers – The Implications for Health.*
LSHTM introduces No Smoking Policy.
New Chairs: John Cleland (Medical Demography); C.F.Curtis (Medical Entomology); Paul Fine (Communicable Disease Epidemiology); M.A.Miles (Medical Protozoology).
Deaths of: A.W.Woodruff; T.P.Eddy; and Erica Wheeler.
Closure of Winches Farm.

1993 April: 3rd Annual Public Health Forum: *Tuberculosis - Back to the Future.*
Formation of 'UK Malaria Consortium' jointly with the Liverpool School and ODA funded.
Retirement of Gerald Webbe.
Alumni Reunions, attended by staff members, in Kuala Lumpur and Thailand.

1994 April: 4th Annual Public Health Forum: *Vaccination and World Health.*
First Science Open Day for sixth formers at the School.
New personal chairs: Nick Black (Health Services Research); Betty Kirkwood (Epidemiology and International Health); Anne Mills (Health Economics and Policy).
Paul Fine (Head, Communicable Disease Epidemiology Unit) opens first Annual Pump Handle Lecture of new John Snow Society.
Death of Sir John Reid, Chair of the Board of Management since 1989.
Death of P.C.C.Garnham.

1995 April: 5th Annual Public Health Forum: *Health at the Crossroads – Transport Policy and Urban Health.*
R.Feachem resigns as Dean to become head of new public health department at World Bank. B.S.Drasar Acting Dean; Keith McAdam, on secondment as Wellcome

PREVENTION AND CURE

Professor of Tropical Medicine, becomes Director of the MRC Laboratories in The Gambia, replacing Brian Greenwood who after 15 years in The Gambia is awarded a personal chair in the Department of Medical Parasitology.

Other new personal chairs: A.Bryceson (Tropical Medicine); R.Hayes (Epidemiology and International Health); Harrison Spencer, Dean (Public Health); A.J.Swerdlow (Epidemiology).

Death of E.T.C.Spooner and of J.D.Gillett.

1996 Professor Harrison Spencer takes office as Dean.
April: 6th Annual Public Health Forum: *Diet, Nutrition and Chronic Disease*.
George McDonald Medal awarded jointly to D.J.Bradley and C.F.Curtis.
Drasar Committee on Restructuring.

1997–8 Implementation of Drasar Committee Report.

INDEX

Abraham, Sir Edward, 181
Adamson, William, 11
Addison, Christopher, 67
Alberman, Eva A., 156
Alcock, Alfred William, 18-21, 239, 257, 258
Algoe, Miss A.E., 141
Anchylostomiasis, 38-40
Applied Nutrition Research Unit, 200
Applied psychology, 187
Arbovirus Unit, 230, 266
Armitage, Peter, 111, 112, 115
Ascaris, 245
Asiatic Cholera Society, 93
Athlone Committee, 68, 70, 73, 74
Athlone, Earl of, 68, 73
Atkinson, A.L., 37, 38
Avery Jones, Sir Francis, 110
Aykroyd, Wallace Ruddell, 202

Bacteriology, 14
  academic discipline, as, 126
Bagshawe, A.W.G., 46
Balfour, Andrew, 16, 20, 65, 69, 78, 82, 113, 240, 329
  background, 84, 85
  suicide, 85
  writings, 85
Bancroft, Joseph, 32
Bancroft, Thomas, 33
Barton, Alberto, 10
Bassett-Smith, P.W., 10, 56
Bastianelli, Guiseppe, 51
Bertram, D.S., 265, 266
Bilharz, Theodor, 32, 35
Bilharzia Mission, 38
Bilharziasis, 35-38
Biometrics, 93
Bird, R.G., 225, 226
Birkinshaw, J.H., 181, 183
Blacklock, D.B., 246
Board of Management, 156
Boerma, A.H., 209

INDEX

Boyce, Rubert, 7, 11, 12, 130
Boyd, Sir John, 45
Bradford Hill, Austin, 98, 99, 102, 104, 106-112, 118, 137, 186
Bradley, David, 306, 307, 309
Brass, William, 114-116
British Institute of Preventive Medicine, 5
British Red Cross, 68
Bromfield, R.J., 302
Brotherston, J.H.F., 159-161, 168
Brownlee, John, 94, 96
Bruce, David, 43-45
Bruce-Chwatt, Leonard, 305-307
Brugia, 249, 250
Buckley, John Joseph Cronin, 243-250, 303
Bureau of Helminthology, 233
Bush, W.T., 302
Busk, George, 31
Busvine, J.R., 265, 266
Buxton, Patrick, 225, 257-265

Cambridge University Diploma in Tropical Medicine and Hygiene, 19
Cameron, T.M.W., 243
Cancer houses, 242
Cantlie, James, 4, 14, 16, 19
Cardiovascular disease, 328
Carpenter, G.D.H., 47
Castellani, Aldo, 16, 43, 285-289
Caton, Richard, 12
Central Institution of Hygiene and Public Health
  proposal for, 75, 76
Centre for Agriculture and Biosciences International, 234
Centre for Population Studies, 116, 172
Certificate in Public Health, 160
Chadwick, Edwin, 93, 150
Chain, E.B., 183
Chamberlain, Joseph, 5, 6, 8-10, 13
Chamberlain, Neville, 78, 80, 81
Charles, Sir Richard Henry Havelock, 20, 68
Chave, Sidney, 166
Chemistry, academic discipline of, 179-185
Chemotherapy, 311-314

INDEX

Cholera, prevention of, 15
Christophers, Sir Rickard, 53-55, 254, 255, 284, 295, 299
Christopherson, J.B., 85
Christy, Cuthbert, 43
Clay, H.H., 152
Clinical Nutrition Unit, 212
Clinical tropical medicine, 267-273
Cochrane, A.L., 102
Cohen, J.B., 179
Colonies
　ill-health of European workers in, 30
Committee for the Relief of Distressed Seamen, 4
Committee on Imperial Defence, Bacteriological Warfare Subcommitttee, 130
Conference on Tropical Diseases, 74
Cook, Albert, 42
Cook, G.C., 268
Cook, John, 42
Cooper, Willie, 301-303
Court of Governors, 156
Cowell, M.P., 198
Craddock, Stuart, 182
Cranefield, Paul, 5, 6
Crawford, Dorothy, 144
Croft, Simon, 232
Crowden, G.P., 152-154
Cruickshan, J.C., 135
Cryopreservation, 229
Culpin, Millais, 154, 155, 186, 187

Daniels, C.W., 19, 20, 53, 54, 249
Davaine, Casimir-Joseph, 32
Davidson, Andrew, 7, 8
Davidson, G., 266
Dawson, Geoffrey, 81
DDT, 264, 285
Delafield, Max Everard, 152, 181, 184, 185
Delepine, Sheridan, 130
Demrquay, Jean-Nicholas, 32
Department of Biochemistry
　Department of Chemistry merged in, 179

INDEX

  integration of activities in other departments, 184
  main function of, 180
  policy, 183
  war, during, 184
Department of Chemistry as applied to Hygiene, 184
Department of Clinical Sciences, 272
Department of Clinical Tropical Medicine, 267-273
Department of Community Health, 170, 171
Department of Entomology, 257-267
Department of Epidemiology, 115, 116
Department of Epidemiology and Population Health, 267
Department of Epidemiology and Population Sciences, 116, 172, 173
Department of Helminthology, 222, 227, 241-251
Department of Human Nutrition, 169, 197-213
  creation of, 197-199
  diversification of interests, 212
  Gambian enterprises, connection with, 199-201
  Public Health and Policy, submerged in, 212
  research and teaching activities, 209-211
  secondments, 211
Department of Infectious and Tropical Diseases, 144, 267
Department of Medical Demography, 115, 116
Department of Medical Helminthology, 251
Department of Medical Parasitology, 144, 267
Department of Medical Statistics and Epidemiology, 169
  achievements of, 108
  creation of, 104
  smoking and cancer, work on, 109, 110
  stature and influence, 107
  tropical epidemiology, incorporation of, 113, 114
  1960s and 1970s, work in, 112
Department of Medical Statistics, 115, 116
Department of Microbiology
  creation of, 140
  teaching, 142, 143
Department of Occupational Health, 188, 189
Department of Parasitology, 229, 241
Department of Public Health, 105
  Chronic Disease Control Unit, 167
  cooperation wiht other Schools, 159
  development policy, 163-165

INDEX

Human Genetics Unit, 167
increase in staff, 159
Jameson, appointment to Chair, 152
library, 153, 154
London School of Economics, links with, 167
M.Sc. course, transition to, 166, 167, 169
opening of, 150
organisation, 152
post-war, 158-165
research, 161, 162
Social Medicine Unit, 168
teaching, 153, 154
units, 172
war, during, 155
Department of Public Health and Policy, 267, 325
Department of Tropical Hygiene, 116, 307
Devoto, Luigi, 185
Diploma in Applied Parasitology and Entomology, 181, 304, 305
Diploma in Nutrition, 203
Diploma in Public Health
  curriculum, 152
  history of, 150
Diploma in Tropical Medicine and Hygiene, Cambridge, 150
Diploma in Tropical Public Health, 305
Disease
  European travellers, effects on, 1, 2
  impact on society, 1
Division of Bacteriology, 84
Division of Bacteriology and Immunology, 65
  Department of Microbiology, change of name to, 140
  establishment of, 92
  post-war years, in, 135-144
  Spooner as Director of, 135
  teaching, 128-130
  Topley as professor in, 96
Division of Clinical Tropical Medicine, 241
Division of Epidemiology and Vital Statistics, 65, 84
  Department of Medical Statistics, becoming, 104
  development of, 101
  establishment of, 92
  Greenwood as Professor in, 96

INDEX

location, 96, 97
research, 97, 98
teaching assistants, 98
teaching, 97-99, 101
war, during, 103
Division of Public Health. See Department of Public Health
Doll, Sir Richard, 109, 111, 112
Done, James, 200
Donovan, C., 56
Drasar, B.S., 143, 144, 308
Dubini, Angelo, 40
Duncan, Andrew, 16
Duncan, J.T., 135
Duncan, William Henry, 3
Dutton, J.E., 44

Ebola virus, 141
Eddy, Trewavas Pearce, 202, 203, 205
Edge, P.G., 100, 101
Edsall, Geoffrey, 140-142
Elephantiasis, 4, 31, 32
Ellis, David, 141, 226
Emergency Public Health Laboratory Service, 131, 132
Endsleigh Palace Hotel, acquisition of, 68
Entomology, 257-267
Environmental cancers, 328
Epidemics, control of, 1
Epidemiologicl Society, 93
Epidemiology
  chronic, non-commincable diseass, 113
  classical, 92
  experimental, 126, 127, 136
  mathematical, 94
  medical ecology, as, 108
  poor relations within, 116-118
  psychiatric, 113
  radical change in, 93
  socially conscious orientation, 110
  theorists, 93
European Commission programmes, 329
Evaluation and Planning Centre for Primary Health Care, 307

INDEX

Evans, David Gwynne, 138-140
Evans, Griffith, 44

Fantham, H.B., 48
Farr, William, 92, 93, 150
Feachem, Richard, 118, 308, 309, 330
Fedchenko, A.P., 34
Fibiger, Johannes, 242
Filariasis, 31-33
Findlay, Carlos, 50
Fletcher, Sir Walter, 156
Flexner, Alexander, 68
Flexner, Simon, 82, 108, 126
Food Systems and Society study, 210, 211
Fowden, Leslie, 200
Frost, Wade Hampton, 108
Fulton, Forrest, 132, 136, 137, 142

Gage Brown, Sir Charles, 6, 7
Galloway, T. McL., 159
Galton, Francis, 93
Gardner, Dame Frances, 156
Garnham, P.C.C., 253, 294, 295, 297-299, 301-305
Gastrodiscoides, 245, 246
Gates, Frederick, 39, 66
Gauvain, Dr Suzette, 189
General Paralysis of the Insane, 299
Gessarol, 264
Giles, G.M., 56
Gillett, J.D., 259, 261
Gold Coast
  mortality rate, 8
Gordon Smith, C.E., 137, 142, 143
Gorgas, William C., 43
Government health policy, 325, 326
Grassi, Giovanni Battista, 51
  Topley, alliance with, 126
  acting dean, eprceived need for, 103
  background, 95, 96
  Leiper, comments on, 103, 104
  National Institute for Medical Research, comments on, 101

INDEX

Professor of Epidemiology and Vital Statistics, as, 96
  reports, 97, 99, 104
Greenwood, Major, 65, 92, 94, 116-118, 152
Griffiths, Mary, 207
Griseofulvin, 183
Gruby, David, 44
Guinea worm, 34, 251
Guinea worm disease, 33-35
Gye, W.E., 182, 183

Hamer, William Heaton, 93
Hamilton Fairley, Neil, 269-271, 303, 313, 314
Hamilton, Patrick, 114, 171, 170
Harriss, Barbara, 210, 211
Hartley, Percival, 181
Health care, economics of, 330
Health of Munition Workers Committee, 95, 185
Healy, M.J.R., 115, 116
Heilbron, Ian, 264
Heilin, D., 312
Heiser, Victor G., 65, 68, 69, 74
Hewlett, Tanner, 73, 239
Hill, Leonard, 94, 95, 186
Hillary, William, 2
Hinds, Stuart, 162, 163
Hley-Hutchinson, Sir Walter, 45
Holt, Julius, 211
Holt, Lewis B., 182
Hookworm disease, 38-40, 68, 69
Hopkins, G.H.E., 258
Hopkins, Gowland, 180
Hospital Feeding Survey, 203, 204
Hospital for Tropical Diseases, 68
Howard, C.H., 301
Human experimentation, 262, 263, 301-304
Human Nutrition Research Unit, 198, 199, 205
Hunter, John, 245

Immunology, 126, 127
Imperial Hospital for Tropical Diseases
  proposal for, 80, 81

INDEX

Industrial Fatigue Research Board, 95, 186
Industrial Health Research Board, 186
Infectious diseases, research into, 326-328
Influenza pandemic, 125
Institute of Agricultural Parasitology, 222-224
International Health Board, 67
Intestinal flukes, 31
Iyer, P.V.S., 298

James, S.P., 54, 240, 298, 300
Jameson, William Wilson, 84, 85, 105, 131, 150, 151, 186, 187, 187, 325
  Court of Governors, etc, relationship with, 156
  government plans, defence of, 157
  indivisibility of offices, 157
  strategy for national public health, 151-158
Jefferys, Margot, 157, 160, 161
Johns Hopkins School of Hygiene and Public Health, 1
Johns Hopkins Medical School, 66, 67, 82, 168
Jones, Alfred, 7, 11, 12
Journal of Helminthology, 233, 250

Kala-azar, 55, 56, 254, 255
Kazantzis, G., 191
Kenwood, Henry, 150, 151
Kilpatrick, Sir James, 138
King, Albert F.A., 50
Kirk, John, 45
Knowelden, John, 188
Koch, Robert, 93
Koino, Ahimesu, 245
Kuala Lumpur Institute for Medical Research, 248, 249

Lainson, Ralph, 231, 232
Lancisi, Giovanni Maria, 50
Landsborough Thomson, A., 133
Lane, Ronald, 188
Lankester, Ray, 45
Laveran, Alphonse, 50, 293
Ledger, Charles, 49
Leiper, John W.G., 223

INDEX

Leiper, R.T., 17-21, 33-40, 65, 68-74, 79, 83, 103, 152, 197, 220-223, 232-234, 239, 242, 295
Leishamnn, W.B., 56
Leishman, Joyce, 243
Leishmaniasis, 231, 232
LeQuesne, Professor L.P., 191
LeRoux, P.L., 307
Leuckart, Rudolf, 41
Lewis, Timothy, 44
Lister Institute, 5, 18, 100
Liverpool School of Tropical Medicine
  Chair of Tropical Medicine, 12
  establishment of, 11, 12
  expeditions, 12, 13
  opening of, 7, 12
  private support for, 11, 12
Livingstone, David, 45
Lloyd-Williams, Katharine G., 156
Loa Loa, 34
Lockwood Stevens, Major H., 286, 287
Logan, Douglas W., 106
Logan, R.F.L., 167
London School of Hygiene & Tropical Medicine
  amalgamation, proposals for, 70-73
  Board of Management, 78
  building of, 78
  centenary, 324
  committees, 81
  cost of, 9
  courses, 17-20
  Court of Governors, first Annual Report to, 81
  creation of, 10
  criminal and pre-clinical departments, 106
  Dean, 20
  design, 81
  difficulties in establishing, 10
  draft Charter, 77
  expeditions, 13
  financial position, 13, 70
  first students, 10
  Great War, during, 239, 240

INDEX

Hospital, physical separation of, 80
Institute of Agricultural Pathology, 82, 83
internal structural reorganisation, 143
intioal teaching staff, 17
Keppel Street buildings, 65, 77, 78
lack of communication within, 116-118
lady graduates, 16
lectures, 19
library, 79, 232, 233, 274, 275
Manson's School, absorption of, 80
mission statement, 332
new premises, 68, 69
new sites, consideration of, 114, 115
official opening, 13, 14
opening of, 6
original, 1
outside agencies, work with, 329-332
planning and completion, delays in, 7
practical laboratory course, 19
preferred location, 9, 11
prevention policies, emphasis on, 15
Public Health Division, 84
re-emergence of School as, 21
refectory and kitchens, 274, 275
reorganisation, 115, 116
reports, 18
research laboratories abroad, exchnages with, 20
Rockefeller influence, extent of, 66
sanitary creed, 14, 15
School Committee reports, 15
second classs of students, 10
structure of, 73, 83
subjects to be covered, 72
teachers, appointment of, 16
teaching and research, organisation of, 82
travelling scholarships, 13
University of London, recognition as part of, 16, 18
World War II, during, 102
Looss, Arthur, 36, 38, 39
Louis, P.C.A., 92
Lovell, Sir Francis, 20

INDEX

Low, George Carmichael, 10, 33, 43, 51, 52, 268, 269
Lung cancer, 109, 110
Lyttleton, Alfred, 13

Mabey, David, 272
McAdam, Keith P.W.J., 272
Macauly, Zachary, 4
Macdonald, George, 293, 294, 297, 298, 304, 305
McDonald, John Corbett, 190
Macdonald, John Smyth, 293
McDonald, William, 38
McDonald, W.A., 302
Macdonald, Wiliam Weir, 265, 266
McKay, Robert, 239, 302
MacKenzie, D.W.R., 141
MacKinnon, Sir William, 6
Mackintosh, James Macalister, 104, 106, 137, 158-160
McLeod, Sir Charles, 287
McRobert, Sir George Reid, 271
Malaria Commission, 13
Malaria, 48-55
  bird, 298
  Centre for the Evaluation of Antimalarial Drugs, 231
  Ceylon, epidemic in, 262
  chemotherapy, and, 311-314
  Chinese medicine, 314
  Cinchona bark, control by, 49
  continuing problem of, 310
  Control Course for Laymen, 293
  control of, 315
  Diagnosis Stations, 284
  epidemiology, 297
  eradication, hopes for, 49
  falciparum, 301
  Great War, outbreak in, 283
  human experimentation, 301-304
  liver, effect on, 300, 301
  mosquito inoculation, 300
  mosquito transmission, 33
  MRC Unit, 295, 296
  Nobel Prizes concerning, 283

INDEX

origins of, 49
prevalence of, 6
prevention of, 15
Reference Centre, 329
Reference Laboratories, 307, 308
research after 1950, 296-305
research and study of, 326
research in 1970s and 1980s, 305-310
Ross Institute, 285-295
Ross, work of, 50-53
Royal Society commissions, 53
species sanitation, 291
stages of, 299
synthetic drugs, search for, 312-314
troops, among, 314
vaccine, wait for, 310, 311
Winches Farm Laboratories, work at, 230
Malaria Consortium, 330
Malbsorption, 207
Mallanby, Sir Edward, 103, 104, 156
Manson, Patrick, 4-9, 10, 12, 14, 16, 17
  Amoy and Hong Kong, experiences in, 31
  microfilariae, finding, 32
  mosquito, study of, 32, 33
  mosquitoes, study of, 50
  schistosomias, study of, 36
Manson-Bahr, Sir Philip, 268, 269, 284
Marshall, T.H., 159
Measles, 205
Medical bactierology
  rise of, 31
Medical education
  post-war review, 65
Medical ethics, 111, 112
Medical imperialism, 30
Medical Research Committee, 67
  Emergency Public Health Laboratory Service, administration of, 133
  policies, 131
Medical Research Council, 94, 100, 105
Medical sociology, 160
Medical Statistics Unit, 116

Medical Zoology Division, 65, 83, 241
Mellanby, Kenneth, 131, 197, 262, 263
Menon, K.P., 298
Meynell, Elinor, 157
Michelli, P.J., 8, 9, 69-71, 74
Miles, M.A., 256
Military personnel
　concerns for, 2
Milk, safety in, 134
Minchin, E.A., 18, 252
Ministry of Health, creation of, 67
Mond, Alfred, 67, 75
Morley, David, 205
Morris, Jeremy N., 163, 165-170, 188
Muller, P.H., 264, 285
Murgatroyd, Frederick, 270, 271, 312
Murray, Robert, 189

Nabarro, D.N., 43
Nagana, 44, 45
Nairne, Sir Perceval, 8
Napoleonic Wars, 3
Nash, R.H., 188

National Health Service
　development of, 105
National Institute of Biological Standards and Control, 138, 139
National Institute of Medical Research, 84, 100, 101
Neal, Ralph, 231
Nelson, George, 227-229, 250
Newhouse, Muriel L., 156, 189
Newman, Sir George, 67, 98, 156
Normand, Charles, 172
Nutrition Policy Unit, 207, 208
Nutrition, study of 197-213

O'Neill, John, 41
Obseity, 207
Occupational health, academic discipline of, 185-192
Onchocerciasis, 40-42, 229, 246, 247
Ormerod, W.E., 180, 181, 224, 226

INDEX

Osler, William, 67
Overseas Development Administraiton, 330
Owen, Sir Isambard, 6

Parasitology, 143, 220
Parkinson, George Singleton, 102, 103, 152, 157
Pasteur, Louis, 93
Payne, Philip, 207, 210
Pearce, Richard M., 69
Pearson, Karl, 93, 95, 116
Penicillin, 181, 182
Perry, Sir Cooper, 156
Peruvian fever tree, 49
Peters, B.G., 243
Peters, Wallace, 231, 232
Peto, Richard, 111
Plague, prevention of, 15
Platt, B.S., 198-205
Pneumoconiosis Research Unit, 189
Porter, J.D.H., 272
Professor of Public Health, 104
Protozoology, 251-257
Public health
  academic discipline of, 324, 325
  concerns with, 1
  policies, formulation of, 3, 111, 112
Public Health Laboratory Service, 130-135

Rabies
  Pasteur's treatment, 5
Raistrick, Harold, 311
  background, 179, 180
  Department of Biochemistry, running, 181
  premature publication of results, 182
  work of, 181-183
Read, Herbert, 5, 7, 9, 72
Reed, Walter, 43
Rees, David C., 18
Rees, Verder, 79
Refugee health care, 273, 307
Registrar-General of Births, Deaths and Marriages

INDEX

establishment of, 92
Reid, Donald Darnley, 104, 107, 112, 113, 115
Reid, Sir John, 143
Renwick, J.H., 167, 168
Rester, F.N.N., 302
Ridley, Frederick, 182
Ritchie Simpson, W.J., 16
River blindness, 40-42
Rivers, John, 209
Roberts, Miss E., 287
Robinson, Arthur, 79, 80
Robinson, Sir Arthur, 65
Robles, Rodolfo, 246
Rockefeller Foundation, 39, 65, 66, 67, 71, 75, 164
Rockefeller Institute for Medical Research, 67, 82
Rockefeller Unit of Occupational Health, 164
Rockefeller, John D., 39, 66
Rogers, Leonard, 44, 55, 56, 254
Rondle, Dr, 141
Rose, G.A., 112, 115
Rose, Wickliffe, 39, 40, 67, 69-71, 74, 75, 77, 80, 82
Ross Institute, 285-295, 309
Ross, Ronald, 12, 94, 283-288, 298
  malaria parasites, work on, 33
  malaria, work on, 50-53
Rossiter, Charles E., 191
Rous, F.P., 243
Rowland, H.A.K., 272
Royal Commission on Medical Education, 165
Royal Statistical Society, 93
Rue, Dame Rosemary, 170
Russell, F.F., 65
Ryle, John, 169

Sambon, Louis Westenra, 16, 36, 242, 243
Sandwith, Fleming Mant, 18, 39, 40
Sanitary Commission, 39, 67
Sanitation, 308, 309
Scabies, 262, 263
Schilling, R.S.F., 164, 188
Schistosoma, 32, 35-38

INDEX

Schistosomes, 227-229
Schistosomias, 35-38
Scott, W.M., 133
Scott Macfie, J.W., 311, 312
Scurvy, 2
Seamen
  concerns for, 2
  distressed, relief of, 4
  problems of, 3
Seamen's Hospital Society, 4, 5
  Albert Dock Branch Hopital, 6
  London School, contribution to, 13
Self-inoculation, 245, 248
Sheppard, R.L., 70
Sherwood, R.J., 188
Shetty, Prakash, 213
Shortt, H.E., 223, 225, 253-255, 284, 295, 298, 299, 303
Shute, R.G., 300
Simon, John, 3
Simpson, W.J. Ritchie, 19, 20, 73, 239, 285, 286, 288
Sinton, J.A., 300
Sleeping sickness, 16, 42-48, 252
  aetiology of, 45
  Commissions, 43
  control of, 47, 48
  epidemic of, 42
  filaria, role of, 43
  Gambia, coming from, 42
  human tsetse-fly disease, as, 46
  prevalence of, 6
  strains of, 48
  studies of, 46
  trypanosomes, role of, 44
Sleeping Sickness Bureau, 46
Smallpox, 141, 142, 308
Smith, Gordon, 114
Smith, John H., 331
Smith, P.G., 116
Smith, Sir Joseph, 131
Snow, John, 93
Society for Tropical Medicine and Hygiene, 19

INDEX

Spencer, Harrison C., 308, 331
Spooner, E.C.T., 135, 136, 138, 140
Standfast, A.F.B., 184
Stanton, Sir Thomas, 156
Statistical Society, 93
Stephens, J.W.W., 48, 53, 54, 255
Steward, John S., 246
Steward, M.W., 143, 144
Stiles, Charles W., 39, 66
Streptomycin, tests on, 110
Surra, 44
Swellengrebel, Nicolaas Hendrik, 290, 291, 294
Syphilis, 299, 300

Tanner Hewlett, Richard, 14, 16
Targett, G.A.T., 230, 232, 315
Thomson, John Gordon, 38, 253
Topley, W.W.C., 14, 92, 95, 96, 152
  ARC, secretary to, 127
  background, 125, 126
  Emergency Public Health Laboratory Service, heading, 132
  Greenwood, alliance with, 126
  hospital pathology, position in, 127
  Professor of Bacteriology and Immunology, as, 96
Topping, Andrew, 106, 107, 137, 160
Tropical diseases
  concern for, 3
  immediate threat, posing, 43
  training in, 6, 7
  use of term, 2
Tropical Division, 65, 82, 83, 241
Tropical Epidemiology UNit, 116
Tropical Health Epidemiology Unit, 309
Tropical medicine
  armed forces, courses for, 102
  concern for, 3
  formal introduction of, 8
  sub-divisions, 19
  use of term, 2
Tropical Medicine and Hygiene Division, 65, 83
Tropical Medicine School, position of, 79

INDEX

Trypanosoma brucei rhodiense, 142
Trypanosomes, 224-227, 252, 256, 299
Trypanosomiasis, 42-48
Tsetse-flies
  Carpenter's studies of, 47
  nagana, carrying, 44, 45
  sleeping sickness, carrying, 46
Tuberculosis
  control of, 108
  treatment of, 110
TUC Centenary Institute of Occupational Health, 189-192
Typhus, 263

United Nations Development Project, 309
University College Hospital, 271, 272

Vaccination strategies, 327
Varma, M.G.R., 266
Vaughan, Patrick, 172
Villerme, L.R., 92
Vincent, G.E., 68, 74
Virchow, Rudolf, 92
Virology, 138, 143

Waddy, B.B., 305
Waksman, S.A., 110
Walford, Dr Diana, 131
Walton, W.S., 162, 163
Waring, Sir Holburt, 156
Warren, M.D., 162, 169
Waterlow, J.C., 198, 205, 206, 208-210
Watson, Sir Malcolm, 288-293, 295
Watts, Dr A.S., 163
Webb, R.A., 198
Webbe, Gerald, 228
Weiner, J.S., 190
Wellcome Bureau of Scientific Research, 69
Wellcome, Henry, 113
Wellcome Trust, 113, 329
Wenyon, Charles Morley, 18-21, 251-253
West Africa

INDEX

medical personnel, salaries, 9
Wheeler, Erica, 205
Wigglesworth, V.B., 258-263, 265
Wilberforce, William, 4
Wilson, Graham Selby, 14, 129, 132-134, 198
Winches Farm Laboratories, 83
  Arbovirus Research Unit, 230, 266
  closing down of, 220, 232
  development programme, 223, 224
  establishment of, 221, 222
  history of, 221, 222
  leishmaniasis research, 231, 232
  malaria, work on, 230
  onchocerciasis, study of, 247
  protozoology research, 256
  schistosomes, work on, 227-229
  trypanosomes, work on, 225, 226
  work at, 224-234
Wolfson Molecular Parasitology Unit, 256
Woodruff, A.W., 270-273
Woods, Miss H.M., 97
World Bank, 308, 309
Wright, Almroth, 116
Wucherer, Otto, 32

Yellow fever, 43
  prevalence of, 6
Yorke, Warrington, 300, 312

Zoonoses, 250
Zuckerman, A.J., 141-143